HEALTH CARE AND POOR RELIEF IN COUNTER-REFORMATION EUROPE

The role of religion was of paramount importance in the change of attitudes and approaches to health care and charity which took place in the centuries following the Council of Trent. *Health Care and Poor Relief in Counter-Reformation Europe*, edited by Ole Peter Grell and Andrew Cunningham with Jon Arrizabalaga, examines the effects of the Counter-Reformation on health care and poor relief in Southern Catholic Europe in the period between 1540 and 1700.

As well as a comprehensive introduction discussing issues of the nature of the Catholic or Counter-Reformation and the welfare provisions of the period, *Health Care and Poor Relief* sets the period in its social, economic, religious and ideological context. The book draws on the practices in different localities in Southern Europe, ranging from the Republic of Venice and the Kingdom of Naples to Germany and Spain. These examples establish how and why a revitalised and strengthened post-Tridentine Catholic Church managed to reshape and reinvigorate welfare provisions in Southern Europe.

HEALTH CARE AND POOR RELIEF IN COUNTER-REFORMATION EUROPE

Edited by

Ole Peter Grell and Andrew Cunningham with Jon Arrizabalaga

ROUTLEDGE

London and New York

First published 1999
by Routledge
2 Park Square, Milton Park, Abingdon, Oxfordshire OX14 4RN

Simultaneously published in the USA and Canada
by Routledge
711 Third Avenue, New York, NY 10017

First issued in paperback 2014

Routledge is an imprint of the Taylor and Francis Group, an informa company

Typeset in Times by
M Rules

British Library Cataloguing in Publication Data
A catalogue record for this book is available from the British Library

Library of Congress Cataloguing in Publication Data
Health care and relief in Counter-Reformation Europe/[edited by]
Ole Peter Grell and Andrew Cunningham, with Jon Arrizabalaga
p. cm.
Includes bibliographical references and index.

1. Poor – Medical care – Europe, Southern – Religious aspects – Catholic Church – History. 2. Public welfare – Europe, Southern – Religious aspect – Catholic Church – History. 3. Counter-Reformation – Europe, Southern – History. I. Grell, Ole Peter. II. Cunningham, Andrew, Dr III. Arrizabalaga, Jon.
RA418.5.P6H3874 1999
362. 1′094′09032–dc21

ISBN 13: 978-0-415-17844-0 (hbk)
ISBN 13: 978-0-415-75739-3 (pbk)

CONTENTS

LIST OF FIGURES

LIST OF CONTRIBUTORS

Jon Arrizabalaga, C.S.I.C., Barcelona, Spain

Andrew Cunningham, Wellcome Unit for the History of Medicine, University of Cambridge

Silvia De Renzi, Wellcome Unit for the History of Medicine, University of Cambridge

Martin Dinges, Institut für Geschichte der Medizin der Robert Bosch Stiftung, Stuttgart, Germany

Isabel M.R. Mendes Drumond Braga, University of Lisbon, Portugal

David Gentilcore, Leicester University

Ole Peter Grell, Wellcome Unit for the History of Medicine, University of Cambridge

John Henderson, Wellcome Unit for the History of Medicine, University of Cambridge

Jonathan I. Israel, Department of History, University College, London

Colin Jones, Warwick University

María Luz López Terrada, University of Valencia, Spain

Richard Palmer, Lambeth Palace Library, London

Brian Pullan, Manchester University

Bernd Roeck, Rheinischen Friedrich-Wilhelms-Universität, Bonn, Germany

ACKNOWLEDGEMENTS

This volume results from a conference organised by the Cambridge Wellcome Unit for the History of Medicine (Early Modern Programme), and the C.S.I.C., Barcelona (History of Medicine), held in Barcelona in 1996. We are grateful to the Societat Catalana d'Història de la Ciència i de la Tècnica for providing us with a suitable meeting place, in a seventeenth century hospital, the Casa de Convalescencia, dedicated to St Paul. The organisers are most grateful to the Wellcome Trust, the D.G.I.C.Y.T. (Spanish Ministry of Education and Science) and the C.S.I.C., for their generous funding of this conference. We are grateful too to Howarth I. Penny for his help in preparing the text for the press.

1

THE COUNTER-REFORMATION AND WELFARE PROVISION IN SOUTHERN EUROPE

Ole Peter Grell and Andrew Cunningham

This volume offers a comparative survey of the welfare provisions available to the sick and poor in Catholic Southern Europe during the Counter-Reformation period, 1540–1700. It seeks to highlight the relationship between a revived and dynamic Catholicism and welfare reforms on one hand, and the changes in health care, that is 'professional' medical care, nursing and hospitals, on the other. It draws attention to the fact that the major context for health care in the early modern period was poor relief and that welfare provision has to be seen within the context of the predominant religious ideology, in this case the Counter-Reformation. Together the thirteen chapters in this volume provide ample examples of how and why a revitalised and strengthened post-Tridentine Catholicism managed to reshape and reinvigorate welfare provisions in Southern Europe, while simultaneously emphasising the extent to which this restructuring depended on, and based itself on, earlier reforms initiated as a consequence of the civic humanist and Catholic reform movements of the fifteenth century.

Geographically this volume deals with the Mediterranean Catholic countries of Italy and Spain, plus Portugal, France and southern Catholic Germany. From the outset the editors sought to include a chapter on Austria, covering the so-called Habsburg inherited lands, in order to achieve the fullest geographical coverage, but since no scholar, to our knowledge, is or has been working in this field recently, this unfortunately proved impossible. The little attention paid to health care and poor relief in the recent social history of Austria further emphasises the lack of scholarly interest in this area.[1]

Within these geographical parameters the book will seek to establish how, why, and where, a revitalised and strengthened post-Tridentine Catholic Church managed to reshape and reinvigorate welfare provisions in Southern Europe. The use of the historiographically much debated and contested term 'Counter-Reformation' in the title of this volume is deliberate. Rather than opting for terms such as 'Catholic Reformation' or 'Catholic renewal', the term Counter-Reformation still seems the most appropriate and precise. This is a view which to some extent is borne out by the recent historiographical debate in Germany. Here Catholic historical scholarship, in the wake of the seminal work by H. Jedin, *Katholische Reformation oder Gegenreformation?*, published in 1946, rather than contesting the term Counter-Reformation has sought to elevate the concept to being on a par with that of the Reformation.[2] Today it is generally accepted that post-Tridentine reforms to a considerable extent were rooted in earlier moves towards reform generated by humanism and the Catholic reform movements of the fifteenth century. But so was the Reformation. The drive towards reform, *reformatio Ecclesiae*, had officially been a part of the agenda of the Catholic Church since the days of the Great Schism (1309–1417). These ideas were pursued by the conciliar movement first at the Council of Constance (1414–17) and later at the Council of Basle (1431–49) where a wholesale reform of the papacy as well as of local ecclesiastical forms and structures had been envisaged, but failed to materialise. The general urge and expectation of an immediate renewal of religious life and Christian society, with little hope of being fulfilled from within the Church, gave rise to a number of apocalyptic and millenarian movements in the fifteenth century. They, in turn, served to prepare the way for the evangelical reformers in northern Europe, while inspiring reformist preachers such as the Dominican Girolamo Savonarola in the south. For Savonarola and his followers Florence became the new Jerusalem, where a reform of piety and morals were urgently needed in order to prepare the way for the millenium. Vigorous campaigns against a variety of perceived sins such as gambling and prostitution were initiated, while repeated calls for reforms of the many lay confraternities were issued. But of a far more enduring nature and of considerably greater significance in our context was Savonarola's contribution to welfare reforms. He was instrumental in creating a system of public health care and poor relief in Florence which brought together existing and newly founded institutions and hospitals, such as the Monte di Pietà, for the benefit of the city's sick and poor.[3]

While the Reformation was gathering momentum in northern Europe, where the mendicant orders and the lay confraternities were the prime target for some of the most venemous attacks by the evangelical reformers,[4] the Catholic Church in Italy showed remarkable vitality, and a considerable number of new religious orders and confraternities were created, from where they later spread to Spain and France. Most, if not all, had their roots in the vibrant urban environment of the large cities of northern and central Italy. It remains somewhat of a paradox to historians why this renewal should have taken place in Italy far away from where the Protestant challenge was strongest, i.e. in Germany, central Europe and the Netherlands. That, however, may well be a typically anachronistic interpretation. It is, in our opinion, far more likely that the evangelical movement in northern Europe in the 1520s was ideologically much closer to the movement for reform in Italy which generated the new religious orders than we realise today, despite the different paths they eventually took. Take, for instance, the Capuchins, who began as a renegade movement within the Franciscan Observant community in Italy, eventually receiving papal recognition in 1528. They sought to renew the spirituality and piety of their Franciscan forefathers and endeared themselves to the urban population of Italy, through their charitable works, especially caring for the sick while preaching the Gospel. At the height of their success from around 1575 to 1650 they, together with the Jesuits, became the standard-bearers of the Counter-Reformation.[5] However, it is noteworthy that the first Vicar-General of the Capuchins, Bernardino Ochino (1487–1564), became one of the most prominent evangelical Italian reformers when he together with another cleric, Peter Martyr Vermigli, fled Italy for Geneva in 1542.[6] Thus one of the leading, new religious orders of the Counter-Reformation is intrinsically bound up with the Reformation through its first Vicar-General. Further evidence of how closely interlocked the Reformation and the Counter-Reformation remained until the 1540s can be seen from the fact that Pier Paolo Vergerio (1498–1565), the nuncio sent to Germany to meet Luther in 1535 by the first Counter-Reformation pope, Paul III, eventually followed Ochino and Martyr into exile in 1549 and publicly converted to Protestantism.[7]

Despite the fact that the Capuchins were transformed into an order in the service of the militant Counter-Reformation, especially in Germany, the order continued to distinguish itself in works of charity in Italy in particular, where it played a major role in caring for plague victims. In 1576–77 the Capuchins assisted the great

Counter-Reformation bishop Carlo Borromeo in nursing many of the thousands who fell victim to the plague in Milan. Similarly in 1629 when Italy was hit by another major epidemic they stepped in, running charities, providing medical care while comforting the dying: a front-line commitment which saw droves of Capuchins die. However, their involvement in welfare provision was not restricted to periods of epidemics. In many cities they established so-called *bottega di Cristo*, shops where food and grain was sold to the poor at subsidised prices, or took over the running of the Monti di Pietà which provided cheap loans for the poor.[8]

The new orders and confraternities, such as the Clerks Regular of Somascha founded in Venice by the layman Girolamo Emiliani for the care of orphans in particular, shared certain characteristics. They sought to remedy the ills of the urban society where they emerged, ministering primarily to the poor, destitute women and orphans, not only spiritually but also materially, more often than not promoted by significant lay, noble and patrician patronage. Similar ambitions characterised the new female orders and sisterhoods, such as the Ursulines founded in Brescia in 1535, living in mixed lay-clerical communities or with their families, who concentrated their efforts on hospitals, orphanages and half-way houses for prostitutes. Initially they recruited their members from among artisan and mercantile families in the towns. These women then became patrons of poor and orphaned girls, gradually expanding their charitable work to hospitals and poor and sick women in general. Their active charitable work saved them from the post-Tridentine drive towards enclosure of female orders. The Counter-Reformation Church's concern with improving the moral standards of the clergy caused it to see the enforcement of clerical celibacy as a central task. Linked to that it came to consider chastity as ranging above all other attributes for female religiosity, something which enclosure, or isolation from the world, sought to guarantee. This also helps to explain the post-Tridentine Church's obsession with prostitutes as a group in need of a particular and determined effort on the Church's part in order to possibly save the souls of such women who had squandered their chastity and whose souls were about to be lost.[9] It is in this context we should see the two new types of religious houses for women or girls established in Rome by Ignatius Loyola – the Santa Marta and the Vergini Miserabili. As opposed to the already well-known nunneries for penitent prostitutes, these institutions offered half-way houses for women wanting to escape prostitution or poor girls who were thought at risk of falling into prostitution (see Chapter 2).

In his opening survey chapter (Chapter 2), Brian Pullan emphasises that the Catholic reform movements remained localized geographically, as well as organisationally until the 1530s, and that only from the 1540s did any central, papally directed reform initiatives materialise. Pullan considers sixteenth-century Catholicism to have been composed of three ingredients, early Catholic reform, the Counter-Reformation, and an older, unreformed folk religion. This latter component appears to be similar to the magical paganism which Jean Delumeau claims characterised medieval Christianity and which Counter-Reformation Catholicism, according to him, sought to obliterate through its attempt to Christianise society.[10] Post-Tridentine Catholicism was, in Pullan's view, never concerned with tackling poverty per se, but only with poverty as a possible danger to people's souls. As such, poor relief and welfare provision served as an avenue along which a considerable number of souls might be saved by the Church.

Catholic societies of the 1540s inherited two major welfare institutions created by the Catholic reform movement of the fifteenth century – the general hospital and the Monti di Pietà. These consolidated hospitals provided refuge for pilgrims and care for the sick and orphans. Their re-organisation and centralisation began in northern Italy in the mid-fifteenth century and spread to the rest of the peninsula, France and Spain during the sixteenth century. The Monti di Pietà, cheap loan shops for the poor generally supervised by local clergy and urban administrators, also spread across Italy from the cities in the north, and later to Spain and France, where they set out to impose morality on the process of lending.

Among the other institutions in the welfare domain inherited by Counter-Reformation Catholicism were the relatively new hospitals for incurables, dedicated primarily to the treatment of the pox – a new and frightening disease which had begun to make a dramatic impact from the mid-1490s. Many of these new hospitals for incurables were created by a new and different type of confraternity – the Oratory or Company of Divine Love – which, as opposed to the older confraternities, was not concerned with mutual support, except for the inner spiritual renewal of its members, but geared to serve the local Christian community through charitable work for the sick and poor. It spread rapidly from Genoa, where the first hospital for incurables was founded in 1499, to the other major Italian cities, and it also inspired the creation of other similar lay brotherhoods across Italy, such as the Roman Confraternita della Carita established in 1519, the confraternity of San Girolamo della Carità in

Vicenza, and the confraternity of Saints Philip and Paul in Milan.[11] All these new confraternities with their new spiritual ethos and social commitment became essential servants of the Counter-Reformation Church, increasingly controlled and directed from Rome. Attending the sick in hospitals became an essential duty in the post-Tridentine Church not primarily for social and medical reasons, but in order to win the struggle for the endangered souls of the poor sick and dying, as Brian Pullan emphasises in Chapter 2.

In Chapter 3, Jonathan Israel claims that the introduction of a new mechanistic and experimental medicine and health care system was delayed by nearly a century in southern Catholic Europe, in Italy, Spain and Portugal in particular, as a consequence of the Counter-Reformation and general economic decline. Economically both Spain and Italy experienced a long and severe decline, beginning at the end of the sixteenth century and continuing until the beginning of the eighteenth century, which affected the major cities in particular, resulting in drastic falls in population sizes and commercial and financial stagnation, if not collapse. Thus the means needed to introduce the new medicine and health care were simply not available in the south. No new and enlarged teaching hospitals were built, nor other facilities such as anatomical theatres, botanical gardens, laboratories and medical museums and collections.

This retardation in medical and health care renewal in the Catholic south was undoubtedly ideologically affected by the Counter-Reformation. In this context it matters less whether this was a direct consequence of Counter-Reformation Catholicism which sought to root out all forms of heresy, or whether it was an indirect intellectual effect of ecclesiastical measures, as claimed by Israel in Chapter 3. Even if the influence in southern Europe of the reorganised and revitalised Roman Inquisition (1542) is still being debated, there can be little doubt it generated a climate of fear. The Church's discouragement of Catholic students from attending universities in Protestant countries quickly took effect and Italian students stayed at home, while Spanish students only attended good Catholic universities in Italy.[12] Similarly, even if it is still debated how much the creation of the Roman Index of Prohibited Books in 1549 affected cultural life in Italy in particular, it is generally accepted that it had a negative effect especially over time: many books published in Protestant countries were simply not read and discussed by the intellectual elite in the south, while the lack of learned journals meant that an intellectual forum and exchange of new ideas was missing in Italy and Spain.[13]

Four chapters dealing with Counter-Reformation welfare provisions in Tuscany, Venice, Rome and the kingdom of Naples offer detailed examples of how reforms in health care and poor relief were initiated in the major Italian localities.

In his chapter on early modern Tuscany (Chapter 4), John Henderson underlines the fact that there were significant differences between the system of charity in operation in sixteenth century Tuscany as compared with the preceding century. The system may have become more hostile towards the poor and begging, as a consequence of the growing levels of poverty, but that reaction was supplemented by a moral and religious renewal generated by the Catholic Church, which actively sought to combat poverty because of its perceived negative moral consequences. Taking his departure from the many new orders and confraternities which nearly all had a significant lay input, such as the Company of Divine Love and the Ministri degli Infirmi, which came into existence in sixteenth century Italy, and their dedication to the care of the sick and poor, especially those seen to suffer from incurable conditions such as the pox, or the French disease as it became known in Italy, Henderson points towards the religious and moral imperative which lay behind this social involvement, namely the urge to save the souls of those imperiled by destitution and disease. The welfare reforms of the Medici Duke, Cosimo I, centralising and improving the administrative machinery through the appointment of the Buonomini – the twelve good men – served to solve some of the financial problems encountered by some of the major Florentine hospitals in the wake of the siege of the city, but it also served to streamline a system which was coming under increasing strain from the growing numbers of poor. Likewise, the creation of a hostel for abandoned boys in the 1540s may have been brought about by the explosive increase in the number of foundlings taken in by the hospital of the Innocenti, which made it impossible for that institution to cater for older children, but it was the religious rationale, first providing the boys with proper religious instruction and only secondly teaching them a useful trade in order to become God-fearing Christians, which was the driving force behind this scheme. In the second half of the sixteenth century, four conservatories for girls, dedicated to the moral protection, education and training of orphaned young girls, were established by committed lay Florentine Catholics, but supported by the Medicis as well as local clerics. This was a classic example of the Counter-Reformation obsession with female chastity, seeking to prevent young women from falling into prostitution which would endanger their salvation (see Chapter 4).

In Venice the ethos of the 'new Catholicism' was making an impact as early as the end of the fifteenth century, when the city leaders began regulating prostitution not only in order to control disease, but also to prevent souls from being endangered. From the start of the sixteenth century the city also benefited from the charitable work for the sick and poor undertaken by the new orders and societies which were motivated by this drive for piety. The Company of Divine Love, with its mixture of laymen and priests, established hospitals for incurables, mainly victims of the pox, during the 1520s, while other new orders such as the Theatines, founded in 1524, and the Somaschi were active in the Republic's hospitals (see Chapter 5). In Venice this Catholic revival also included the episcopate, which otherwise remained unaffected in most of southern Europe until after Trent. According to Richard Palmer in Chapter 5, the bishop of Verona, Gian Matteo Giberti, provided an early model for Counter-Reformation bishops such as Carlo Borromeo. As already pointed out by Brian Pullan, this emphasis on serving Christ by caring for and nursing the sick poor which became so prominent in early sixteenth century Italian Catholicism received further impetus via post-Tridentine Catholicism's urgent concern for the redemption of sinners and salvation of souls.[14] In this respect hospitals offered particularly useful 'missionary' fields, where the physical and medical needs of the poor sick mixed naturally with their spiritual needs, and access to deathbeds was more readily available.

As in Tuscany, the care of foundlings was a prime concern in sixteenth century Venice and by the middle of the century twelve hundred children were in the care of the city's foundling hospital, while smaller towns such Brescia and Bergamo may have cared for as many as a thousand. Again, the motivation for this charitable work was to hinder mortal sins and to save souls, by preventing infanticide and saving abandoned infants who might otherwise die without being baptised. As pointed out by Richard Palmer this obsession with charitable work launched in the decades before Trent was accelerated and augmented by the Counter-Reformation to reach a comprehensive system of charity around 1600, or a 'holy perfection' of good works, which eventually involved a significant element of social control (see Chapter 5).

Considering the central role played by the papacy in the re-shaping of the Catholic Church both ecclesiastically and theologically in the period after Trent, it is hardly surprising that Rome or the Papal State itself went through thorough administrative and political reforms from the end of the sixteenth till the beginning of the seventeenth century. This was all part of the dynamics which served to assert the power of a triumphant Counter-Reformation Church, and in which new poor relief initiatives served the double purpose of providing a measure of social control while promoting the triumphalist message of the post-Tridentine Church. It is in this context that Silvia De Renzi analyses the role of the hospital of Santo Spirito and the careers of some of its physicians (Chapter 6). By 1600 this incredibly wealthy hospital was able to cater for more than twelve hundred sick people mainly from the poorer section of Roman society, looking after their individual medical needs. No patients suffering from diseases such as the pox, which was deemed incurable, were admitted and the Santo Spirito dealt mainly with people suffering from a variety of fevers and wounds. Simultaneously, the hospital offered excellent medical training for young physicians and surgeons, who benefited from the teaching provided by the senior physicians and surgeons and the many dissections and post mortems which took place. By the early seventeenth century the hospital appears to have provided its patients with round-the-clock nursing by members of the Order of the Holy Spirit and committed laymen all motivated by the post-Tridentine ethos of serving Christ through the care of the sick and the poor. Appointment as physician to the Santo Spirito was, according to De Renzi, highly sought after by Counter-Reformation physicians in Rome, despite the poor pay, because it was a near certain way of enhancing one's personal career. Public service, treating the sick poor, served to demonstrate a physician's commitment to the new Catholicism, as when Johannes Faber treated a seriously ill peasant who been bitten by a viper and called a priest to hear his confession because he was as concerned about the peasant's soul as about his physical well-being. But simultaneously it served to further a physician's reputation and career.

Even if Naples, one of Europe's most populous cities in this period, had one of the richest and most imposing hospitals of the age – the Casa Santa dell' Annunziata – the city never experienced the unification and centralisation of hospitals which took place in so many major Italian cities during the late fifteenth and early sixteenth century. Neither were the Spanish viceroys able to centralise these institutions later in the century on a par with what took place in Spain. Similarly, poor relief in Naples remained decentralised and medieval in character, even if the Counter-Reformation provided it with renewed momentum. As pointed out by David Gentilcore (Chapter 7) it is impossible to separate hospitals founded before

Trent from those founded after, even if it is unquestionable that the Counter-Reformation gave rise to significant new hospital charity in Naples. The strengthening of episcopal power after Trent also meant that the religious dimension of the hospitals were reasserted. Since they were ecclesiastical institutions bishops naturally sought to exercise jurisdiction over them. The large clerical body which was attached to the Annunziata in Naples after Trent is evidence of the considerable religious role the hospital played. Thus in 1575 the hospital established its own seminary while Jesuit preachers made it a centre for Tridentine sermons, and the splendour of its religious ceremonies was widely admired.

The Annunziata, however, also spent large amounts of its considerable wealth on charity, maintaining more than 8,000 foundlings on an annual basis. It also provided medical care for the sick poor, separated into several wards according to their disease, while providing out-door assistance to the shamefaced poor. Those suffering from incurable diseases were not admitted to the Annunziata, but treated in the hospital for the incurables, established in Naples, as in so many other Italian cities, during the early sixteenth century. On a par with other Italian cities Naples also saw a number of new confraternities dedicated to the service of the sick poor come into existence in the Counter-Reformation era.

Of the new Counter-Reformation orders the Camillians proved particularly active in the hospitals in Naples from the start of the seventeenth century. This male nursing order founded by Camillo de Lellis in 1586 attended the sick according to the physicians' orders. They were to assist the sick in all practical matters, wash them and make their beds and most importantly help them die a 'good death'. In Naples their activities were not restricted to the city's hospitals, but they also visited the sick at home and during epidemics their service to the community proved invaluable. Their willingness to care for plague victims caused many members of the order to die from this disease during outbreaks in Naples in the seventeenth century. Among other Counter-Reformation initiatives in the city was the proliferation of loan facilities for the poorer sections of society, the so-called Monte di Pietà, in the closing decades of the sixteenth century.

With regard to the increasing number of poor who flocked to Naples during the sixteenth century, the city's Spanish viceroys never sought to institute a centralised policy dealing with the problem, as did other Italian states of the period (see Chapter 7). No large-scale beggars' hospitals were created and no attempts were made to enclose the poor in Naples, something which set the kingdom apart not only from other Italian states, but from Spain and Portugal too.[15]

Developments in the Iberian peninsula followed a somewhat similar pattern to that of Italy even if most initiatives tended to come a generation or two later, as can be seen from the three chapters dealing with Castile, Aragon and Portugal.

In his survey of welfare provision in Counter-Reformation Castile, Jon Arrizabalaga (Chapter 8) emphasises that attitudes to the poor and begging were changing in Castile, like the rest of Europe, during the sixteenth century. The government's response to the growing number of beggars consisted of attempts to enclose the poor, a policy which was abandoned by the early seventeenth century due to the severe economic difficulties of the Spanish empire. The social crisis generated by the famine of 1539 caused the government of Emperor Charles V to issue a new poor law which sought to regulate begging, restricting it through a licensing system to the deserving poor. Despite the relatively mild changes introduced, the new poor law gave rise to a vigorous debate on poor relief in Castile between the Dominican Domingo de Soto and the Benedictine Juan de Robles. De Soto wanted to uphold the traditional freedom to beg without distinguishing between deserving and undeserving poor and with no interference from civic authorities. Robles, defending the recent poor law, wanted to regulate begging further. Evidently inspired by Juan Luis Vives he wanted the deserving poor to receive some form of public charity administered by lay civic officials under episcopal supervision.

The economic and social crisis which affected the Spanish monarchy from the last decades of the sixteenth century until the middle of the seventeenth eventually resulted in the emergence of two major proposals on how to deal with the growing problem of poverty. The canon Miguel Giginta suggested that a central fund be established which could finance the construction of a network of beggars' hospitals across the Spanish kingdoms. Giginta's plans, that all cities should have only two hospitals, one for beggars and another for the sick poor, were not only supported and promoted by the powerful Counter-Reformation bishop of Segovia, but also by the Jesuits. A couple of decades later another plan for the 'General Reformation' of the system of welfare in Spain was produced by Philip II's court physician Pérez de Herrera. Herrera's aims were far more modest than Giginta's. He wanted to establish shelters or hostels for the poor in fifty major Castilian towns, where the poor would be provided with accomodation for the night only and spiritual guidance.

These shelters were to be administered by a group of clerical and lay officials who would register the needy and discriminate between the deserving and undeserving poor. As a true son of the Counter-Reformation, Herrera was deeply concerned with female chastity and the danger of prostitution and wanted female workhouses to be established in the major cities in order to 'recover' such lost souls.

The amalgamation and consolidation of hospitals which had begun in Italy and the Crown of Aragon in the fifteenth century did not take place in Castile until the late sixteenth century when it was strongly promoted by Philip II. However, the consolidation never became universal nor permanent in Castile. Interestingly, the consolidation which took place coincided to some extent with Giginta's reform proposals. By 1592 moves were undertaken to split up some of the consolidated, large-scale hospitals because their amalgamation were felt to have had a negative effect on welfare provision. Meanwhile some of the proposals of Pérez de Herrera were acted upon and shelters for the poor were built in a number of Castilian cities, but with the death Philip II in 1598 who had been personally committed to the reforms, and the growing financial difficulties of the Spanish empire, Herrera's project was left to fade away (see Chapter 8).

Overall, money appears to have been pouring into charities in Spain in the late sixteenth century. The laity was evidently totally committed to the post-Tridentine ethos. Hospitals benefited from large donations from wealthy merchant-bankers such as Simon Ruiz in Medina del Campo, as did orphanages and other religious foundations. Ultimately, however, this was a quest to save souls, as can be seen from the colossal sums which were invested in the dead and dying. Masses for the dead proliferated. In Cuenca the number of masses specified in wills tripled between 1605–35, while in Barcelona there was an eightfold increase in masses for the dead between the sixteenth and seventeenth century.[16]

In her survey of welfare provision in the Crown of Aragon, María Luz López Terrada (Chapter 9) emphasises the involvement and control of lay urban officials in poor relief and medical care in the cities of Valencia and Barcelona during the early modern period. Focusing on the hospital system in the three major cities of Saragossa, Valencia and Barcelona, she draws attention to the fact that consolidation of revenue and services of numerous small hospitals into one large, central institution began in the fifteenth century, more or less simultaneously with developments in Italy. First among these consolidations were the foundation of the Santa Creu Hospital in Barcelona in 1401, followed by the Royal General Hospital in Saragossa in 1425, and finally by the amalgamation of the hospitals of Valencia in 1512. As opposed to the Castilian hospitals, which remained decentralised and under the direct control of the Church, these three large general hospitals in the Aragon cities were controlled by a mixed committee, consisting of clerics, chosen from the local cathedral chapters, and members of the local urban elites. These new central hospitals were primarily dedicated to the cure of the sick, occasionally dealing with out-patients too, providing guidance for public health initiatives in times of epidemics, and caring for both foundlings and the insane. Their sizes were considerable as can be seen from the Saragossa hospital which had 500 sick beds apart from wards for foundlings and the insane. All three hospitals employed a considerable medical staff, not only physicians, surgeons and apothecaries, but also nurses, not to mention a considerable number of employees who provided essential services such as cooks, bakers, cleaners, etc. Despite the lay, civic input in their running the three hospitals also maintained an ecclesiastical presence. This clerical input grew considerably towards the end of the sixteenth century under the influence of the Counter-Reformation. Thus in Valencia the hospital had only had two priests attached to it before 1585, from that date, however, another four chaplaincies were added, and by the seventeenth century the hospital could draw on the services of no less than nine priests (see Chapter 9).

The Counter-Reformation in Portugal, like most of the Catholic south, benefited and built on the achievements of an earlier movement for Catholic reform. As Isabel Mendes Drumond Braga demonstrates in Chapter 10, this resulted in the creation of a new type of confraternity – the Misericórdia – in Lisbon in 1498 – from where it rapidly spread across the rest of Portugal and its overseas dependencies. Under the direct protection of the crown these confraternities, which were not geared to the need of their own members, but to the general needs of the local communities, initiated a reform of poor relief and hospitals in Portugal. The Misericórdias became instrumental in the consolidation of hospitals in the country in the sixteenth century and they quickly accumulated considerable wealth. This may be considered to have led to a laicisation of health care and poor relief in Portugal, but considering the intermediate position of the confraternities, somewhere between the lay and ecclesiatical sphere, this would be a misconception, especially since the Misericórdias came into existence because of the impact on the laity of the piety of Catholic reform.

Gradually during the sixteenth century the Misericórdias annexed more charitable roles. In most urban centres they took over the responsibility for foundlings from local authorities. They also provided female orphans with dowries to prevent them from being drawn into prostitution, while local safe houses were established for women at risk. This obsession with female chastity was, as we have already seen, generated by post-Tridentine Catholicism. Obviously the Misericórdias were firmly rooted in the Catholic reform movement of the late fifteenth century, but their increasing role and influence within all aspects of health care and poor relief in Portugal from the late sixteenth century onwards clearly would not be comprehensible without the new religious and ideological commitment of post-Tridentine Catholicism (see Chapter 10).

In France there was initially 'competition' by each confessional group to cope with its poor, according to Colin Jones (Chapter 11). But under the pressure of the Wars of Religion, the crown gained control of poor relief and hospitals from the municipalities (of whatever confession), and found itself competing with a revitalised Catholic Church. Jones sees here what he calls a 'charitable imperative', a moral obligation to give. To take an active role in the care of the poor came to be a sign of a renewed Catholic, seeking to put into practice an *imitatio Christi*. New religious orders built and ran hundreds of new institutions in France, including *hôpitaux généraux*. And at the parish level the 'Company of the Holy Sacrament' was active: 'good angels' fighting prostitution and famine, and developing confraternities for home relief and medical care for the needy poor, the disorderly poor, as well as the sick poor, constantly promoting the spirituality and the work ethic of inmates. Even with the strong centralising monarchy seeking to control such institutions, it is clear from Jones's account that the ideology of renewed Catholicism was crucial to developments in health care and poor relief in France.

Martin Dinges, in his chapter discussing Southern France more closely (Chapter 12), is concerned to see just how the Catholic Church managed to remain a major player in the field of health care and poor relief, even though challenged by other confessions and by state enterprise. Moreover, he sees the Catholic Church as regaining in Southern France in the seventeenth century influence over health care and poor relief it had lost in the sixteenth century, and doing so through Counter-Reformation impulses. At grass-roots level, while Counter-Reformation influence on self-help and mutual help was probably minimal, at the institutional level it was great. The hospitals which in the sixteenth century came to be reformed under lay (municipal) influence, by the seventeenth century are perfect examples of the Catholic spiritualisation of daily practice. The hospitals became full of religious: that is of priests, to tend the altars and of new female and male nursing orders to care for the sick. Dinges argues that the spirituality of nursing sisters seeking spiritual cleansing also resulted in the better physical cleansing of the wards, and hence their greater hygienic standards.

The formal church in Bordeaux too had a major input into poor relief on Counter-reformation models. Imitating Carlo Borromeo (Charles Borromaeus) the leading Roman cardinal who dedicated himself to caring for the poor, the local bishop of Bordeaux also tried to defeat malaria, build institutions for cripples, distribute alms regularly and create workhouses for the care and physical and spiritual retraining of the poor. Catholic elites, similarly inspired by reform ideology, helped found the new *hôpitaux généraux*. In general, Dinges shows that the impulse of Catholic reform led to initiatives in all areas of health care and poor relief. In the small Calvinist communities in the south of France, poor relief was also a main concern of church elders.

Finally, we turn to the situation in Catholic southern Germany. This area has not been greatly researched as yet, with the major exception of Cologne. However, Bernd Roeck (Chapter 13) argues that health care and poor relief had a deeply religious character. In this way this area resembles other areas of Catholic Europe during the Counter-Reformation. The variety of confessional positions on offer in the region did not undermine this: as Roeck writes, 'confessionalisation was simultaneously Christianisation'. While the economic crises of the sixteenth century meant greater secular involvement in poor relief, this resulted in a competitive relationship between church and state. Vives was taken as the guide for the relief of the poor in these new circumstances, in which the goal was not just the relief of poverty as a holy duty, but the elimination of poverty altogether as a Christian duty. But where the Protestants thought that the elimination of poverty was a communal, state, duty, the German Catholics who followed Vives found him saying that it should be an individual duty, an obligation of Catholic charity. Over the treatment of beggars Protestant and Catholic policy differed most clearly, with Protestants banning begging and seeking to institutionalise beggars, and Catholics in general continuing to tolerate beggars and giving to them as acts of Christian charity. In general, and for all the intricacies of the confessional and geographical situation in Catholic Germany, what holds true is what we have seen to be the case just about everywhere in Counter-Reformation Europe, that the Counter-Reformation gave an impetus and a direction to the care of the sick and healthy poor, to the creation of new institutions for their welfare, to the dedication of new religious orders to their care.

Notes

1 E. Bruckmüller, *Sozialgeschichte Österreichs*, Vienna, 1985, see pp. 157–8 and 268–70 in particular.
2 See H. Jedin, *Katholische Reformation oder Gegenreformation? Ein Versuch zur Klärung der Begriffe*, Lucerne, 1946. See also, E.G. Gleason, 'Catholic Reformation, Counterreformation and papal reform in the sixteenth century', in T. Brady *et al.* (eds), *Handbook of European History 1400–1600*, vol. 2, Leiden, 1995, pp. 317–45. Some recent scholars such as Wolfgang Reinhard and R. Po-Chia Hsia, however, find all denominational terms inadequate and prefer the concept of confessionalisation which in their view makes it possible to analyse the impact of Lutheranism, Calvinism and Catholicism simultaneously without any preconceived confessional bias, W. Reinhard, 'Gegenreformation als Modernisierung? Prolegomena zu einer Theorie des konfessionellen Zeitalters', *Archiv für Reformationsgeschichte*, 68, 1977, pp. 226–52, and R. Po-Chia Hsia, *Social Discipline in the Reformation: Central Europe 1550–1750*, London, 1989. In certain comparative constructs, such as social discipline, this may be a useful concept, but generally it is in danger of steamrollering the historical and religious landscape making every confession look the same.
3 See L. Polizzotto, *The Elect Nation: The Savonarolan Movement in Florence 1494–1545*, Oxford, 1994.
4 See O.P. Grell, 'The Protestant imperative of Christian care and neighbourly love', in O.P. Grell and A. Cunningham (eds), *Health Care and Poor Relief in Protestant Europe 1500–1700*, London, 1997, pp. 43–65, especially pp. 48–9.
5 R. Po-Chia Hsia, *The World of Catholic Renewal 1540–1770*, Cambridge, 1998, p. 29.
6 For Ochino, see D. Cantimori, *Eretici italiana del Cinquecento*, 3rd edn by A. Prosperi, Turin, 1992.
7 For Vergerio, see A. Jacobson Schütte, *Pier Paolo Vergerio: The Making of an Italian Reformer*, Geneva, 1977.
8 Hsia, *Catholic Renewal*, pp. 29–30. See also, F. Cuthbert, *The Capuchins: A Contribution to the History of the Counterreformation*, 2 vols, reprinted New York, 1971.
9 Hsia, *Catholic Renewal*, pp. 36–41. See also R. P. Liebowitz, 'Virgins in the service of Christ: the dispute over the active apostolate for women during the Counter-Reformation', in R. Ruether and E. McLaughlin (eds), *Women of Spirit: Female Leadership in the Jewish and Christian Traditions*, New York, 1979, pp. 132–52.
10 For Pullan's view, see Chapter 1 of this volume. See also J. Delumeau,

Catholicism between Luther and Voltaire: a New View of the Counter-Reformation, London, 1977; for another interpretation of the role of the Counter-Reformation and the content of medieval Christianity, see J. Bossy, *Christianity and the West, 1400–1700*, Oxford, 1985. Bossy does not see the Middle Ages as pagan, instead he considers pre-Tridentine Catholicism as rooted in the natural and local allegiances of late medieval society.

11 See J.C. Olin (ed.), *The Catholic Reformation, Savonarola to Ignatius Loyola: Reform in the Church, 1495–1540*, New York, 1992, Chapter 2.

12 Gleason, 'Catholic Reformation', p. 327.

13 For a discussion of this, see A. Borromeo, 'The Inquisition and inquisitorial censorship', in J.W. O'Malley (ed.), *Catholicism in early Modern History: A Guide to Research*, St Louis, 1988, pp. 253–72.

14 See B. Pullan, '"Support and redeem": Charity and poor relief in Italian cities from the fourteenth to the seventeenth centuries', *Continuity and Change*, 3, 1988, pp. 177–208.

15 For Italy and beggar hospitals see pp. 177–208 Chapters 2, 4, 5 and 7 of this volume; for Spain and Portugal see Chapters 8 to 10. See also L. Martz, *Poverty and Welfare in Habsburg Spain. The Example of Toledo*, Cambridge, 1983, pp. 66–76.

16 Hsia, *Catholic Renewal*, pp. 52–3.

2

THE COUNTER-REFORMATION, MEDICAL CARE AND POOR RELIEF

Brian Pullan

Most historians would probably agree that a Counter-Reformation occurred in most Catholic countries, but few would now think the words an adequate description of the many changes of direction and emphasis in the beliefs and practices of the Catholic Church in the Early Modern centuries. For the term inevitably suggests a reactive movement responding to the different versions of Protestantism and designed to halt their advance – to reverse the triumphs of heresy, to reconquer contested regions of France, Germany and Central Europe, to compensate for the loss of souls in Europe by sweeping missionary campaigns to convert pagans and infidels in overseas countries, to reaffirm Catholic values by insisting on the truth of those dogmas that had been most bitterly attacked. Critics of the concept argue in favour of a much lengthier and less defensive process, best called Catholic reform or restoration, which arose spontaneously in the later Middle Ages and continued throughout the sixteenth century and beyond. It stood, among much else, for a more introspective Christianity founded on meditative prayer and the systematic examination of conscience, for a moral discipline which extended to clergy and laity alike, for a systematic lay piety shaped by participation in confraternities – in societies devoted to ceremony and good works, and designed to encourage people who could not withdraw from everyday life to follow a modified religious rule based on the practice of charity in all senses of the word.

Arguably, however, until the 1530s Catholic reform movements for the most part remained localised and uncoordinated, arising within particular dioceses or religious orders. They owed little to a Papacy preoccupied with exploiting the Papal States as a major source of revenue, heavily involved in Italian politics and in pursuing its own dynastic schemes, increasingly secularised. Popes were generally wary of summoning any general council lest it raise the issue of the location of sovereignty within the Church and theories of conciliar supremacy be revived. Only from about 1540 did a centrally directed campaign develop, in response, at least partly, to a threat from so-called rebels now believed to have distanced themselves irrevocably from the Church by obstinately defying its authority and taking their stand on the absolute primacy of the Bible.

It may be best to think of sixteenth-century Catholicism as woven of three strands, of Catholic reform, of the Counter-Reformation, and perhaps of an older, unreformed folk religion, that began to intertwine from about 1540 onwards. The missionary forces of the Catholic Church were directed, not only against Protestant or Reformed heresy, but also against more prosaic and commonplace enemies of salvation – against ignorance of the most rudimentary tenets of Christianity (even of the creed, the Hail Mary and the Our Father); against sins, including sexual promiscuity, disorderly conduct and blasphemy; and against superstition, or foolish and false religion, as the ecclesiastical hierarchy and the Holy Office chose to define it. Their target was not poverty as such, and certainly not the poverty which spurred ordinary labouring folk to earn their living. Rather, it was the tendency of certain kinds of poverty to imperil souls by tempting their victims into prostitution, vagrancy, or even incest in families who could not afford to own separate beds and were forced to sleep together. As Ludovico Antonio Muratori would eventually declare, *circa* 1720, in one of the more conventional parts of his controversial treatise on charity, 'it is not only riches but deep poverty that can act as a dangerous temptation in a person's life and a powerful instigator of a great many sins'.[1] 'How many sins are committed for lack of bread, and how many for want of a bed?' demanded Giovanni Battista De Rossi in 1730, in a letter to a friend in charge of the village parish of Rocca di Papa.[2] Poor relief, inspired by the traditional notions of corporal and spiritual mercy both to the soul and to the body, drawing much of its strength from the taking of the Eucharist by its charitable practitioners, and invoking the sacrament of penance as one of its most formidable weapons, was enlisted in the struggle for the conquest of the greatest possible number of souls.[3]

About 1540, a traditional date for the beginning of the Counter-Reformation, Catholic societies were not starting from scratch. They had inherited many institutions from the past, for there was no general attempt to dissolve hospitals, almshouses, convents and confraternities, even though some of these (as in Ypres and Lyons) were instructed to channel their almsgiving through centrally controlled common chests, general almonries or *bureaux des pauvres*.[4] Two organisations, in particular, can be traced to the Catholic reform movements of the fifteenth century. These were the great general hospitals and the Monti di Pietà. Both were championed, at least in Italy, by eloquent and gifted preachers from one order especially, the Observant or strict Franciscans.

General hospitals were formed by creating unions of most, but seldom all, of the existing hospitals in a city. They were not always brought together under one roof, but it was usual to subject quite large numbers of small, struggling or actively corrupt foundations to one flourishing and relatively large one. This would now, through a board of governors representing the more important social 'conditions' in the city, both lay and clerical, rule over the lesser institutions, in so far as they had not been suppressed.[5] It would do so somewhat in the manner of the famous super-hospital of Santa Maria della Scala in Siena, whose tentacles stretched throughout Tuscany and even into the Florentine state. This Sienese hospital and several of its imitators combined the functions of a refuge for pilgrims, a hospital for sick people, and an organisation for bringing up abandoned and orphaned children.[6] Unlike the hospitals of the sixteenth and seventeenth centuries they had no particular concern with the internment of beggars and no disposition to specialise in the treatment of a particular disease or category of illnesses. This process of concentrating and consolidating hospitals, in the interests of greater efficiency, was under way in northern Italy in the mid-fifteenth century and was to continue in the peninsula at least until the 1580s.[7] It was carried out in some French cities, such as Toulouse, in the early sixteenth century, and in Spain the process spread from Aragon to Castile after 1500, involving many cities, including Salamanca, Medina del Campo, Seville, and Madrid.[8] Resistance often sprang from descendants of the founders, who had no wish to see their family hospitals, cherished items of patronage, disappearing into the anonymity of a large municipal organisation, and from the wardens or priors of small foundations, who feared the loss of modest but valuable sources of income.

When they began, Monti di Pietà were generally public pawnshops, usually supervised by the commune with some guidance and co-operation from local churchmen.[9] They were designed to lend money, either gratuitously or at very moderate rates of interest intended to cover administrative costs but not to make a profit. Their intended clients were local people of all social ranks except the poorest, who had no possessions to pledge, no gold rings or cheap jewellery or spare items of clothing or household linen.[10] To finance the operation they drew to some extent upon charitable gifts, but even more upon deposits of money made by individuals, by government magistracies, and by other institutions. Initially designed to serve as substitutes for Jewish bankers (though some communes hedged their bets and resorted to both Jewish and Christian establishments), the Monti di Pietà set out to regulate and impose morality on the processes of borrowing and lending, if only by limiting the sums lent, refusing to lend to children of the house without parental approval, and making pointed inquiries as to why the borrower wanted the money. One of many charges against Jewish bankers, as in the city of Savona near Genoa in 1479, had been that by asking no questions and providing cash too readily, they had encouraged clients to ruin themselves through drink and gambling.[11] Foundations of new Monti di Pietà were to continue in Italy well beyond 1540, and they were certainly known in France and Spain, although they may have been less prominent in those countries. In 1561, for example, an Arca de Misericordia y Monte de Piedad (literally, a 'mercy chest') was founded in Toledo, with the threefold aim of lending money and grain to the poor, giving alms to needy parishioners, and selling cheap bread in times of dearth.[12] Similar institutions, under the name of Prêts Charitables, were to be promoted by zealous, aggressive organisations such as the Compagnie du Saint Sacrement in Lyons and Grenoble in the late seventeenth century.[13]

Since the great hospitals of the fifteenth century seldom absorbed every foundation in their towns and frequently strained at new ones, the Catholic societies of the 1540s inherited other items. There were pesthouses or *lazzaretti*, part hospitals for those thought to be stricken with plague, part quarantine centres for people and goods from suspect places, and part convalescent homes for survivors of the terrible illness.[14] And hospitals for incurables, or hospitals prepared to treat the pox, were common to Italy, Spain and France from the turn of the fifteenth century onwards. Sandra Cavallo, the historian of poor relief in Turin, has warned against the assumption that charitable foundations always originated in generous attempts to confront economic or natural crises, promptly directing assistance to the regions of most pressing need.[15] But it is difficult to discard the belief that the pesthouses and pox hospitals were direct responses to the challenge of acute and frightening disease, even though other uses were subsequently found for both of them. *Lazzaretti* surely sprang from the growing recognition that plague might be caused by contagion, especially among the poor, as well as, or rather than, a general corruption of the air which would affect people of every social order. Hospitals for incurables were a response to the horrors of the *morbus gallicus*, the sexually transmitted disease that broke out in the 1490s and presented hospitals with a new problem on an alarming scale. For they were now confronted, not with fevers or injuries that could be cured or run their course in a matter of days or weeks, but with a disease resembling the almost-extinct leprosy in that it brought to its far more numerous victims, not immediate death, but life in pain, coupled with grotesque disfigurement and sometimes with progressive and permanent loss of physical abilities.[16] Several, but by no means all, of the hospitals for incurables in Italy were inspired by the Company or Oratory of Divine Love, which originated in Genoa and represented a new and fashionable type of confraternity of laymen and clerics, often associated with Catholic reform. It was not, as were many of the older confraternities, a society for mutual support, concerned with the organisation of processions and ceremonies and the presentation of religious dramas or *tableaux-vivant*. Members combined personal piety of a more inward-looking nature with works of mercy and charity directed outwardly towards poor people, often abjectly miserable, who were not and could never have been members of the confraternity itself.[17]

After 1540 permanent pesthouses, in the lengthening intervals between epidemics, represented unused plant, and were sometimes pressed into service as places of isolation and confinement for the most abjectly poor folk in the city – especially in Genoa, between about 1580 and the mid-1650s.[18] They were well suited to the campaigns for good order and discipline, assigning special places to repulsive or undesirable groups of people, that arose from the Counter-Reformation's campaigns against sin and ignorance. On occasion city governments would command all homeless and destitute persons to report at a designated assembly point, with a view to their being accommodated in a disused monastery or in other enclosed premises which had often been used as a pesthouse. Sometimes the authorities would conduct a 'Triumph of Charity', in which all the local beggars, visible *en masse* for the first and last time, were marched or carried off in procession to their new quarters, accompanied by some of their benefactors.[19] Reading accounts of such rituals, one wonders whether the pesthouses were being used to contain the beggars simply because they represented available, vacant space. Or were the very poor regarded as potential sources of infection who needed to be isolated, and were deeper analogies being drawn between social disorders and the disorder of disease?[20]

As for the incurables, by the 1540s the great physician Fracastoro was already commenting on the senility of the disease which he had named 'Syphilis', though other names would long be preferred. His expectation that the ageing malady would not only lose its virulence but expire altogether was not to be fulfilled, and there would be one especially fierce outbreak in Seville in 1568.[21] Most of the hospitals remained, their attention shifting to other chronic conditions and protracted diseases, such as tuberculosis, hernia, and sores that refused to heal.[22] It was generally accepted, however, at least in Italy, that only at the Incurabili could one obtain the expensive treatment, using decoctions of guaiacum or *lignum* that promised to cure the pox, or at least to palliate its symptoms; in Seville, the hospital of St Cosmo and St Damian was known unflatteringly as Las Bubas, 'the pustules', because it would treat the illness. In Naples and Venice especially, such hospitals were closely identified with the Counter-Reformation's campaigns against sin and its consequences, for they put forth branches and concerned themselves with rescue work among prostitutes and children in danger of being sold into whoredom or otherwise betrayed by their parents and relatives.[23]

As will appear later, work in any hospital, attending the sick, was in the age of the Counter-Reformation a vital exercise for those bent on mastering themselves and struggling for the souls of the sick and dying. Work among the so-called incurables was particularly important as an ascetic exercise and a technique for mortifying the senses, given the exceptionally repellent, Job-like nature of the patients' afflictions. Inevitably, though, the term 'incurable' changed its meaning through time. Already, by the mid-sixteenth century, it had come to mean 'requiring prolonged treatment' rather than 'beyond all hope of a cure'; in Florence the guaiacum regime lasted between thirty and fifty days.[24] Even so, the turnover of patients in hospitals such as San Giacomo degli Incurabili in Rome was surprisingly rapid; many, it seems, were given medication and discharged, rather than kept in the wards indefinitely.[25] By the early eighteenth century, in Turin and possibly also in Crema, the term 'incurable' was associated with old age rather than with any specific affliction, Turinese citizens endowing beds for incurables, acquiring the right to nominate their occupants, and using them to provide for superannuated servants and other dependents.[26]

Many historians will associate the 1540s with well-known events or tendencies that heralded the Counter-Reformation – with the incorporation of the Society of Jesus, with the death or eclipse of the moderate reformers who had urged dialogue with the Protestants and believed in justification by faith alone, with the establishment of the revived Roman Inquisition, with the opening sessions of the Council of Trent. Can a historian of poor relief point to an equally significant series of events in the same decade? Possibly not, but the exercise is worth trying.

In Italy the 1540s saw the establishment of an Ufficio dei Poveri in Genoa as a public institution which would compensate for the inadequacies of existing charities; the Company of Divine Love, which had long been promoting various charitable initiatives in the city, made sure of representation on the governing body.[27] Its actions as a pressure group for the promotion of Catholic values through the practice of charity were to be paralleled, if not imitated, by equally versatile confraternities in other cities in future decades, such as the Azzurri in Messina or the Compagnie di San Paolo in Lodi and Turin.[28] Medicean Florence and papal Bologna, in 1542 and 1548 respectively, launched schemes for the repression of begging.[29] In Venice, systematic attempts were made to enforce the poor law which had been on the statute book since 1529 and to give the local board of public health responsibility for controlling, not just beggars and vagabonds, but prostitutes as well.[30] Both the Florentine and the Bolognese schemes proclaimed the significant principle that beggars must be kept out of churches, hitherto favourite pitches for those playing on the charity of the pious, on the grounds that proper conditions for worship could never be guaranteed unless these unholy intruders were prevented from interrupting services and disturbing the faithful. The conditions on which prostitutes could enter churches were minutely prescribed by Venetian ordinances. According to a brief issued by Cardinal Pucci in 1542, Cosimo de' Medici, Duke of Florence, had turned his attention to orphans and other poor beggars who 'go about like brute beasts rather than rational creatures, without the knowledge of any divine commandment or of good behaviour'.[31] This was an early instance of an indictment against beggars, portraying them as bestial creatures who could only be made human through knowledge of Christian doctrine, a charge-sheet which was to become lengthier and more colourful over the next century and a half.[32] In 1541, in the Italian city of Modena, there was an especially bitter dispute over a ruthlessly imposed scheme to force all the existing hospitals together into one Sacred Union under a well-paid manager.[33]

These measures may be attributed in part to changes in the religious climate. But some may also have been reactions to the widespread shortages of 1539–40, to the same famine that in Spain drove hundreds of peasants and shepherds into the cities of Zamora and Burgos, and prompted the city government of Zamora to assign responsibility for the care of the poor to affluent city families, stipulating that 'the paupers, who are to be given all that they need to eat, are not to go from door to door, and all of them must wear badges over their chests with the names of the persons who are giving them food'.[34] However, such regulations were not merely responses to crises, since attempts were also made to use the giving or withholding of alms as instruments of religious discipline. An ordinance approved by the theologians of Salamanca prescribed that regular support should be denied to idlers, evil-livers, and irreligious characters who failed to confess and take communion as the Church required.[35]

These and other poor laws, restricting begging and making giving to deserving cases virtually compulsory, were soon to inspire the famous debate between the Dominican Soto, sometime chaplain to Charles V, and the Benedictine abbot Juan Robles de Medina – Soto maintaining that to beg was a fundamental human right with which no-one should interfere, and Medina treating the need to beg as a burden of which all abjectly poor people ought to be relieved.[36] It was Medina who invoked Christ's example to justify a new remedial charity, administered by hospitals and directed towards supporting and curing the sick and afflicted, which would be more effective and more profoundly Christian than one based on casual, face-to-face transactions between a beggar and an almsgiver. 'No-one of sense should doubt', he argued, 'that it is better to cure the afflicted man than to give him every day a *blanca*, and better to maintain the pauper than to give him every day a *maravedí*'.[37] He would later add that 'we do not read that the Son of God extended to beggars any charity other than to take away from them the occasion to beg – giving them health, so that they could earn without the shame and toil of begging'.[38] The theologians' controversy contributed to a protracted discussion in Catholic countries, which was to extend over many decades, as to whether the very poor ought to be kept visible and accessible to the general public of compassionate almsgivers, or whether they ought to be shut away in institutions, managed by boards of governors and other officials, which stood some chance of curing them of their spiritual shortcomings as well as their physical afflictions.

It was during the 1540s, too, that Rome itself began to develop as a paradigmatic city, providing leadership and example in the sphere of charity as in other fields. Every kind of known charity ought to exist and be practised in the papal city, rather than merely enjoy distant papal approval. Rome had been slow to respond to some new fashions, and had established a Monte di Pietà only in 1539.[39] But during the 1540s at least two new types of religious house or conservatory for women and girls were established in Rome by Ignatius Loyola and subsequently spread, frequently through Jesuit influence and often under other names, to other cities of Italy. They were the houses of Santa Marta and of the Vergini Miserabili, both of which were dedicated to the preservation and restoration of female honour and to the salvation of souls. Santa Marta provided the model for many temporary refuges for compromised or dishonoured women who might be charged with adultery and even exposed to vengeance from angry relatives, the Vergini Miserabili for institutions which would protect girls from being sold as child whores by mercenary and uncaring relatives.[40]

Nunneries for penitent prostitutes, dedicated to the Magdalen or to St Mary of Egypt, had long been known in French and Italian cities, and were being revived and expanded afresh in the sixteenth century.[41] But Loyola's houses were new departures, in that they offered a less drastic solution, a half-way house or breathing-space, to women anxious to escape from prostitution, and in that the Vergini Miserabili concentrated on prevention of the fatal sin by attempts to protect young people rather than on its cure through a lifetime of austere discipline and repentance on the part of adults. In Seville, towards 1600, there was a Casa Pia founded by the Jesuits, where women eager to abandon prostitution sometimes stayed for as little as two or three days.[42] By the middle and late seventeenth century, similar institutions would be introduced to French cities. These were designed to accommodate professional prostitutes, unmarried mothers and women suspected of having extra-marital relations, and bore such names as the Filles Pénitentes (as in Amiens and Lyons) or La Providence, the Company of the Holy Sacrament's equivalent to the Vergini Miserabili, established in Lyons in 1707.[43]

Rome's influence over charities, superficially standardised but usually adapted to local circumstances, was exerted not only through the power of example, but also through the establishment of archconfraternities and archhospitals, to which similar charities abroad could be affiliated.[44] These bodies sometimes recognised superiors in Rome out of a sincere desire to imitate them and share in their spiritual privileges, but occasionally did so from a disingenuous wish to free themselves from local ecclesiastical control.[45] At intervals pious authors attempted to immortalise Rome's achievements, through breathlessly eulogistic accounts of everything done for the poor in the holy city – statements which sometimes conveyed the impression that charity and hospitality were the principal industries of Rome. Gregory Martin, translator of the Vulgate for English Catholics, sang Rome's praises in 1580–81;[46] Camillo Fanucci followed him in 1602;[47] the *Pietas Romana* of Theodor von Meyden, written in 1624, was translated for the benefit of English readers in the reign of James II;[48] then came the encyclopaedic volumes of the Abbot Carlo Bartolomeo Piazza, which were divided into numerous shorter treatises or discourses, and ran through more than one edition at the close of the seventeenth century.[49]

Something has been said about the beginnings of the new Catholic charity and its debt to earlier Catholic reformers. But what were its deepest characteristics? Its highest ideals lay in self-sanctification through heroic personal service to the poor, rather than in the acquisition of merit through casual or impersonal almsgiving. Its central objectives lay in the conquest of souls by means of organised charity in which the use of the sacraments, especially communion and confession, the channels of grace and the means to salvation, played a prominent part. At the most humdrum level, regular giving to the poor was made to depend on their good and devout behaviour – on proof of attendance at mass or at schools of Christian doctrine, a firm requirement of Julius Echter of Mespelbrunn, prince-bishop of Würzburg,[50] whereas the rectors of the General Almonry at Lyons in 1613 wanted a catechism conducted at each distribution of bread in order to remedy poor people's ignorance of the rudiments of Catholic belief.[51] More ambitiously, Catholic charity chose to deal with sin and ignorance by imposing the total discipline of a closed institution, which narrowly resembled a convent or monastery, upon the children and adults who were confined within it, sometimes forcibly. Such establishments ranged from the relatively refined conservatories for orphans and endangered girls, the *Zitelle*, to the harsher and more coarse-grained hospices for beggars or Mendicanti.[52] These distinctions were underlined in Venice in the 1590s, when administrators employed by the beggars' hospital were accused of treating their charges as if they were *Zitelle* and feeding them on meat – an imputation which they strenuously denied.[53]

Prominent targets were habitual sinners, not respectable folk guilty of occasional lapses: delinquents whose entire culture was one of disorder and irreligion, implying not only ignorance of the sacraments, but a determination to do without them. Beggars and vagrants were, in the rhetoric of those who justified their confinement in hospitals in Italy and France, in the language of pamphleteers such as the Jesuit Andre Guévarre, portrayed as lost souls. No-one frequented churches more than they, but no-one was more profoundly unaware of Christian doctrine or more disruptive of devotion. Professional beggars who posed as cripples or blind men, or told fictitious hard-luck stories, were guilty of depriving the genuinely poor of their rightful share in a limited supply of alms. Equally common was the charge that they were not so much cunning, work-shy petty criminals as sinners spawned in sloth and ignorance, who cohabited outside wedlock, who gambled and cursed and brawled and slept rough, who corrupted their own bastard children, and spent their ill-gotten gains in taverns and brothels and other unsavoury places.[54] One pamphlet of the Company of the Holy Sacrament in France, the most militant seventeenth-century organisation for the pursuit of sinners, alleged that 'The poor contract a marriage with threepence and a ring, and they dissolve the union without any other ceremony than by breaking the ring and returning the threepence'.[55]

The earliest beggars' hospitals, which sprang up in Bologna, Cremona and elsewhere in northern Italy from about 1560 onwards, were much like hospitals for incurables under another name, in that entrants to them were supposed to be genuinely crippled, destitute, homeless, solitary, or young. Sturdy adult beggars were punished or set on work in other places.[56] Spanish reformers such as Cristóbal Pérez de Herrera, chief physician to the Spanish galleys, seem to have favoured a similar arrangement, although his hospices or *albergues* did not aim at totally enclosing the impotent poor – only at providing them with shelter, and leaving them to go out and beg during the day and take their meals where they would.[57] But Italian institutions of the seventeenth and eighteenth centuries drew inspiration openly from the hospital which enclosed the poor of Lyons in 1614 and more furtively, perhaps, from the workhouse for disorderly young people and 'bestial' men established in Amsterdam in the 1590s. In Genoa, Rome, Naples and Palermo, they were called Alberghi dei Poveri or Ospizii rather than hospitals. One of their functions was to impose discipline on recalcitrant, disorderly and irreligious people. They had their infirmaries, but the emphasis had shifted from bodily to spiritual sickness, which could only be treated by prolonged exposure to an all-embracing regime. At least in theory the effective remedy for the disorders connected with begging was the monotonous regularity of a quasi-monastic life. This was to be based on a separation of sexes to combat promiscuity; on a segregation of different age groups to prevent the corruption of children; on a working day designed to cure idleness and measured out precisely by a clock which chimed every quarter of an hour (as in Genoa); on movements from one part of the premises to another, from workshop to refectory, that were organised into religious processions, each column of inmates marching two-by-two behind a cross to the sound of the litany and under priestly surveillance, as though to counter the ill-effects of a godless and disorderly existence.[58] Whereas Protestant Europe attacked monasticism and withdrawal from the world, Catholic Europe discovered new uses for it and made at least symbolic attempts at separating the disorderly poor from the rest of society – though there is reason to doubt that Foucault's 'great internment' was ever actually realised. It was an ambition and a threat rather than an achievement. To incarcerate poor people other than the elderly, the crippled and the young proved too strenuous and costly an undertaking in most parts of western Europe. Every spell of dearth and every hard winter was likely to bring hordes of beggars into the towns, and to defy the attempts of hospitals and their inadequate police forces to enclose them.[59]

Very likely the attack upon habitual and disorderly sinners, and particularly upon beggars, vagrants and prostitutes, was partially prompted by the fear of disease. Sin and sickness were linked in the official statements made by the Church, and the Church presented the sacrament of penance as a sovereign remedy for both. Confession boxes, built into the walls, were prominent features of the churches in the beggars' hospitals of Naples and Palermo.[60] Both the plague and the pox were regarded as general scourges called for by the sins of the community at large, as much as by the misconduct of particular victims, but it was also argued that the first need and duty of every sick person was to make a confession. This was not merely a means of preparing the soul against the possibility of death, but a step towards the physical recovery of the patient. Hence the ecclesiastical demand that doctors should refuse, at least after a time, to attend patients who had failed to confess.

This subject takes us back to the 1540s. Another event of that decade was the dispute in Rome between the clergy and the medical profession over the revival and enforcement of one of the acts of the Fourth Lateran Council of 1215, the canon '*Cum infirmitas*' of Pope Innocent III. His legislation had stated that physical sickness 'sometimes' sprang from sinfulness, on the strength of Christ's words to the cripple he had healed at the pool of Bethesda – 'Go, and sin no more, lest something worse befall you.' Hence the 'doctors of bodies', on being summoned to the bedsides of sick persons, must immediately advise them to call the 'doctors of souls', in the belief that once provision had been made for the spiritual health of the sick there could be a more useful resort to 'physical medicine, since when the cause ceases the effect ceases also', the removal of guilt and fear producing more favourable psychological conditions for the recovery of the body. Should any doctor neglect this obligation, he must be excluded from church until he made satisfaction for his fault.[61]

Attempts were made by the reformers in the sixteenth century to interpret the decree as meaning that doctors should actually be forbidden to attend patients who had turned a deaf ear to their exhortations and refused to confess. A determination to assert the primacy of the soul over the body, to contend that the saving of souls must take priority over all other forms of attention to the sick, was now of crucial importance. The older decree had merely suggested that every kind of remedy, including the spiritual, should be explored. Constitutions issued by Gian Matteo Giberti, the reforming bishop of Verona, ordered all rectors of churches to admonish their parishioners that if they fell sick they must call a priest before they summoned a doctor, and then proceeded to threaten doctors with severe penalties if they paid more than two visits to any patient who had refused or failed to make a confession.[62] In Rome Ignatius Loyola, who had noticed that many sick persons received the sacrament only with their last breath, attempted to get the legislation of Pope Innocent, construed in this way, enforced by Pope Paul III. Understandably opposed by the medical profession, who were jealous of their autonomy and insisted that they had a duty only to encourage patients to confess and not to deny them attention, the founder of the Society of Jesus carried the day. Efforts to enforce the decree were certainly made outside Rome, in the dioceses of Faenza and Modena (by the bishops) and in the island of Sicily generally (by the Spanish Viceroy, Don Juan de Vega).[63]

Nobody knows for sure how successfully the Church imposed its views, or whether the 'doctor of bodies' and the 'doctor of souls' were accustomed to collaborate or to regard each other as rivals, adopting different approaches to the patient. It seems certain, however, that many hospitals, catering mainly for poor people unable to afford medical attention in their own homes, became missionary fields and battlegrounds for the salvation of souls approaching death. As studies of sixteenth-century Florentine hospitals have shown, it would be wrong to imagine that sick wards were simply places where people went to die.[64] Most patients left the wards alive, though one may well wonder how many made a successful convalescence after their discharge. But the possibility of death in hospital was ever present, and patients entering Roman establishments in the late sixteenth or early seventeenth centuries were supposed to be immediately prepared for confession and communion.[65] One duty undertaken by Camillo de Lellis's male nursing order, founded at the Incurabili in the late sixteenth century, was to ensure that the sick had not only made a good confession but were also properly prepared for communion and actually swallowed the wafer, not allowing it to stick to their palates.[66] Metaphors from the battlefield came easily to those who described the achievements of the Camillans, who were expected to combine pastoral duties with the intimate, menial tasks of nursing for which tact and forbearance were most needed. In an early account of the Camillans their founder's biographer, Father Cicatelli, fervently portrayed them as crusaders against the Devil and his angels, saying that:

> all other religious, lords, and knights who wear the cross on their left side, bear it as a defensive weapon like a shield to defend themselves from the blows and temptations of enemies from hell. But our congregation has the special task of helping souls in their final battle at the time of death, and so we wear the cross on the right side, as if it were the blade of a sword and an offensive weapon to subdue the devils who are the most deadly enemies of so powerful a symbol'.[67]

Hospital wards were also the scenes, in the sixteenth century and afterwards, of a struggle for self-sanctification on the part of devout people seeking both to find Christ in the poor and to imitate Christ and the apostles directly by going forth and healing the sick. It was as if they were being Christ themselves, and finding him in somebody else. In the pious literature of the sixteenth century and afterwards, the dedicated orders of hospitallers of the late Middle Ages seem to have mysteriously disappeared and been replaced by a brutal, callous staff of 'mercenary' workers unmoved by any sense of religious dedication to the service of the poor and bent only on making gains for themselves. From the sixteenth to the eighteenth century, their deficiencies were countered – partially at least – by Jesuit novices, by students at the English seminary in Rome, by groups of part-time volunteers inspired by such ardent reformers as Filippo Neri in Rome or Matteo Guerra in Siena, and by new nursing orders vowed to the service of the sick, such as the Camillans, or the Fatebenefratelli, or, in France, most famously, the Daughters of Charity. Should the volunteers be people of social standing, their acts of self-humiliation as servants of querulous and malodorous patients would be all the more poignant.[68] The service of the sick, mortifying the senses and calling for mastery over the shrinking flesh of the genteel visitor to the wards, was a form of ascetic practice. Gregory Martin, the English priest who extolled the charities of Rome in 1581, took one of his texts from St Jerome's account of the heroic deeds of Fabiola, the rich Roman matron who had personally brought the sick poor off the streets and into her own hospital. In papal Rome, he continued:

> for one woman count a multitude of men and wemen that shewe their charitie, and very many in their own persons, making it a spiritual exercise of their humility, and a satisfaction for their sinnes, and a mortifying of their bodies, and a repressing of vice and concupiscence, to goe to this Hospital or that, to serve the sick and sore, bringing them their meate, swipping their floor, making their beddes, and more or lesse according to their measure of charitie.[69]

It is tempting to imagine that this kind of penitential exercise was intended to be a substitute for the older forms of austerity, but this was not entirely so in Siena. Here followers of Matteo Guerra, all of them involved in administration or nursing at the hospital of Santa Maria della Scala, formed a company of flagellants of a kind which would have been familiar to citizens of fifteenth-century Florence. From 1579 onwards, the rector permitted Matteo to hold meetings in the chapel of the Holy Nail, which preserved the remains of one of the spikes by which Christ had been fastened to the cross. In the presence of this powerful reminder of the Saviour's passion, members of the devout circle completed their day of strenuous service to the poor by re-enacting the sufferings of Christ through 'a long and bloody application of the discipline' in the darkened room, after reciting the seven penitential psalms and the litanies and hearing either a suitable sermon or a series of readings from sacred texts.[70]

Characteristic of Catholic reform and the Counter-Reformation, or at least of their official rhetoric, was an insistence that charity should be as much spiritual as physical. Its highest end was the salvation of the soul; its most prominent targets were the souls of habitual sinners and of all sick persons approaching the moment of death when the demons might be expected to renew their assault; its fiercest enemy was the kind of poverty that threatened to lead souls to damnation. Its weapons included the imposition of a quasi-monastic discipline upon the most gravely endangered souls, and the systematic use of the sacrament of penance, partly as a means of curing physical illness, but also as a way of securing service to Christ's most unprepossessing representatives, the sick and sore. It was true that its affirmation of the supremacy of the soul could well lead charitable activity away from the living poor and towards the souls of the dead who were suffering in purgatory. Large sums were invested in the so-called Monti dei Morti by confraternity members and others bent on securing large numbers of masses for the souls of the departed.[71] These contributed incidentally to the support of the priests employed to say or sing them, who in some people's view could be numbered among the Poor of Christ, and it could therefore be argued that they were not solely preoccupied with the dead at the expense of the living.

By the early eighteenth century, however, Ludovico Antonio Muratori, librarian to the Duke of Modena and parish priest of Santa Maria Pomposa, was in trouble for protesting against excessive investment in charity to the souls of the dead and in the lavish decoration of churches.[72] He had been moved to plead for a simpler kind of practical Christianity which would concentrate above all on the service of the living poor and on the seven works of corporal mercy. Muratori may be claimed as a herald of the Enlightenment, but his ample treatise on charity was in many ways a traditional document, which drew heavily on patristic authority and harked back to the days of Filippo Neri in sixteenth-century Rome. His own practical measure was to establish in Modena a Compagnia della Carità strongly reminiscent of the organisations disseminated throughout the diocese of Verona by Gian Matteo Giberti towards the year 1540.[73] And his arguments included a very traditional complaint about the poor quality of hospital staff, 'worse than dogs', whose harshness was such that:

> the unhappy crowd of patients, abandoned to their misfortunes, wish that they had been left to suffer on the straw in their cottages, under the eyes of their loved ones (who at least do all they can to help them), rather than fall into the hands of these cruel creatures, bent solely upon their own

> gain, in a place dedicated, not to charity, but to barbaric acts.[74]

He called, once more, for the intervention in hospitals of ascetic volunteers, preferably persons of noble rank, who would pursue self-sanctification through the loving service of sick people by performing menial tasks. 'The higher and more noble the charitable persons who stoop to the service of the languishing poor, the greater their merit in the sight of the most high'.[75] Through the service of the sick you recognised God's gift of good health; in the misery of others you saw what might well happen to yourself. Did these sentiments mark the dawn of the Enlightenment, or were they, rather, a plea for a revival of the true and original spirit of Catholic reform and the Counter-Reformation?

Notes

1 L.A. Muratori, *Trattato della Carità Cristiana e altri Scritti sulla Carità*, ed. P.G. Nonis (Rome, 1961), p. 303. This work was first published in 1723.

2 P. Fragnelli, '"Carità operativa" e cura d'anime nelle lettere di Giovanni Battista De Rossi, 1730–1744', *Ricerche per la Storia Religiosa di Roma*, 7 (1988), p. 313.

3 For some of the characteristics of Catholic poor relief, see B. Pullan, 'Catholics and the poor in early modern Europe', *Transactions of the Royal Historical Society*, 26 (1976), pp. 15–34; B. Pullan, '"Support and redeem": charity and poor relief in Italian cities from the fourteenth to the seventeenth century', *Continuity and Change*, 3 (1988), pp. 177–208.

4 For Ypres, see J. Nolf, *La réforme de la bienfaisance publique à Ypres* (Ghent, 1915), especially pp. 47–9; for Lyons, see N.Z. Davis, 'Poor relief, humanism and heresy: the case of Lyon', in her *Society and Culture in Early Modern France* (Stanford, CA 1975), p. 39.

5 For one important example, see F. Leverotti, 'Ricerche sull' origine dell' Ospedale Maggiore di Milano', *Archivio Storico Lombardo*, 110 (1984), pp. 77–113.

6 For a description of the hospital in the mid-fifteenth century see F. Leverotti, 'L'ospedale senese di Santa Maria della Scala in una relazione del 1456', *Bullettino Senese di Storia Patria*, 91 (1984), pp. 276–91. A valuable monograph on the hospital and its estates is S.R. Epstein, *Alle Origini della Fattoria Toscana. L'Ospedale della Scala di Siena e le sue Terre (metà '200 – metà '400)* (Florence, 1986).

7 A late example is that of Udine, capital of the Venetian province of the Friuli, in 1584, when a merger between the two large hospitals of the Misericordia and Santa Maria Maddalena created a single organisation whose income outstripped that of the commune. See A. Tagliaferri, *Struttura e Politica Sociale in una Comunità Veneta del '500 [Udine]* (Milan, 1969), pp. 113–17.

8 See J. Soubeyroux, *Paupérisme et rapports sociaux à Madrid au XVIIIème siècle* (2 vols, Lille and Paris, 1978), I, pp. 316–25; M.E. Perry, *Crime and Society in Early Modern Seville* (London, 1980), pp. 172–3; L.M. Martz, *Poverty and Welfare in Habsburg Spain: the Example of Toledo* (Cambridge, 1983), pp. 34–8, 61–5, 77–86; M. Flynn, *Sacred Charity. Confraternities and Social Welfare in Spain, 1400–1700* (Basingstoke, 1989), pp. 102–5.

9 Important collections of papers on the history of the Monti di Pietà are *Archivi Storici per le Aziende di Credito* (2 vols, Rome, 1956), by various authors, and *Banchi Pubblici, Banchi Privati e Monti di Pietà nell' Europa Preindustriale. Amministrazione, Tecniche Operative e Ruoli Economici. Atti del Convegno Genova, 1–6 ottobre 1990*, in *Atti della Società Ligure di Storia Patria*, new series, 31 (1991), fascicle i and ii (continuously paginated). For a general survey which concentrates on the origins of Italian Monti di Pietà rather than their subsequent development, see V. Meneghin, *I Monti di Pietà in Italia dal 1462 al 1562* (Vicenza, 1986).

10 For the kinds of goods pledged with Monti di Pietà see, for example, M. Martelli, *Storia del Monte di Pietà in Lugo di Romagna (1546–1968)* (Florence, 1969), pp. 87–8; I. Capecchi and L. Gai, *Il Monte di Pietà a Pistoia e le sue origini* (Florence, 1976), pp. 83–5, 128–9, 223–47; P. Massa Piergiovanni, 'Assistenza e credito alle origini dell' esperienza ligure dei Monti di Pietà', in *Banchi Pubblici*, pp. 602–3; C. Bresnahan Menning, *Charity and State in Late Renaissance Italy: the Monte di Pietà of Florence* (Ithaca and London, 1993), pp. 92–4.

11 Massa Piergiovanni, 'Assistenza', p. 596.

12 Martz, *Poverty*, pp. 135–7. On Spain see J. Lopez Yepes, *Historia de los Montes de Piedad en España. El Monte de Piedad de Madrid en el siglo XVIII* (2 vols, Madrid, 1971).

13 J.P. Gutton, *La société et les pauvres: l'exemple de la généralité de Lyon, 1534–1789* (Paris, 1971), pp. 383–4; K. Norberg, *Rich and Poor in Grenoble, 1600–1814* (Berkeley, Los Angeles and London, 1985), pp. 83, 91.

14 See A.G. Carmichael, 'Plague legislation in the Italian Renaissance', *Bulletin of the History of Medicine*, 57 (1983), pp. 519–21; A.G. Carmichael, *Plague and the Poor in Renaissance Florence* (Cambridge, 1986), pp. 118–21.

15 S. Cavallo, *Charity and Power in Early Modern Italy. Benefactors and their Motives in Turin, 1541–1789* (Cambridge, 1995).

16 For a general survey of hospitals for incurables, see A. Malamani, 'Notizie sul mal francese e gli ospedali degli incurabili in età moderna', *Critica Storica*, 15 (1978), pp. 193–216. On them and on the *morbus gallicus* in general, see the new work by J. Arrizabalaga, J. Henderson and R. French, *The Great Pox. The French Disease in Renaissance Europe* (New Haven and London, 1997). See also C. Quétel, *History of Syphilis* (Cambridge, 1990).

17 On the general theme of a change in the character of confraternities, see B. Pullan, 'Aid to brothers and charity to all Christians', to appear in the proceedings of the conference *Corpi, 'Fraternita', Mestieri nella Storia della Società Europea*, held at Trento, 30 May–1 June 1996.

18 See E. Grendi, 'Pauperismo e Albergo dei Poveri nella Genoa del Seicento', *Rivista Storica Italiana*, 87 (1975), pp. 630–8; R. Savelli, 'Dalle confraternite allo stato: il sistema assistenziale genovese nel Cinquecento', *Atti della Società Ligure di Storia Patria*, new series, 24 (1984), pp. 196–9, 204, 208.
19 See N. Terpstra, *Lay Confraternities and Civic Religion in Renaissance Bologna* (Cambridge, 1995), pp. 203–4 (Bologna in 1563); D. Lombardi, *Povertà Maschile, Povertà Femminile: l'Ospedale dei Mendicanti nella Firenze dei Medici* (Bologna, 1988), pp. 58–9 (Florence in 1591 and 1621); the extract from E. Tesauro's *Istoria della Compagnia di S. Paolo*, Turin, 1701, in A. Monticone, (ed.) *La Storia dei Poveri: Pauperismo e Assistenza nell' Età Moderna* (Rome, 1985), pp. 102–3 (Turin in 1628).
20 See G. Fracastoro, *De contagione et de morbis contagiosis*, in his *Opera omnia* (Venice, 1555), f. 125, 127v.; Quétel, *History*, pp. 50–52.
21 Perry, *Crime*, p. 227.
22 Cf. M. Vanti, *S. Giacomo degl'Incurabili di Roma nel Cinquecento. Dalle Compagnie del Divino Amore a S. Camillo de Lellis* (Rome, 1938), pp. 37, 56–67; S. Ravicini, *Sulla Universalità dell' Opera Ospedaliera della S. Casa degl' Incurabili in Napoli. Memorie e Documenti Storici* (Naples, 1899), p. 273.
23 G. Vitale, 'Ricerche sulla vita religiosa e caritativa a Napoli tra Medioevo ed età moderna', *Archivio Storico per le Province Napoletane*, 86–87 (1970), pp. 226–35, 265–73; B. Pullan, *Rich and Poor in Renaissance Venice: the Social Institutions of a Catholic State, to 1620* (Oxford and Cambridge, Mass., 1971), pp. 235–8, 264–7, 376–9, 386.
24 B.J. Trexler, 'Hospital patients in Florence: San Paolo, 1567–68', *Bulletin of the History of Medicine*, 48 (1974), p. 49; cf. M. Del Lungo, 'Aspetti dell' organizzazione sanitaria nella Genova del Settecento: la cura delle malattie veneree', *Società e Storia*, 22 (1983), p. 772.
25 Vanti, *S. Giacomo*, p. 28; Arrizabalaga *et al.*, *The Great Pox*, pp. 200–1.
26 Cavallo, *Charity*, pp. 141–6; Malamani, 'Notizie', p. 211.
27 Savelli, 'Dalle confraternite', pp. 191–4.
28 See Pullan, 'Aid', forthcoming.
29 See L. Passerini, *Storia degli Stabilimenti di Beneficenza e d'Istruzione Elementare Gratuita della Città di Firenze* (Florence, 1853), pp. 27–8, 802–12; the extracts from the Bolognese scheme of 1548 printed in P. Camporesi, (ed.) *Il Libro dei Vagabondi* (Turin, 1973), pp. 409–12; Terpstra, *Lay Confraternities*, p. 204.
30 Pullan, *Rich and Poor*, pp. 297–309, 380–2.
31 See Document F in Passerini, *Storia*, pp. 802–3.
32 See, for example, the charges against beggars listed in *La mendicitàa proveduta nella città di Roma, coll' Ospizio Publico fondato dalla pietà, e beneficenza di Nostro Signore Innocenzo XII Pontefice Massimo* (Rome, 1693), pp. 9–10.
33 P. di Pietro, 'Sulla Santa Unione degli ospedali e delle opere pie della città di Modena nel 1541', in *Atti Primo Congresso Italiano Storia Ospitaliera* (Reggio Emilia, 1957), pp. 217–27.
34 Flynn, *Sacred Charity*, pp. 82–3, 88.
35 Ibid., pp. 90–4.
36 For discussions of the debate see, for example, Pullan, *Rich and Poor*,

pp. 281–6; Martz, *Poverty*, pp. 22–30; Flynn, *Sacred Charity*, pp. 90–95; B. Geremek, *Poverty: a History* (Oxford and Cambridge, Mass., 1994), pp. 196–9. Also on Soto see M. Fatica, 'Le voci contrarie alla *nova pauperum subventio*: (1) Christiaan Kellenaar. (2) Domingo de Soto', in his *Il Problema della Mendicità nell' Europa Moderna* (secoli XVI–XVIII) (Naples, 1992), pp. 77–118.

37 J. Medina, *De la orden que en algunos pueblos de Espana se ha puesto en la limosna: para rimedio de los verdaderos pobres* (Salamanca, 1545), folios B4v.–B5r.

38 Ibid., folios Ev.–E2r.

39 See G. Balis-Crema and R. Lunardi, 'Cenni storici sul Monte di Pietà di Roma', *Archivi*, I, pp. 561–71.

40 See P. Tacchi Venturi, *Storia della Compagnia di Gesù in Italia* (4 vols in 2, Rome, 1950–51), I i, pp. 384–5; I ii, pp. 284–94; II ii, pp. 166–82, 185–9; also J.W. O'Malley, *The First Jesuits* (Cambridge, Mass., and London, 1993), pp. 178–88. For a comprehensive account of women's institutions, see S. Cohen, *The Evolution of Women's Asylums since 1500. From Refuges for Ex-prostitutes to Shelters for Battered Women* (New York and Oxford, 1992).

41 See P. Pansier, *L'oeuvre des Répenties à Avignon du XIIIe au XVIIIe siècle* (Paris, 1910).

42 M.E. Perry, 'Deviant insiders: legalised prostitutes and a consciousness of women in early modern Seville', *Comparative Studies in Society and History*, 27 (1985), pp. 153–4.

43 P. Deyon, *Étude sur la société urbaine au 17e siècle: Amiens, capitale Provinciale* (Paris/The Hague, 1967), pp. 354–5; Gutton, *La Société*, pp. 389–92; Norberg, *Rich and Poor*, pp. 20–3.

44 On archconfraternities in general see C.F. Black, *Italian Confraternities in the Sixteenth Century* (Cambridge, 1989), pp. 72–4.

45 For examples, see M. Bascapè, 'Confraternite cittadine e pietà dei laici agli inizi dell' età moderna', in A. Caprioli, A. Rimoldi and L. Vaccaro, (eds) *Diocesi di Lodi* (Brescia, 1989), pp. 276–7, 279–81; A.L. Sannino, 'Le confraternite potentine dal XV al XIX secolo', *Ricerche di Storia Sociale e Religiosa*, new series, 19 (1990), pp. 125, 135, 136.

46 G. Martin, *Roma Sancta* (1581), ed. G.B. Parks (Rome, 1969).

47 C. Fanucci, *Trattato di tutte l'opere pie dell' alma città di Roma* (Rome, 1602).

48 T. von Meyden, *Pietas romana (a faithful relation of several sorts of charitable and pious works eminent in the city of Rome)* (Oxford, 1687).

49 C.B. Piazza, *Eusevologio romano; overo, Delle opere pie di Roma* (2 vols, Rome, 1698).

50 See R. Jütte, *Poverty and Deviance in Early Modern Europe* (Cambridge, 1994), p. 138.

51 W.J. Pugh, 'Social welfare and the Edict of Nantes: Lyon and Nimes', *French Historical Studies*, 8 (1973–4), p. 355.

52 Cf. F. Giusberti, 'La città assistenziale: riflessioni su un sistema piramidale' in *Forme e Soggetti dell' Intervento Assistenziale in una Città di Antico Regime* (Bologna, 1986), pp. 13–29.

53 Pullan, *Rich and Poor*, pp. 367–8.

54 See B. Pullan, 'Poveri, mendicanti e vagabondi (secoli XIV – XVII)', in

C. Vivanti and R. Romano (eds) *Storia d'Italia. Annali 1. Dal feudalesimo al capitalismo*, (Turin, 1978), pp. 1008–20.

55 Norberg, *Rich and Poor*, pp. 33–4.

56 See M. Fantarelli, *L'Istituzione dell' Ospedale di S. Alessio dei Poveri Mendicanti in Cremona (1569–1600)*, ed. G. Politi (Cremona, 1981), document 8, pp. 60–8.

57 See M. Jiménez Salas, *Historia de la Asistencia Social en España en la Edad Moderna* (Madrid, 1958), pp. 103–8; Martz, *Poverty*, pp. 86–90.

58 For a comparative study of beggars' hospices, see A. Guerra, E. Molteni and P. Nicoloso, *Il Trionfo della Miseria. Gli Alberghi dei Poveri di Genova, Palermo e Napoli* (Milan, 1995) – for foreign influences on these Italian institutions, see the 'Introduction' by B. Pullan, p. 12. On Genoa, see also Grendi, 'Pauperismo', pp. 640–59; E. Belgiovine and A. Campanella, 'La fabbrica dell' Albergo dei Poveri. Genova 1656–1696', *Atti della Società Ligure di Storia Patria*, new series, 23 (1983), pp. 133–91. On Rome, *La Mendicità Proveduta*, and M. Fatica, 'La reclusione dei mendicanti a Roma durante il pontificato di Innocenzo XII (1692–1700)', in his *Il Problema*, pp. 161–216.

59 For the famous thesis about the *grand renfermement* of social undesirables in seventeenth-century France, see M. Foucault, *Folie et déraison: histoire de la folie à l'âge classique* (Paris, 1961). Cf. O. Hufton, *The Poor of Eighteenth-century France*, 1750–1789 (Oxford, 1974), pp. 140–3, 155–8; Pullan '"Support"', pp. 198–9.

60 Guerra, Molteni and Nicoloso, *Il Trionfo*, pp. 116, 167–70.

61 IV Lateran, c. 22, in J.D. Mansi, *Sacrorum conciliorum nova et amplissima collectio* (56 vols, Florence, Venice and Paris, 1759–1927), XXII, coll. 1010–11. The biblical reference is to John, v, 14.

62 G.M. Giberti, *Constitutiones, titulus iv, c. 11,* in his *Opera*, ed. P. Ballerini (Ostiglia, 1740), pp. 58–9.

63 See Tacchi Venturi, *Storia*, II ii, pp. 190–5.

64 Trexler, 'Hospital patients', p. 54; K. Park, 'Healing the poor: hospitals and medical assistance in Renaissance Florence', in J. Barry and C. Jones, (eds) *Medicine and Charity before the Welfare State* (London and New York, 1991), pp. 34–7; K. Park and J. Henderson, '"The first hospital among Christians": the Ospedale di Santa Maria Nuova in early sixteenth-century Florence', *Medical History*, 35 (1991), pp. 164–88.

65 See the description of the procedures at the Santo Spirito by Fra Domenico Borgarucci in R. Grégoire, '"Servizio dell' anima quanto del corpo" nell' ospedale romano di Santo Spirito (1623)', *Ricerche per la Storia Religiosa di Roma*, 3 (1979), pp. 239–41. In general, Martin, *Roma Sancta*, pp. 66, 69.

66 Clauses 41 and 42 of the Rules of the Compagnia dei Servi dei Poveri, composed by Camillo de Lellis in 1584–5, in Vanti, *S. Giacomo*, p. 134.

67 Quoted in C. Longo Timossi, *Pauperismo e Assistenza. I Camilliani a Genova nel Primo Seicento* (Genoa, 1992), p. 38.

68 See L. Ponnelle and L. Bordet, *Saint Philippe Néri et la société romaine de son temps (1515–1595)* (Paris, 1929), pp. 126, 157–9, 172–3, 205, 350; Martin, *Roma Sancta*, p. 114; Grégoire, '"Servizio"', p. 244; F.D. Nardi, 'Matteo Guerra e la Congregazione dei Sacri Chiodi (sec. XVI-XVII). Aspetti della religiosità senese nell' età della Controriforma', *Bullettino*

Senese di Storia Patria, 91 (1984), pp. 23–30, 36; C. Jones, 'Vincent de Paul, Louise de Marillac, and the revival of nursing in the seventeenth century', in his *The Charitable Imperative: Hospitals and Nursing in ancien régime and Revolutionary France* (London and New York, 1989), pp. 89–121; O'Malley, *The First Jesuits*, pp. 171–3.

69 Martin, *Roma Sancta*, pp. 182–3.

70 Nardi, 'Matteo Guerra', pp. 30–2.

71 For examples see E. Grendi, 'Morfologia e dinamica della vita associativa urbana. Le confraternite a Genova fra i secoli XVI e XVIII', *Atti della Società Ligure di Storia Patria*, new series, 5 (1965), pp. 285–8; S. Musella, 'Dimensione sociale e prassi associativa di una confraternita napoletana nell' età della Controriforma', in *Per la Storia Sociale e Religiosa del Mezzogiorno d'Italia*, ed. G. Galasso and C. Russo (2 vols, Naples, 1980), I, pp. 357–8, 370, 375–8; Sannino, 'Le confraternite', p. 129.

72 For the publishing history of the treatise, see pp. 33–48 of Nonis's 'Introduction' (separately paginated) to Muratori's *Trattato*, cited above, note 1.

73 For the statutes of Muratori's Compagnia della Carità, see Muratori, *Trattato*, pp. 799–808, and cf. the *Trattato* itself, pp. 481–92. For Giberti's Compagnia, Pullan, *Rich and Poor*, pp. 272–6.

74 Muratori, *Trattato*, pp. 549–50.

75 Ibid., p. 582.

3

COUNTER-REFORMATION, ECONOMIC DECLINE, AND THE DELAYED IMPACT OF THE MEDICAL REVOLUTION IN CATHOLIC EUROPE, 1550–1750

Jonathan Israel

By 1750, the overthrow of the old medicine of humours, based on Hippocrates and Galen and its replacement with what the Italians called *medicina meccanica sperimentale*, the revolutionising of medical instruction and clinical practice after the pattern which began to be introduced in northern Europe during the third quarter of the seventeenth century, the systematic replacement of the old remedies and medicines with new treatments, and general reorganisation of the hospitals and public health care policy if still far from complete, was well under way throughout the whole of Catholic southern and central Europe. Both in terms of ideas, and the practical application of the new methods and procedures, the revolution had progressed to the point that it had the upper hand and dominated the scene from Paris to Palermo and from Seville to Vienna.

The leaders of the medical revolution in southern Europe – a revolution emanating, in the main, from the north – saw much to celebrate and take pride in but also considerable grounds for dissatisfaction and complaint. In 1727, the professor of practical medicine at Padua, Carlo-Francesco Cogrossi, on contemplating the contemporary Italian medical scene, lavishly praises those Italians who had contributed to the victory of the new medicine over the old but also regrets that, in some respects, the northern countries and (France) were ahead of Italy and that, in general, northerners were disinclined to acknowledge the earlier role of Italian men of science and medical men in building the new mechanistic, experimental philosophy of medicine, and principles of medical teaching, and in inventing the new instruments, such as the microscope and thermometer, which had contributed so much to the recent advances in medical science.[1] In the medical faculties of many an Italian university, the full blast of the late seventeenth-century medical revolution was not felt until the 1750s and 1760; or even later.[2]

In Spain, the commencement of the revolution can be dated precisely enough – to the year 1687 when the Valencian professor of medicine Juan de Cabriada published his epoch-making *Carta filosófica médico-chymica*,[3] a work which roundly rejects the entire corpus of the old medicine and replaces it with the new ideas, and especially the iatromechanistic doctrines of Leiden professor Franciscus De Le Boe Sylvius (1614–72).[4] But the resistance, both theoretical and practical, of *medicina Galénica-Arábiga*, as Spanish modernists liked to call it, was to prove long and tenacious and, as late as 1768, one of the leading lights of the medical revolution in Spain, Andrés Piquer (1711–72), could lament that 'for a large part of the present century' Spanish medicine had remained sunk in 'decadence'.[5] Nor was this a residual phenomenon to be found only in the outlying posts of Spanish culture. In 1766, the medical faculty at Salamanca was severely criticised for its backwardness by a royal commission set up by Carlos III, and it was not until 1771 that the medical revolution triumphed, with the texts of Boerhaave and the commentaries thereon of van Swieten and Haller being adopted as the basis of medical instruction, obligatory courses in chemistry and physics based on the text-books respectively of Boerhaave and the Utrecht professor Petrus van Musschenbroek (1692–1761), and proposals for a range of new facilities, in particular an anatomical theatre, a medical museum and anatomical display and a botanical garden.[6]

Nor was the position much different in Catholic Central Europe, despite the fact that one of Boerhaave's pupils and closest associates, the French physician, Jean-Baptiste Bassand, had been appointed court physician of the Emperor Karl VI in 1729. The powerful Austrian minister, Kaunitz, one of the chief architects of the Enlightenment in the Austrian lands, had visited Leiden as a young diplomat, in 1732, and met Boerhaave and other leading medical figures.[7] But it was not until Boerhaave's most famous pupil, Gerard van Swieten (1700–72), who had been brought up as, and always remained, a devout Catholic, was appointed 'Premier Médecin et

Bibliothecaire' at the court of Maria Thérèsa, in 1745, that the real medical revolution in Central Europe began.[8] Van Swieten began lecturing on Boerhaavian physiology, pathology and the general doctrines of the new medicine in the Vienna Hofbibliothek, of which he was director, in 1746. As his position became stronger, and his influence at court grew, he brought in a whole team of medical men from the Netherlands to assist with setting up the new facilities and equipment and to help with the new medical teaching.[9] Of particular importance was the creation in 1753 of an academic teaching clinic, known originally as the 'Medicinisch-und Chyrurgischen Kranken-Curirungs-Schul', with daily bedside instruction, which was placed under the direction of another influential pupil of Boerhaave, likewise of Dutch Catholic background, Antonius de Haen (1704–76).[10]

Cogrossi was, of course, right that many of the new instruments, above all thermometers and microscopes, had begun in Italy even if their further development and propagation, after the middle of the seventeenth century, had taken place chiefly in, and from, the Netherlands and, to a lesser extent, Britain and France. It is equally true that such large-scale facilities as botanical gardens and anatomical theatres had begun in sixteenth-century Italy and that some of the principal developments had continued to be in Italy down to the 1630s. But after around 1640, further development had taken place mainly in Protestant countries and in Paris. The anatomical theatres built at Copenhagen (1643), Groningen (1655) Kiel (1666) and Frankfurt-an-Oder (1689) were based on the Leiden model while that installed in the Gustavianum, at Uppsala, in 1662, was more influenced by the Padua model, but either way the new activity took place mainly in the Protestant north.[11] After the famous theatre at Bologna, constructed in the 1630s, there was a long pause in most of Catholic Europe (apart from Paris) which lasted nearly a century. The principal wave of construction in these countries began only in the second quarter of the eighteenth century when, among other places, anatomical theatres were acquired by Würzburg (1725), Ferrara (1731), Ingolstadt (1735), Prague (*c.*1745) and Vienna (1750s).[12] In Spain, the acquisition of such facilities, as we have seen, came later still.

Thus even though Italy had led the way in the sixteenth century and some of the Italian universities, most notably Padua, had acted as a magnet to Protestant medical students coming from northern countries at any rate down to the 1640s,[13] it seems to be the case that from the middle of the seventeenth century, Catholic southern and

Central Europe, including Italy, resisted the fundamental changes in medical thought, teaching and practice more strongly, and accepted the medical revolution emanating from the north, more slowly and reluctantly, than Protestant Europe and, to an extent, France. If we accept that this was so, we are confronted by a rather important and wide-ranging historical phenomenon which invites a broad discussion, broad both geographically and chronologically, of the general cultural context of the progress of medical science in Early Modern times.

In explaining the relative retardation of southern and Central Europe after 1640, it would clearly be a mistake to place much emphasis on the Catholic–Protestant divide as such. Any suggestion that the Catholic Church and its institutions had formed an intrinsically closer link with the old Aristotelian *philosophia recepta*, and as an intellectual adjunct of this *medicina Galénica*, would seem to have little foundation since the presiding figures of orthodox Calvinism, in the Netherlands as much as in Switzerland,[14] and still more Lutheran orthodoxy in Germany and Scandinavia,[15] were no less wedded to *philosophia recepta* than those of the Catholic world. If there was a great deal of resistance to the medical revolution of the late seventeenth century in Italy, Spain and the Catholic German-speaking lands, precisely the same is true of large parts of Protestant Europe. In Sweden–Finland, for example, it is undeniable that the academic medical establishment was heavily dominated by Dutch training and ideas at a much earlier stage than any Catholic country, at least as early as the 1660s and that Swedish medicine remained under a 'modernizing' Dutch and North German influence, without interruption down to the late eighteenth century. Nevertheless, the theological and, in part, the philosophical faculties continued to be dominated by conservative anti-Cartesians down to around 1700[16] and both before, and after, 1700, there was a good deal of resistance at the institutional level to some of the main changes associated with the medical revolution. Despite the construction of the Uppsala anatomy theatre in 1662–3 there was no regular dissecting there for many decades, owing to opposition,[17] while the introduction of Leiden-style bedside academic diagnoses, recording of case histories, and post-mortems championed above all by Lars Roburg, met with all kinds of obstruction. Roburg, who acquired his own training in Holland in the 1680s, briefly succeeded in establishing an academic ward on the Leiden model in the second decade of the eighteenth century.[18] But there was to be no permanent teaching hospital, or regular clinical instruction for medical students, in Sweden until the middle of the eighteenth century.

One of the central strands of the medical revolution was the phasing out of bleeding and purging, both of which were deeply embedded in the old medical doctrines, as principal remedies for a wide variety of illnesses and indisposition. But this proved an uphill task in Britain and Germany scarcely less than in Italy, Spain or Austria and even some of the Dutch leading lights, including van Swieten, advocated the use of bleeding in certain contexts, albeit giving new reasons for its use. If from the mid-seventeenth century onwards we encounter, with increasing frequency, spirited assaults on the whole culture of bleeding and purging not only in the Netherlands and Protestant Germany but also in Catholic lands such as France and Spain where Cabriada opened the attack in his *Carta filosófica* in 1687,[19] both the practice and the intellectual defence of bleeding remained extremely tenacious in Britain and many other parts of Protestant Europe, as well as Catholic lands, until far into the eighteenth century. Walter Harris, writing in 1699, regarded it strictly as a peculiarity of the Dutch that they 'bleed so sparingly and seldom as they do', finding it difficult to 'comprehend, considering how profusely the French and the more southern Nations do use venesection upon most occasions'.[20]

The religious split between the Catholic and Protestant worlds then can hardly be said to be the direct cause of the generally sluggish reception of the medical revolution in southern Europe. Rather it seems best to assume that a variety of other, mostly indirect, factors were at work, some of which had more relevance to what might be termed the intellectual or theoretical side of the medical revolution and others – while affecting both, inevitably, since the two aspects can never be entirely separated – of more particular relevance to the practical aspects. If the medical revolution was clearly an integrated package of intellectual *and* practical changes, each interacting closely on the other, it may nevertheless be possible to identify specific factors causing retardation which would tend to hamper one rather than the other set of changes.

On the intellectual side, the medical revolution flowed, we have seen, from the displacement of the old system of doctrines based on Hippocrates and Galen with what in mid-eighteenth-century England were called the 'principles of the mechanical physicians', the most celebrated of whom was Boerhaave who was universally reputed, from Glasgow to Moscow and from Stockholm to Seville, to have 'gone farther than any one in applying the science of mechanicks to medicine'.[21] Originally, this mechanistic medicine had been essentially Cartesian, Cartesian philosophy having achieved a general dominance in the Dutch universities by the 1650s,[22] and then, after 1660, often through contact with the Dutch universities, rapidly become entrenched and sporadically dominant in large parts of Protestant Germany, Switzerland, Scandinavia and Scotland where Cartesianism swept the board in the 1670s.[23] Later, partly owing to the impact of Newton and Locke (to begin with chiefly in Britain and the Netherlands), and partly owing to the anti-Cartesian reaction in the Dutch universities, of which Boerhaave himself was a leading proponent, Cartesianism, as such, rapidly faded from the picture. Given this framework in which 'our notions of physick change with our philosophy', as one contemporary English observer put it, it seems plausible that the same factors which caused the slower reception of mechanistic philosophy in general in southern and Catholic Central Europe also played a significant part in impeding the reception of mechanistic medicine. My argument would then be that it was less any intrinsic divide between Protestant and Catholic Europe, rooted in theology or religious culture, but rather the indirect intellectual effects of the Counter-Reformation which are important here, in particular the tendency for academic and book censorship to be exercised by the ecclesiastical arm rather than the secular authorities, strong discouragement to attending universities in Protestant countries, and absence of erudite journals able to advertise, review and discuss books published in Protestant countries.

At the same time, and equally, the medical revolution of the later seventeenth century, involved the application of a series of inventions, devices and new procedures to create or improve facilities for the practice of medicine as well as for medical research and instruction. Especially significant we have seen, was the introduction of bedside teaching,[24] the recording of case histories using direct observation and new instruments such as thermometers to note changes in the condition of patients,[25] more systematic use of anatomical dissections and demonstrations,[26] chemical analysis of medicines; the phasing out of bleeding and purging, and the creation of medical collections and museums featuring diseased and healthy soft as well as hard organs. This latter development only became possible with the invention, notably by Frederik Ruysch at Amsterdam, of new chemical preparations capable of preserving soft organs for display.[27]

No doubt some of the factors impeding intellectual change mentioned above would also have contributed to hindering the spread of new inventions and procedures, but here it seems at least as likely, and probably more, so that the chief factor was lack of investment and resources with which to lubricate the wheels of the medical revolution.[28] Even a commanding lead in medical science, as the Dutch experience in the middle decades of the eighteenth century clearly demonstrates, could rapidly be undermined, and transformed into dilapidation and decay by economic decline, contraction of the cities, and a general loss of urban vitality.[29] If economic deterioration is so severe that towns substantially shrink and remain smaller than they had previously been over a long period of time, this means that there is neither the demand, nor the opportunity, nor the means, to build new hospitals, to renovate and enlarge medical premises, to invest in new facilities such as anatomical theatres, laboratories, botanical gardens, and medical museums and collections. Neither are the resources available to keep medical libraries up to date or to pay the high salaries required to attract leading exponents of the new medicine from abroad.

In this connection, the economic decline of both Italy and Spain from the end of the sixteenth century down to the beginning of the eighteenth, and especially the contraction of the leading cities of Italy and Spain, is, I would argue, a factor of no small importance. Spain's economy collapsed essentially due to the undermining of the urban industries and commerce of Castile, chiefly caused by a flood of imports from northern Europe in the early seventeenth century. The economic decline of Spain after around 1590 had a great many consequences but the most dramatic and obvious to the visitor was the decay and shrinkage of the cities of Castile. Toledo, a thriving commercial and industrial centre with a population of around 60,000 in 1590 by 1650 had been stripped of practically all its industry and had a population of only around 20,000, a level at which it remained down to the middle of the eighteenth century.[30] This picture of dramatic collapse with (contrary to what it has lately become fashionable to claim) scarcely any signs of recovery either in the last quarter of the seventeenth or the first quarter of the eighteenth century, applies also to most of the other formerly vibrant urban centres of Castile – Burgos, Valladolid, Cordoba, Granada and Segovia.[31] Despite some recovery in the middle decades of the eighteenth century, the population of Segovia still stood at only about 80 per cent of its level of 1590 as late as 1750.[32] Of the major cities of Spain, only Seville and Madrid retained the bulk of their late sixteenth-century population levels and, during the first half of the eighteenth century, only these cities and, rather more impressively Valencia and

Barcelona,[33] showed any capacity for growth and development. Not surprisingly these four cities were also the centres of the medical revolution in Spain.

Similarly in Italy, commercial and industrial failure in the seventeenth century led to the decay and shrinkage of the cities. This was a general phenomenon after around 1600 throughout the Italian peninsula though in the Tuscan cities the process began earlier. Venice with a population of 170,000 in 1550 fell to only around 120,000 by 1650 and had risen from this level only marginally, perhaps to around 140,000, by 1750.[34] Florence, from around 80,000 inhabitants in the 1590s had contracted by about a quarter by 1650 and had still not regained its late sixteenth-century level by 1750.[35] Milan with a population of approximately 130,000, in 1600 shrank to well under 100,000 in the middle of the seventeenth century and staged only a painfully slow recovery, to around 120,000, by 1750.[36] Naples, Verona, Pavia, Como, Sienna and many other Italian cities likewise lost a large proportion of their population during the seventeenth century and failed to recover all – and in some cases any – of the lost ground during the first half of the eighteenth. Turin was the only Italian city which staged a vigorous expansion of population and activity in the late seventeenth and early eighteenth century and only Turin was the scene of large-scale urban renewal, planning and building, before the middle of the eighteenth century.[37] But here too, owing to the disruption of the War of the Spanish Succession (1702–13), during which Turin was besieged by the French and heavily bombarded, in 1706, significant reorganisation of poor relief and health-care institutions and substantial rebuilding and new construction began only in the second decade of the eighteenth century.[38]

During the sixteenth century, Italy and Spain had both witnessed some of the most imposing hospital construction to be found anywhere in Europe. Clearly there was a strong stimulus, social as well as religious, and no lack of means, for investing lavishly in civic health-care in the age of the High Renaissance and Counter-Reformation. If the health-care culture of sixteenth-century Italy and Spain was infused with a profound religious sensibility, this served to sanction and encourage the pride the main cities took in establishing impressive health-care institutions. The movement of consolidating small medieval hospitals into large general hospitals, already well under way in Italy in the fifteenth century, continued and accelerated in many parts of Italy during the early and mid sixteenth century but appears to have generally stopped around 1580.[39] In Spain, the wave of construction of large civic hospitals, inspired by the Italian example, began slightly later and continued somewhat longer but here too the process ceased with the decline and contraction of the cities. In Seville, the Hospital de Cinco Llagas begun in 1546 was finished in 1613, marked the end of the period of hospital reconstruction and expansion. In Toledo, two immense hospitals were constructed in the sixteenth century, buildings intended to be, and which were, among the most imposing in the city, easily eclipsing most of the aristocratic palaces. These were the Hospital de Santa Cruz[40] with its splendid Renaissance façade and vast wards, built in the years 1524–44 and the more obviously Italianate Hospital de Afuera, designed by the famous architect Alonso de Covarrubias (1488–1570) who had also worked on the final stages of Santa Cruz. The latter establishment took more than half a century to complete (1541–99) and only a few years after its completion had already become redundant as rapid economic decline and shrinkage of the city dramatically reduced the need for hospital space. The seventeenth-century fate of Covarrubias' hospital was itself to be converted into an aristocratic palace.

In both Italy and Spain then what might be termed the 'long seventeenth century' was an age of prolonged stagnation and indeed contraction in the building and refurbishing of hospitals and other civic and academic medical facilities, including anatomical theatres and 'pharmaceutical' gardens. But during the middle decades of the eighteenth century, first Italy and then Spain, like Austria and Catholic southern Germany, became the scene of an impressive new wave of construction and refurbishment of hospitals and medical facilities. Italy, for the first time since the 1630s, acquired a new series of large hospitals, anatomical theatres and botanical gardens as well as up-to-date medical laboratories.[41] Beginning in the 1750s, a series of five botanical gardens were established in different Spanish cities.[42] Among the most impressive of the new medical buildings erected in Spain was Ventura Rodriguez's functional but yet splendid lecture and operating theatre for the new royal college of surgery in Barcelona, of 1761.[43]

Economic factors then combined with a set of cultural factors to produce the phenomenon of a retarded medical revolution in southern and Habsburg central Europe. The problem was therefore in no sense one of theological, ecclesiastical or philosophical barriers as such. Despite the papal Inquisition and a strict censorship in Italy, the censorship exercised by the religious orders in the Austrian empire,[44] and the Spanish and Portuguese Inquisitions, mechanistic philosophy was everywhere able to penetrate, and, eventually, editions of Boerhaave and other modern medical authors of the north poured from Italian, Austrian and Iberian presses.[45] As early as the 1680s, the intellectual elite in various parts of Italy, ranging from Naples to Venice, were engulfed in a war of philosophies scarcely less intense than that being waged in France and northern Europe.[46] In certain restricted circles – small groups of academics, bibliophiles, courtiers, physicians and lawyers – knowledge of Cartesianism, Gassendi's atomism, Leibnizianism, Spinozism and just about every other strand of thinking being debated in the north had a deep impact. In Spain and Austria too, though the process had advanced less far in those countries than in Italy it had clearly begun.[47] If in all these countries there was a pervasive and frequently expressed fear,[48] evident among both opponents of change and most of the 'modernists', that the unrestricted spread of the New Philosophy would inevitably stimulate the growth and propagation of deism, atheism and irreligion of every kind, precisely this same dread pervaded the intellectual life of northern countries and not least the Netherlands and Britain.[49]

It may be true that the Reformed churches of Switzerland and the Netherlands, and the Lutheran churches of Germany and Scandinavia, were, by the 1680s, deeply divided in their responses to the sort of mechanistic philosophy, most notably Cartesianism, which was, or was perceived to be, compatible with belief in a providential God, the Creation, and the immortality of the soul. But precisely the same was the case with the Catholic Church, most obviously in France where rival Cartesian blocs – the Malebranchists, followers of Arnauld, and those who followed Pierre-Sylvain Régis – as well as Aristotelian anti-Cartesians battled for supremacy in the universities and academies but also, even at the highest ecclesiastical levels, in Italy.

Arguably, then, the slower penetration, and propagation, of the new medical culture in Catholic central and southern Europe was due, like the slower spread of the early Enlightenment in general – less to theological opposition to new ideas than the prevailing lack of awareness of the new science and new medicine in society generally. The slow and relatively weak diffusion of new ideas placed the Aristotelians, Galenists, and, according to van Swieten, also medical quacks and charlatans, in a stronger position to influence and manipulate the general public and by this means resist the advance of the medical revolution than was the case in northern countries.[50]

As the root cause of a social phenomenon such as this it is perhaps most convincing to point to a whole array of cultural barriers which were by-products and essentially indirect consequences of the Counter-Reformation. Commenting on the lack of a regular erudite journal in Italy, comparable with those then playing such an important part in the intellectual life of northern Europe, the editors of the first volume of the new Italian journal, the *Giornale de' Letterati d'Italia*, (successor to several previous attempts to establish such an organ in Rome, Parma and Modena) stressed, launching their venture in Venice in 1710, the backwardness and isolation to which, to the dishonour of Italy, absence of such a periodical contributed. It also highlighted and reinforced the failure to spread the new thinking and knowledge of new inventions made abroad, among the general reading public.[51] They claim that lack of readers and access to foreign books had caused the collapse of the previous series of the *Giornale de' Letterati*. But Italy's failure to acquire such a basic tool of cultural life also condemned the Italian cultured classes not only to ignorance of what was being published abroad but even to being more ignorant than northern Europeans about what was being published in the various parts of Italy.[52] In the early decades of the eighteenth century, Austria and Spain, like Italy but in sharp contrast to Protestant Germany, Scandinavia and France as well as the Netherlands, lacked a regular journal which was in a position to review a broad cross-section of scientific and erudite literature produced abroad.

Lack of awareness of, and access to, books published in Catholic as well as Protestant lands was one factor then. Another was the strong discouragement applying throughout Spain, Portugal, Italy and, to a lesser extent, in Austria (but not to France) to studying any subject at all in Protestant countries. However important books and periodicals may have been as vehicles of the early Enlightenment, it is evident that the medical revolution spread above all through academic study abroad and direct contact with key teachers and innovators. The ascendancy of the medical ideas of Le Boe Sylvius, Craanen, Bontekoe, De Graef, Ruysch, Overkamp and Blankaart in Sweden–Finland from the 1660s onwards, for example, and later, of Boerhaave, in early eighteenth-century Scotland, seems to have been chiefly due to the presence of growing numbers of Swedish and Scottish medical students in the Dutch universities. The large numbers of Protestant Germans in the Dutch medical faculties ensured the early spread of the medical revolution not only in Germany itself but, eventually, in the Baltic provinces and St Petersburg.[53] By contrast, relatively few Austrians studied in the Dutch universities and there were scarcely any Spaniards, Italians or Portuguese. In 1737, Boerhaave's class in Leiden comprised ninety-seven students of whom thirty-seven were Dutch; of the foreigners, twenty-eight were British, and there were ten Germans, four Scandinavians, three Irish, two Swiss, two Russians, one Greek and one Frenchman but apparently no-one from Italy, Spain, or Portugal.[54] The medical school at Franeker had nothing like the international allure of Leiden or Utrecht. Nevertheless, during the century 1650–1750 forty-four Germans received doctorates in medicine there along with five Scandinavians, five Hungarians, and five Frenchmen but only one from Spain, Portugal and Italy combined.[55]

One of Boerhaave's most able and influential pupils, António Nunes Ribeiro Sanches, was Portuguese. But he is the kind of exception which proves the rule. After studying at Coimbra and Salamanca, he spent the years 1727–30 studying at Leiden. But he appears to have come from a New Christian family and to have been a crypto-Jew. Certainly he never returned to southern Europe. He settled first in Russia and, by 1740 had become a court doctor and one of the most senior medical men in St Petersburg where, ever since his arrival, in 1731, he had been one of the leading lights of the medical revolution.[56] Later he lost favour, after being denounced as a Jew, and settled in Paris where he spent the last thirty-six years of his life and published a number of influential medical works in French.

To sum up, it would appear that the impact of the long economic recession in Spain and Italy combined with a considerable measure of cultural and intellectual isolation to impede the progress of the medical revolution in southern and Habsburg central Europe over many decades. This intellectual isolation was not insisted on by the Church, and gradually diminished, but it was buttressed by strong mechanisms of censorship originally introduced to prevent theological contamination by Protestant books, and curb irreligious ideas, but which came to have the additional effect of excluding a great deal of scientific and philosophical debate emanating from Protestant countries. As a consequence, outside influences were minimised and the pace of change was slow, compelling the 'modernist' physicians of Spain and Italy to wage a long and very arduous polemical war against the tenacious resistance of Aristotelians and *Galenistas*. The intellectual strategy of the 'modernists', inevitably was to lay great stress on the compatibility of the new medicine and medical doctrines with Catholic orthodoxy while at the same time seeking to demolish the psychological legacy of suspicion and hostility towards cultural influences emanating from France, England and northern Europe in general and, as regards medical knowledge specifically, the Netherlands.

Notes

1 Carlo-Francesco Cogrossi, *Saggi della medicina italiana divisi in due dissertazioni epistolari nelle quali le invenzioni del Santorio con nuove reflessioni, ed osservazioni s'illustrano* (Padua, 1727), pp. 7, 17, 31.
2 See, for instance, Bruno Zanobio, 'Sulla riforma dell'insegnamento della medicina nella università di Pavia al tempo di Gerard van Swieten', in Erna Lesky and Adam Wandruszka (eds) *Gerard van Swieten und seine Zeit* (Vienna, 1973), pp. 109–10.
3 On Cabriada's Carta, see José Maria López Piñero, *La introducción de la ciencia moderna en España* (Barcelona, 1969), pp. 101–8; on the role of Valencia in initiating the medical revolution in Spain, see Emilio Balaguer Periguell, 'Continuidad y ruptura en la renovación científica valenciana', *Anales de la Universidad de Alicante. Historia moderna* II (1982), pp. 251–8.
4 José Maria López Piñero, *Joan de Cabriada i la introducción de la ciencia medica moderna a Espanya* (Valencia, 1994), pp. 58, 89; Le Boe Sylvius played an important part in establishing the European pre-eminence of the Leiden medical faculty in the mid-seventeenth century, laying a particular stress on bed-side instruction and seeking chemical explanations for bodily changes and the effect of medicines, see G.A. Lindeboom, *Geschiedenis van de medische wetenschap in Nederland* (Haarlem, 1972), pp. 91–3.
5 Andrés Piquer, *Dictamen sobre reforma de estudios médicos en España* (1768) in *Obras postumas del doctor Don Andrés Piquer, médico de camera que fue de S.M. y protomédico de Castilla* (Madrid, 1785), p. 163; on Piquer, see also Balaguer Periguell, 'Continuidad y ruptura', p. 255 and Richar Herr, *The Eighteenth-Century Revolution in Spain* (Princeton, NJ 1958), p. 41.
6 G.M. Addy, *The Enlightenment in the University of Salamanca* (Durham, NC, 1966), pp. 93–8, 105–7.
7 F.T. Brechka, *Gerard van Swieten and his World (1700–1772)* (The Hague, 1970) p. 92.
8 Ibid., pp. 97–111; Georg Baumgartner, *Die Pharmakodynamik van Swietens* (Bleicherode am Harz, 1938), p. 6; Erna Lesky, 'Gerard van Swieten. Auftrag und Erfüllung' in Lesky and Wandruszka, *Gerard van Swieten und seine Zeit*, pp. 19–26.
9 Brechka, *Gerard van Swieten*, 137; among these was the botanist Adrianus van Stekhoven who was appointed director of the gardens at Schönbrunn, in 1753.
10 Ibid., p. 137; Lesky, 'Gerard van Swieten', pp. 25–6.
11 Gottfried Richter, *Das anatomische Theater* (Berlin, 1936), pp. 44–9, 51–4.
12 Ibid., pp. 51–4, 62.
13 Arturo Castiglioni, 'Una pagina di storia dell'insegnamento clinico (da

Padova a Leida)', in *Memorialia Herman Boerhaave. Optimi Medici* (Haarlem, 1939), pp. 78–81.

14 On Dutch Calvinist orthodoxy and Aristotelianism, see Theo Verbeek, *Descartes and the Dutch. Early Reactions to Cartesian Philosophy, 1637–1650* (Carbondale, IL, 1992), pp. 6–11, 39, 68–9.

15 On the Aristotelianism of the theological faculty at Uppsala in the late seventeenth century, see S. Lindroth, *Svensk Lärdomshistoria* (4 vols, Stockholm, 1975–81) II, pp. 450–64.

16 Ibid., II, pp. 464–5; E. Rolf Lindborg, *Descartes i Uppsala. Striderna om 'ny filosofien' 1663–1689* (Uppsala, 1965), pp. 347–8.

17 S. Lindroth, *A History of Uppsala University 1477–1977* (Uppsala, 1976) pp. 74–5.

18 Åke Dintler, *Lars Roberg. Akademiska sjukhusets grundare* (Uppsala, 1959) pp. 131–5.

19 López Piñero, *Introducción de la ciencia moderna*, 101–3; a fierce French assault on blood-letting was [Louis Cusac] *Reflexions sur la theorie et la pratique d'Hippocrate et de Galien* (Paris, 1692).

20 Quoted in J.I. Israel, 'Dutch influence on urban planning, health care and poor relief in the North Sea and Baltic regions of Europe (1567–c.1720)' in A. Cunningham and O.P. Grell (eds) *Health Care and Poor Relief in Protestant Europe 1500–1700*, London, Routledge, 1997, p. 76.

21 John Barker, *An Essay on the Agreement betwixt Ancient and Modern Physicians* (London, 1747), p. 176.

22 Verbeek, *Descartes and the Dutch*, pp. 86–90; J.I. Israel, *The Dutch Republic. Its Rise, Greatness and Fall, 1477–1806* (Oxford, 1995), pp. 889–916.

23 On the triumph of academic Cartesianism in Scotland in the 1670s, see Paul Wood, 'The scientific revolution in Scotland' in Roy Porter and M. Teich (eds) *The Scientific Revolution in National Context* (Cambridge,1992) p. 266.

24 On the introduction of this innovation in central and southern Europe see: Brechka, *Gerard van Swieten*, pp. 135, 137; Lesky, 'Gerard van Swieten', pp. 25–6; Castiglioni, 'Una pagina di storia', pp. 79–80.

25 This was one of de Haen's chief innovations in Vienna in the early 1750s (Brechka, *Gerard van Swieten*, p. 137).

26 Zanobio, 'Sulla riforma', p. 110; Addy, *Enlightenment in the University of Salamanca*, p. 106

27 Richter, *Das anatomische Theater*, pp. 63–4.

28 Such a view is partly suggested and partly rejected in Mario Biagioli, 'Scientific Revolution, social bricolage, and etiquette' in Porter and Teich, *Scientific Revolution in National Context*, pp. 14–15, 21–2.

29 Israel, *Dutch Republic*, pp. 1049–51.

30 Antonio Domínguez Ortiz, *Sociedad y estado en el siglo XVIII español* (Barcelona, 1976), pp. 192–3.

31 Juan Gelabert, 'Urbanisation and deurbanisation in Castile, 1500–1800' in I.A.A. Thompson and Bartolomé Yun Casalilla (eds) *The Castilian Crisis of the Seventeenth Century* (Cambridge, 1994), pp. 188–204.

32 Ibid., p. 189; Bartolomé Yun Casalilla, *Sobre la Transición al Capitalismo en Castilla. Economía y Sociedad en Terra de Campos (1500–1830)* (n.p., 1987) pp. 415, 431.

33 Pierre Vilar, *La Catalogne dans l'Espagne moderne* (3 vols Paris, 1962) ii, pp. 44, 47–8.
34 Dino Carpanetto and Giuseppe Ricuperati, *Italy in the Age of Reason, 1685–1789*, (London, 1987), p. 9.
35 Ibid., p. 14.
36 Domenico Sella, *Crisis and Continuity. The Economy of Spanish Lombardy in the Seventeenth Century* (Cambridge, Mass., 1979), pp. 3, 52, 86.
37 Carpanetto and Ricuperati, *Italy in the Age of Reason*, p. 8.
38 Geoffrey Symcox, *Victor Amadeus II. Absolutism in the Savoyard State, 1675–1730* (Berkeley and Los Angeles, 1983), pp. 150–2, 199–200.
39 Brian Pullan, *Rich and Poor in Renaissance Venice the Social Institutions of a Catholic State to 1620* (Oxford, 1971), pp. 202, 206–7; see also Chapter 1 of this volume.
40 George Kubler and Martin Soria, *Art and Architecture in Spain and Portugal and their American Dominions 1500 to 1800* (Harmondsworth, 1959), pp. 4, 10, 351–2.
41 Richter, *Das anatomische Theater*, pp. 36, 51–4, 62; in Florence, renovation and expansion of the hospitals seems to have been chiefly a phenomenon of the third quarter of the eighteenth century, see Eric Cochrane, *Florence in the Forgotten Centuries, 1527–1800* (Chicago, 1973), pp. 430–3.
42 Herr, *Eighteenth-Century Revolution in Spain*, p. 44.
43 Kubler and Soria, *Art and Architecture*, p. 49.
44 Grete Klingenstein, 'Van Swieten und die Zensur' in Lesky and Wandruszka, *Gerard van Swieten und seine Zeit*, pp. 95–8.
45 The late seventeenth-century Dutch medical authors rarely or never appeared in southern or central European editions but, from the 1720s onwards, editions of Boerhaave in particular, became frequent; Boerhaave's *Institutiones Medicae and Opera Omnia*, for example, were published at Venice in 1723; there were an especially large number of editions of Boerhaave in southern Europe in the 1740s and 1750s with Venice, Turin, and Naples being the main publishing centres; the first part of van Swieten's *Commentaries* on Boerhaave's *Aphorisms* was published in 1744–5 in Turin, Venice and Naples, see G.A. Lindeboom, *Bibliographia Boerhaaviana* (Leiden, 1959), pp. 47.
46 Claudio Manzoni, *Il 'Catholicesimo Illuminato' in Italia. Tra Cartesianismo Leibnizismo e Newtonismo–Lockismo nel primo settecento (1700–1750)* (Trieste, 1992), pp. 11, 89, 113.
47 José Maria López Piñero, *Ciencia técnica en la sociedad española de los siglos XVI y XVII* (Barcelona, 1979), pp. 445–6.
48 Arturo Ardao, *La filosofía polémica de Feijóo* (Buenos Aires, 1962) pp. 97–121; Manzoni, *Il 'Cattolicesimo Illuminato'*, pp. 11, 45; R.A. Kann, *A History of the Habsburg Empire* (Berkeley and Los Angeles, 1974) pp. 192–4; Klingenstein, 'Van Swieten und die Zensur', pp. 98–106; one of the most eloquent expressions of this fear is Andrés Piquer, *Discurso sobr la aplicacion de la philosophia a los assuntos de religion para la juventud española* (Madrid, 1757), especially the 'prologo' and pp. 50–1, 97–103; but danger or not, Piquer insisted that the old philosophy had to be discarded: 'ninguna systema philosophica es simpliciter necessario para la theologia', see p. 80.

49 Israel, *Dutch Republic*, pp. 1038–66.
50 Klingenstein, 'Van Swieten und die Zensur', p. 96; R.A. Kann, *A Study in Austrian Intellectual History from late Baroque to Romanticism* (London, 1960), p. 135; Corrado Dollo, *Filosofia e Scienze in Sicilia* (Padova, 1979) pp. 204–6.
51 [Scipione Maffei, Antonio Vallisnieri and Apostolo Zeno], *Giornale De' Letterati D'Italia* I (Venice, 1710), pp. 46–56.
52 Ibid. p. 51.
53 On German Protestant pupils of Boerhaave propagating the medical revolution in Russia, see H. Ackerknecht, 'Boerhaave-Schüler als Medinalpolitiker' in Lesky and Wandruszka, *Gerard van Swieten und seine Zeit*, pp. 123–5; for the statistics of foreign students at Leiden, see H.T. Colembrander, 'De herkomst der Leidsche studenten' in *Pallas Leidensis 1925* (Leiden, 1925), pp. 275–91.
54 J.D. Comrie, 'Boerhaave and the early Medical School at Edinburgh' in *Memorialia Herman Boerhaave*, p. 33.
55 H. de Ridder-Symoens, 'Buitenlandse studenten aan de Franeker universiteit, 1585–1811' in G.Th. Jensma, F.R.H. Smit and F. Weston (eds) *Universiteit te Franeker 1585–1811. Bijdragen tot de geschiedenis van de Friese hogeschool* (Leeuwarden, 1985) pp. 74–7.
56 Ackerknecht, 'Boerhaave-Schüler', pp. 122–3; David Willemse, *António Nunes Ribeiro Sanches élève de Boerhaave et son importance pour la Russie* (Leiden, 1966), pp. 36–40.

4

CHARITY AND WELFARE IN EARLY MODERN TUSCANY

John Henderson

The systems of charity and welfare established in the Italian city-states in the sixteenth century were ostensibly little different from those already in place. That is, the poor were helped through an intermeshing system of public welfare and private charity. The welfare of the State was provided at times of emergency caused by natural or man-made crises, most significant of which were plague, famine and war. Much of the relief of the poor in non-crisis periods remained the province of organisations inspired by Christian charity and run by devout lay men and women. The main types of corporations were the religious confraternity and the hospital, which had dominated poor relief systems ever since the demographic expansion of the thirteenth century had necessitated the foundation of charitable institutions to help the poor members of the new urban centres during periods of individual crisis caused by sickness and life-cycle poverty.[1]

While this intermeshing system had to be partly rethought in the case of countries and regions which joined the Protestant churches, with the abolition of organisations such as confraternities whose financial existence was largely predicated and funded through investment in Purgatory, in those countries still dominated by the Catholic Church this system remained unchallenged. Indeed the Catholic Reformation largely built on and developed the existing system both in its pastoral and charitable work. There were, however, quantitative and qualitative differences in the welfare and charitable systems of the sixteenth century when compared with the preceding 100 years. These have traditionally been seen as stemming, on the one hand, from the increasing levels of poverty and the more intolerant official responses to the poor and, on the other, from the more moralistic character of the reactions of the church hierarchy during the Catholic Reformation. This led to the foundation of institutions designed to protect not only orphaned children and women from the perils of society, but also to help to reform the morals of fallen women. This new emphasis in the character of church responses to the poor cannot all be attributed to the influence of the Council of Trent, but should be seen as characteristic of the whole reform movement of which Trent was the culmination and codification rather than the beginning.[2]

This chapter, which will both summarise current research and begin to look at some areas which need further examination, has three parts. We shall begin by outlining briefly the origins of the Catholic reform movement in Italy in the early sixteenth century, especially the association between the poor sick and the new Orders founded in this period, including the Capuchins, that of S. Giovanni di Dio and the Camilliani. The second and main section examines Tuscany, in particular Florence, and the reforms by the Medicean Dukes of the welfare and charitable systems of their state in the sixteenth century. In this process we shall seek to determine how far the influence of the Counter-Reformation Church might be said to have been an active force in determining the institutional character and response of welfare in Medicean Tuscany.

The French Disease, Companies of Divine Love and the new Orders

Understanding the economic and demographic developments in sixteenth-century Italy, with falling real wages and growing population levels in many urban centres, helps to explain the force behind changing attitudes towards the poor, towards, that is, a more intolerant set of beliefs which tended to divide them increasingly between the deserving and undeserving.[3] The pressure on resources clearly made choices inevitable and led to those features which are seen as so characteristic of early modern attitudes towards the poor, in particular the growing harshness towards those who were regarded as undeserving.[4] But there is also another element which relates to one of the main themes of this volume, namely the attitude towards the poor sick and in particular those sick from epidemic disease. Indeed it has been argued that already from the mid-fifteenth century Italian governments made a growing association between disease and poverty and sought to victimise the poor who were seen increasingly as not just the victims of epidemics, but also the cause.[5] This was predicated on the observations of both the members of health boards and their medical advisors that the poor were those worst affected by plague.

Another important factor which helped to stimulate both this antagonism and the growing intolerance towards the poor, was the appearance and spread of the French Disease, *Mal Francese*, from the mid-1490s.[6] The main problem was that compared with victims of plague who died rapidly, the *mal franciosati* suffered from a chronic illness so that they remained to litter up the streets, creating an unpleasant and unaesthetic sight. But worse still they were also seen as a threat to public health; as a decree of the Venetian Sanità or Health Board of 1522 makes clear, the poor incurables gave off 'a terrible stench . . . [which] may breed infection and disease'.[7] Seven years earlier Pope Leo X in his Bull *Salvatoris Nostri*, complained about Rome becoming inundated with the incurably sick who cannot be accommodated in the city's hospitals and are therefore 'obliged for the whole day to look for food through the city, sometimes dragging themselves along on little trolleys and vehicles, giving offence both to themselves and blocking the way of those whom they encounter'.[8]

It should be stressed that despite the fact that this Bull emanated from both the head of the Catholic Church and the ruler of the city of Rome, the impact of *Mal Francese* did not in itself call forth a series of new government measures to deal with the *mal franciosati*.[9] Rather, I would argue, it helped to create the climate of intolerance towards the poor, and in particular towards the chronically sick, which came to characterise official policies in sixteenth-century Italy, a subject to which we shall return within the context of the Medicean reforms of the welfare system of Tuscany.

But Christian charity also obviously continued as a fundamental influence on sixteenth-century attitudes to the poor. Indeed an active interest in ministering directly to the sick poor was characteristic of the new Orders. This was in contrast to their predecessors, such as the Observants, who had tended instead to encourage others to establish, reform or work in hospitals.[10] Members of these Orders often gained experience in the hospitals of Rome, since many had their headquarters in the city.[11] One of the best known were the Capuchins or Frati Cappuccini, who tended to the sick in hospitals including the Incurabili in Rome, Naples and Genoa.[12] Indeed because the *mal franciosati* had especially unpleasant conditions they provided the Capuchins in particular with an ideal way of imitating their main spiritual example, St Francis, in his concern and care for lepers.[13] Another new Order, the Ministri degli Infirmi, received papal recognition in 1591 and, as their title suggests, dedicated themselves almost exclusively to the service of the sick.[14] This role was extended from the hospitalised sick to looking after the victims of epidemics in their own houses.[15]

Another feature which characterised these Orders, and was to have important implications for the organisation and provision of charity to the sick poor, was their association with the laity. This reflected the origins of many of these new Orders, that is their founders came from outside the Church with close links to groups of devout lay men and women, particularly confraternities, who sought solutions to what they perceived as their century's most pressing social and religious ills.[16]

It was indeed the confraternity which helped to initiate and inspire many of the features of Catholic reform. One type which played a particularly important role was the Company of Divine Love, which originated in Genoa in the late-1490s to put into practice the two main aspects of the Christian ideal of Charity: love of the divine and helping the poor.[17] They combined an ascetic way of life through active penance, frequent communion and helping those rejected by society because of an incurable disease.[18] Within a few years the confraternity had made concrete the second of its aims and raised the money to found a hospital devoted to the treatment of the *mal franciosati*. The 'Ridotto', as it was called, was the first of a series of Incurabili hospitals set up in many of the major cities of northern and central Italy to care for and treat those chronically sick with an incurable condition.[19] One of the most important of the new Incurabili hospitals was that of San Giacomo in Augusta in Rome, which was established by the Roman branch of the Company of Divine Love. In time this hospital became the mother house of all similar hospitals and the largest of its type in Italy, treating as many as two to three thousand patients each year.[20]

The foundation and expansion of these Incurabili hospitals in many of the major cities of northern and central Italy reflects the dual nature of charity in this period: the intolerance of the chronically sick, especially when seen as spreading disease, and the selfless dedication of the members of the new Orders. But underlying both these themes lies a new morality which was so characteristic of charitable initiatives of the sixteenth century.[21] This can be seen behind both secular and ecclesiastical legislation, as in the case of the Venetian Sanità and Leo X's Bull *Salvatoris Nostri*. Morality also inspired another activity associated with some of the Incurabili hospitals, most notably in Naples and Venice, the establishment of convents of Convertite for reformed prostitutes.[22] As we shall see in relation to Tuscany, the preservation of female honour and the rescue of either fallen women or vulnerable girls from the perils of prostitution[23] became an important theme of Catholic reform. However, even though this movement is often associated particularly with the later sixteenth century, these initiatives had already begun in some parts of Italy well before the Council of Trent.

These general introductory comments have traced briefly the origins of the Catholic Church's response to the sick poor in earlier sixteenth-century Italy, and especially the Incurabili hospitals. This has been done in terms of outlining the institutional response, through the charitable missions of the new Orders and their important links with movements of lay confraternities, and also by examining the moral character of these responses. In the rest of this chapter I shall turn to Tuscany to examine how far one can detect the influence of Catholic reform on the changes which were instituted by the Medicean Dukes during the fifty to sixty years following their restoration in 1530.[24] This will, of necessity, include a consideration of how public welfare and private charity intermeshed.

Cosimo I de' Medici and proposals for welfare reforms

When the Medici family returned to Florence in 1530 they inherited a charitable system of which the citizens were proud. The contemporary chronicler Benedetto Varchi wrote the following account of the city's hospitals:

> There are in Florence two types of hospitals, some that receive male and female patients, keeping them apart, treating and looking after them until they have recovered, without charging them anything. The first and major one of these is that of San Gilio, called Santa Maria Nuova . . . [which] spends 25,000 *scudi* each year in looking after the sick. Then there are the hospitals of San Matteo . . . San Pagolo . . . and that of Bonifazio . . . and another which has been founded recently from the alms of many citizens as a result of the persuasive arguments of a worthy preacher; in that hospital they cannot receive anybody who will get better, and for that reason it is called of the Incurabili . . .; and among these, which have large premises, we have not

> counted the hospitals belonging to the guilds . . . and also that for those sick from plague. The other type of hospital is that which receives and gives lodging not only to travellers and other healthy people, but also to the poor of the city, who for a night or two receive food and lodging without paying anything. . . . And on top of these one must not forget the famous Spedale degli Innocenti . . . which has a large building with two large orchards, which feeds, clothes and teaches a profession to all the male and female babies that are left there by anybody and for whatever reason; in addition to the servants they look after over a thousand people.[25]

This description of the city's hospitals makes it clear that Florence provided a series of complementary and specialised services for the poor on the eve of the return of the Medici family. Also included in the term 'hospital' were the institutions providing succour to abandoned babies and those institutions we would call hospices, the traditional role of providing overnight accommodation to travellers and the poor. In other passages Varchi also mentions in passing the charitable role of confraternities, the Compagnia di S. Maria del Tempio, which provided spiritual comfort to condemned criminals, the Buonomini di S. Martino, which specialised in helping the *poveri vergognosi* or shame-faced poor, and the Company of the Misericordia, which played a central role in the identification, transport and burial of those who became infected and died from plague in the city.[26]

In 1530, then, Florence had a system of charity which had not changed substantially since the fourteenth century. There were, however, two notable exceptions, the Lazzaretto and the hospital of the Incurabili. The former had been founded in 1478 and opened during the epidemics of the 1490s.[27] The Incurabili, on the other hand, had been established as a result of pressure from outside, specifically the sermons of the 'worthy preacher' mentioned by Varchi, Don Callisto da Piacenza, a Canon from the Badia Fiesolana.[28] The popularity of the idea is not that surprising, given that it was the Medici Pope, Leo X, who only five years before had supported the foundation of the Incurabili hospital in Rome and may indeed have instructed his brother Giulio, the Archbishop of Florence, to welcome Don Callisto with enthusiasm and further the project of establishing this type of hospital. And here we can also see how the influence of the movement of the Companies of Divine Love reached Florence. Although the confraternity which established the Incurabili hospital was known as 'della Trinità', the ideals and practices were the same.

Despite what seemed to contemporaries as a relatively efficient and generous charitable system, the Medici Duke, Cosimo I, decided to survey and then to institute a reform of the administration of the whole system in the 1540s. It should be emphasised that this does not appear to have been the result of outside influence from the church. It stemmed rather from Cosimo's desire to streamline the bureaucracy of the Tuscan state and forms part of his policy to centralise and to exert greater control over his duchy.[29] In this reform of charitable institutions he was following the example of city governments in other parts of northern Italy over the previous 100 years, when a series of states had reduced the multiplicity of small institutions and centralised their charitable resources on one large hospital.[30] The reason this was not attempted earlier in Florence may have had much to do with the dramatic changes of regime from the mid-1490s and their consequent lack of sufficient political power and will to implement such drastic reforms of a system in which, as has been seen from Varchi's chronicle, Florentines felt such pride.[31]

The attention of Cosimo's predecessor, Alessandro de' Medici, had already been drawn to the financial plight of the city's charitable institutions soon after his return to Florence. This opened the way to the increasingly interventionist policy of Cosimo, his successor from 1537. The problems had been caused during the late 1520s when the Republic had defended itself against the besieging Medicean army. One of the solutions adopted by the Republic in its search for funds to pay for the resistance was to plunder the financial resources of religious and charitable institutions within the city. They were forced to part with both property and cash as well as being subjected to forced loans.[32] Additionally properties belonging to a series of religious institutions, including hospitals, outside and close to the city walls were pulled down in order to prevent them providing cover for the besieging army.[33]

The financial state of S. Maria Nuova apparently caused the most concern to contemporaries, sufficient for the subject to have been mentioned by the chronicler Benedetto Varchi, who recorded that it 'was in the greatest disorder, having lost much during the war and spent much more than in normal times'.[34] More precise information about the reasons for its losses were supplied in a law of March 1533 in which new sources of income were granted to the hospital.[35] In addition to having sustained 'an infinite amount of damage due to the recent war', the Medicean regime blamed the financial losses on the members of the republican government, whom they described as 'men who had little affection for their city'.[36] In particular they were accused of having confiscated money which had been left on deposit with S. Maria Nuova, for over the previous seventy years the hospital had developed a banking service which provided interest on deposits.[37] A commission of enquiry was established to include the Spedalingo (director) of Santa Maria Nuova; it was decided to allow the hospital to suspend payments of its debts for a period of four years, while at the same time the process was speeded up for the reclamation of its own debts.[38]

Although, as we shall see, Cosimo I and his successors did seek to gain greater control over the hospitals of the city and state, the major innovations in Florentine charity added new institutions to the system rather than making changes to the existing structure of charity. This can be seen clearly in Cosimo's edict of March 1542 in which he sought to address the problems of two groups of society for whom existing arrangements were deemed to be inadequate.[39] The first were abandoned children over the age of 3; while there were already a series of institutions which catered for *innocenti*, or foundlings, orphaned children remained a problem. The second, beggars, seem to have provoked a less charitable reaction and one more typical of early modern views of the shiftless poor, a perception no doubt provoked by the influx into Florence of the very poor during the recent dearth.[40] Finally in part at least to raise the money to finance these initiatives Cosimo sought to centralise and control the hospitals outside the city.[41]

This edict was, then, full of good intentions both to reform existing institutions and to tackle what were regarded as some of the major social problems of the day, the existence of destitute children over the age of 3 and the presence of an increasing number of beggars in the city. How far, though, did Cosimo and his administration have either the political will or the resources to implement these proposals?

The administrative machinery of reform was set in motion almost immediately by the election of a commission of five, later extended to twelve, good men or Buonomini, who were given full power to exercise grand ducal authority.[42] What made this initiative particularly remarkable was that the power of the Buonomini was extended not just over the city of Florence, but also over the whole of Medicean Tuscany.[43] They elected local notables to fulfil their orders, which included a complete survey of all hospitals and charitable institutions. Then, given the Buonomini's need for cash to underwrite their reforms, later in the year they adopted what was to be a far-reaching measure. The directors of all the hospitals in the territory, except for those under ecclesiastical control, were required to submit annual accounts of their income and outgoings and then, coming to the nub of the decree, to send their profits to the Buonomini in Florence.[44]

The hostel for abandoned boys

Having established a source of income, it was now possible to tackle what was obviously perceived to be one of the most pressing social problems in the city – abandoned children. This may be related to the long-term effects of the famine of 1539 on the services provided by the foundling hospital of the Innocenti.[45] In that year the hospital had taken in almost 1,000 children, double its average admissions, which meant that it no longer had capacity for older children.[46]

Cosimo's decree talked in emotive terms of 'the misery and calamity in which we find the poor little children of three, five and up to ten years' old, impotent and totally abandoned by their fathers, mothers, relatives, and deprived of any other human and spiritual support'.[47] Indeed by November 1542 the Senato dei Quarantotto noted that 'the number of the poor abandoned children has grown in the city of Florence and is increasing every day'.[48] The problem had, then, become more urgent and the solution proposed was to find an institution in which to house them. The following month the Buonomini took over the extant Spedale dei Broccardi in Via S. Gallo. However, there still remained a shortage of cash and the solution adopted by Cosimo was to suppress the ancient charitable confraternity of the Bigallo, and assign its income to the Buonomini, who henceforth came to be known as the Buonomini del Bigallo.[49] These sums proved insufficient and it was at this point that Cosimo obtained papal permission, through a Bull of July 1543, to appropriate the profits of all hospitals in the *contado* to now include those under ecclesiastical protection.[50]

Once established, the boys' hostel of the Broccardi became an established feature of the city's charitable system receiving support from both public and private sources. Indeed this was a project which must have been seen as particularly worthy of Christian charity since the recipients were more easily controlled and the whole enterprise redounded to the good reputation of the city and its reigning family.

In time the premises proved insufficient for their needs, particularly during the famine of the early 1590s, when the much larger convent of S. Caterina was requisitioned to meet demand.[51]

The Broccardi was designed not just to feed and house its occupants, but also to educate them and to make them into good, moral and useful citizens. The aims of the institution were outlined in the papal brief of June 1542, based on the Buonomini's first statutes,[52] and included the injunction that each child was to be 'instructed in the divine precepts', taught a trade to which they were most suited, and finally once their period of instruction had been completed they were to be found work with an employer who would 'treat them with charity to the honour of God'.[53] The statutes themselves reflect a more strict discipline with punishments for boys leaving the hospice without permission in order that they 'do not have the reason to commit an infinite number of sins and so that they live in fear of God and love of Our Saviour Jesus Christ'.[54]

Beggars

A mixture of Christian charity and discipline also motivated those clauses of the Buonomini's statutes which dealt with beggars.[55] Distinctions were drawn concerning the type of beggar. These distinctions are familiar from legislation in both other parts Italy and Europe at this time and are based on the idea of sorting the moral sheep from the immoral goats. In the former category were those 'poor beggars over ten years of age, impotent and forced to beg in order to live'. They were to be collected in the city's hospitals where they were to 'receive lodging, heat and light'. Those whom the Buonomini decided were 'able to earn their bread through working and labour' were only given shelter and were expected to pay for food through their earnings 'from their own sweat'. Furthermore since this was a measure designed to clear the streets of beggars, only those few licensed by the Buonomini were allowed to beg for a maximum of three days. These included impotent and sick locals and any poor people from outside Florence. The second category for whom the Buonomini had to be on the look-out were swindlers, who simulated sickness and attempted to cheat the public into giving them alms. Once discovered they were punished.[56]

These proposals to deal with beggars would have represented one of the more far-reaching programmes in Early Modern Italy if they had been put into practice. In the event little was done to make them more permanent. Cosimo evidently saw them as unworkable because of the expense involved in administering and financing the scheme. Furthermore since these measures probably represented a reaction to the effects of the 1539 dearth, when significant numbers of beggars had been attracted to the city in search of sustenance, with the amelioration of the situation there was less urgency to institute these plans.

Thus the measures taken to deal with beggars represented reactions to periods of particular shortage rather than a permanent strategy. Indeed with the exception of the dearth of 1555, there were no similarly difficult periods during the rest of Cosimo's life.[57] This improvement was most obviously a reflection of the influence of natural phenomena, reasonable weather and therefore good harvests. However, the ability to maintain a good supply of food to the city was also linked to the increasingly stringent State control of its supply and price in the city.[58] Indeed Cosimo's successor, Francesco I, found it possible to revoke part of the edict in 1577,[59] although in the 1580s Florence began to experience once again a series of shortages, culminating in the famine of the years around 1590.[60]

Thus even if official policies to deal with the poor in the Early Modern period are frequently characterised as intolerant and discriminatory, measures taken to deal with beggars during emergencies cannot be taken as representative of those in force during non-crisis periods. This suggests that existing structures of charity and welfare, and in particular the large number of hospitals and confraternities, upon which the city had relied over the previous 250 years, were apparently seen as sufficient to provide for the poor in non-crisis periods. This does not mean, however, that these institutions were seen as unproblematic in the way in which they were run either in the city or the Tuscan state, as is evident in the following section.

Hospitals in Florence and Tuscany

We have seen that the Medici regime had expressed concern over the financial state of S. Maria Nuova in the early 1530s, following the siege of Florence. Although protectionism in regard to charitable institutions followed on from a long tradition in Florence,[61] the difference now was that the Medici dukes required more in return, that is further control over the way these institutions were run. Through a series of moves they gradually came to exert more control over the election of the Spedalingo of S. Maria Nuova, thus preventing the intervention of the Pope, and later Duke Ferdinand imposed an official who acted as a superintendent of the hospital's administration.[62] Cosimo and his successors, Alessandro and Ferdinando, continued to be particularly interested in control of the large Florentine hospitals.[63] Later the Duke managed to reserve to himself the right to confirm the election of the Director of the Innocenti, another of the city's wealthier charitable institutions.[64] In time many of the larger charities, along with the fraternities of the Misericordia and the Buonomini di S. Martino, came to be seen by the Duke as forming part of the bureaucracy of the Tuscan state.[65]

These moves should not be seen as simply designed to extend Medicean power; official intervention also reflected concern over the state of these institutions, as has been seen in the case of S. Maria Nuova. The same was true of the Spedale di S. Paolo, which had a chequered history in the sixteenth century as a result of the conflicting demands of the hospital, on the one hand, and the needs of those who served the sick. This was especially true once the nursing staff passed from being Tertiaries to nuns. Accusations of indebtedness and falling standards of care for the sick led Cosimo in 1549 to request the Pope to intervene, though here it should be noted that he maintained a distance through respect for ecclesiastical privileges. The papal reforms, which were finally initiated in the 1570s did not resolve all the problems and only in 1592 did the Grand Duke Ferdinand intervene decisively and turned S. Paolo into the city's first hospital for convalescants.[66]

Despite the rhetoric of the 1542 decree and the supporting papal Bull of 1543, it remains unclear at the present state of research how much was achieved by the proposed reforms of the hospitals in the provinces in the immediate aftermath of the establishment of the Buonomini. Whether this was because of the lack of real motivation of the officials appointed to undertake the visitation or because they met the resistance of entrenched interests is still to be determined.[67] We do know, however, that the Buonomini del Bigallo did survey 200 hospitals and charitable institutions,[68] and that they continued to encounter problems in eliciting cash from provincial hospitals to finance their project for the 'poor abandoned boys'. Indeed in 1558 the Buonomini petitioned the Duke for help to enforce the reform of the hospitals of the *contado*. Their righteous indignation led them to describe the conditions there in strong language:

> In these hospitals not only do they not provide hospitality, but they are abandoned and left to be ruined, and the hospital directors in grave offence to God and the greatest

> prejudice and harm of the poor . . . usurp and appropriate the income of the said hospitals.[69]

Almost thirty years later, after Cosimo's successor, the pious Ferdinando, had joined forces with the archbishop of Florence to enforce more rigorous changes and controls on the church of the Medicean state, another more detailed survey of provincial hospitals was put into action. The orders of July 1586 to the captains of the Bigallo and Misericordia, as they were now called, were explicit that the information for each institution should include: an account of what service, if any, they provided to the poor, as well as of the number and quality of beds, and of their income and expenditure 'not only through what they [the Spedalinghi or ministers] said or from their books', but in any way 'in order to discover the truth'.[70]

The presumption in 1586 that the provincial hospitals were being badly run echoes the statements of the Buonomini in 1558. This is partly but far from entirely borne out by the surveys themselves which are more plentiful for this later period for they include accounts of hospitals whose condition satisfied the visitors and others which were in very poor condition. On the one hand, there is the example of the Spedale di S. Jacopo e S. Filippo at Ponte a Rignano which provided 'bed, light and fire' to both male and female paupers, also food to the sick and if they were sufficiently ill they paid for them to be sent to the large general hospital of S. Maria Nuova in Florence. The visitors were moreover satisfied because they declared that the hospital and the Spedalingo's house were in good order as were the beds and linen and the accounts.[71] Very different, however, was the story of the Spedale di S. Michele at Gaville, which boasted only 'a wretched wooden bed with a palliasse and mattress of tow with three sheets, two of which are wretchedly sad and another a bit better . . . and a cover of foreign cloth, used but in a reasonable condition and the said bed is in a room on very humid ground . . .'.[72]

Most of the hospitals surveyed were small institutions, with two to four beds each offering temporary lodging to the travelling poor. Few would have been able to provide much surplus cash to send to Florence; many could at best balance their books and others were in dire financial straits.

Although it would easy to interpret these moves as part of a Medicean strategy to suck dry the charitable corporations of the Tuscan State to the benefit of their own treasury, this would be over-cynical. The dukes did demonstrate a genuine desire to reform these institutions, many of which were short of both personnel and finances, for the benefit of the poorer members of society.

It could also be argued that this was a policy of social control, particularly when taken together with the rather harsh attitudes towards beggars. But while mendicants who came from outside the city may have suffered in particular years,[73] the policy adopted was little different from that which had been enacted in times of crisis by their republican predecessors. Over the following fifty years only periods of crisis saw the reintroduction of these measures. For example, the 1590s, years of severe food shortage throughout Europe, led the Florentine authorities to reimpose their more stringent policies against beggars, particularly in their discrimination against and expulsion of *forestieri*.[74] Then in 1621, when extreme food shortage subsequently combined with an epidemic of petechial fever, a more permanent Beggars' Hospice, the Spedale di Mendicanti, was founded.[75] But even this institution, which appears to smack of Foucaultian repression, changed its policy according to circumstances. When it was established, this Spedale was very much seen as a solution to the problems caused by the diseased poor, who were seen as the generators and carriers of epidemics. In time, though, once the crisis had subsided, the Spedale transformed itself into a Conservatorio for poor women, which provided one of the strategies for helping the poor to deal with particularly difficult periods in their lives.[76] This underlines our earlier suggestion that in Florence at least more intolerant policies taken towards the poor, and especially beggars, should be seen within the context of emergencies rather than as characteristic of all welfare and poor relief in this period.

Conservatories for girls

It was contemporary concern for girls and women that led to the most innovatory developments in Florentine charity in the second half of the sixteenth century, the establishment of four conservatories for girls between 1551 and 1590. Indeed it is here that one can see most clearly the influence of the Catholic reformation on charity, reflecting its moral and social concerns for the education and training of abandoned children and for the preservation of female sexual honour. However, these foundations do not appear to have stemmed either from the direct influence of the ecclesiastical hierarchy or the dukes or grand dukes of Tuscany. Rather they were founded by members of the laity, although one must not forget that they were frequently guided and inspired by individual religious. Thus both the Monastero del Ceppo (1551) and the Monastero di S. Maria e S. Niccolò (1555), to which it was later united, were founded by either groups or female and male members of patrician families.[77] Then in 1554 a group of pious women headed by Margherita Borromei was the main moving force behind the Monastero delle Fanciulle Abbandonate della Pietà, although here one should not forget the profound influence exercised on this group by the Dominican Alessandro Capocchi.[78] Towards the end of the century the Monastero di S. Caterina was established in 1590 by three prominent men: Giovan Battista Botti, who was also closely involved in this period of dearth with initiatives for the institutionalisation of local beggars, together with Giulio Zanchini, a Cavaliere di Malta, and Girolomo Michelozzi, a Cavaliere di S. Stefano.[79]

Even if the moving forces behind the establishment of the Conservatori were members of the patriciate, we cannot divorce them from the influence of the Medici for many would have been involved in government or the court. Michelozzi, for example, was a Knight of the Order of S. Stefano which was established by Cosimo himself.[80] Thus the foundation of the Monastero di S. Maria e S. Niccolò was approved by Cosimo, as was S. Caterina by the Grand Duke Ferdinando who also provided them with a site.[81] Neither can we divorce these initiatives from the influence of the Church, whether this was the general influence of the Council of Trent, local bishops or the more specific influence of individual religious, such as Alessandro Capocchi (d. 1581), who not only inspired the foundation of the Pietà, but also founded confraternities which developed important charitable and educative roles.[82]

It was above all in the aims and morality expressed in the statutes of these four hospices that the influence of the Counter-Reformation can be best detected. Both the statutes of S. Maria e S. Niccolò and S. Caterina emphasize that they were established during periods of crisis which necessitated many girls 'going begging through the streets'; the house was therefore established 'to avoid many bad things and sins'.[83] Clearly, though, while the preservation of female virtue may have acted as the underlying motive for these foundations, periods of dearth usually sparked these initiatives, as in the case of the 1550–1 dearth when S. Maria e S. Niccolò was founded, 1555 when the Pietà began, and S. Caterina during the most severe dearth of 1590.[84]

The statutes of these institutions have similar aims and present a picture of a strict almost monastic way of life; indeed it is no accident that these institutions were known as 'Monasteri'. The prevailing ethos shared much with a conventual way of life, with an emphasis on obedience with rules of silence and good behaviour, summed up in the injunction that the girls have to be 'healthy in body and mind so that nobody through any blemish causes our place to be infected since it is now in such a state of cleanliness'.[85] The mixture of Christian obligation and dutiful obedience is well reflected in the injunctions to the girls of the Monastero di S. Caterina on getting up in the morning. Having been woken at dawn by the ringing of a bell in their dormitory:

> all the girls having first made the sign of the holy cross, they should begin to dress and [then] all assemble in church and having made the sign of the holy cross they make reverence to the most holy sacrament and kneel down . . . [Then] with all speed all should go to make their bed. And [then] . . . the bell is rung for work . . . and they are set to work in silence, praising God, thanking Him in their hearts for the benefits they have received.[86]

They were employed in various ways, each working under a teacher, a Maestra, who taught them to weave or work with silk or gold thread.[87] Emphasis was also placed on literacy; each girl was assigned a literate companion who taught her to read.[88]

Who, then, were these girls? The statutes suggest that they had very strict criteria for admission. The first was an age limit which was usually set between 10 and 12. Secondly, the girls had to be 'truly abandoned', which S. Caterina defined as 'having neither father nor mother nor brothers nor uncles, or other relatives who could take care of them'.[89] S. Maria e S. Niccolò also excluded all those girls who had already been living with or working for somebody for four months or more, even if that person was a neighbour who had provided them with temporary accommodation through charity or employed them as servants.[90] Furthermore the statutes were insistent that all girls should not have some disability, such as being 'blind, deaf, dumb, hunch-backed, crippled', partly because such people 'are not in such danger of something bad happening to them' and partly to avoid encumbering the hospice with either sick or unmarriageable women.[91] But moral criteria were also employed; in a first redaction of S. Caterina's statutes they also refused admission to 'daughters of wicked women, or nieces, or of infamous people'.[92] In this way they hoped that, as in the regulations governing behaviour, to avoid pollution of the conventual atmosphere.

To add flesh to these general statements of intent, we can turn to the admission books of the Pietà for 1555 and that of S. Maria e S. Niccolò for 1571.[93] Both were more or less the same size, with 52 admitted to the first in 1555 and 57 present in the second in 1571. The average age at entry for these two samples appears, however, to have been somewhat higher than envisaged by the statutes, at about 12 years old, with a range of 5 to 20, and only about 35 per cent aged 10 or under. This suggests that a more flexible approach may have been adopted to admission policies than laid down in the statutes, although this may have changed later for over the whole of the seventy-year period from 1558–9 to the early 1620s the majority of girls were between 6 and 10.[94]

Another feature of the admission records in this period which reflects something about the conditions in these hostels is the levels of mortality among these girls. This appears to have been high, at least among the Pietà's first intake of girls; of the 52 who were admitted to the Pietà in 1555, 32 had died before 1564 and 19 during the first year. But this may have been unusual and may reflect less the normal sanitary conditions within the hostel than the presence of an epidemic. Indeed 1554 to 1555 were particularly unhealthy years in Tuscany; they saw an epidemic of petechial fever and, as has been seen, a severe dearth. It is possible that some of the girls may already have been infected on entry and that others who were already weakened by malnutrition might have succumbed to this fever or others associated with intestinal diseases.[95]

Despite the possibility of high mortality, demand must have been high for admission, judging from the numerous petitions received by the guardians of these institutions from people recommending girls who did not even fall into the categories devised by the statutes. There is, for example, the case in 1549 of the girl who was found by Monna Caterina, wife of Papi Tedaldi and daughter of Monna Lionarda di Ginori; she 'had picked up in the middle of the street a poor girl of fifteen years old, who had fled from her own father who wanted to do her harm, as he had already done to the other sister'. The first sister had already been accepted in the Monastero di S. Maria e S. Niccolò and Monna Caterina confirmed the girl's account of the father's bad character.[96] This story indicates, then, that the Abbondate could be flexible over both the age of those accepted and also over whether the child was really an orphan. Although probably the fact that both of the two sisters were described as 'bella' may have helped the petition, just as did the fact that the petitioner, Monna Caterina, was a relative through marriage of the Prioress.[97]

This case, which could be multiplied many times, is representative in that the majority of girls came from relatively humble backgrounds in which the death of one or both parents left the child without financial support. Their social status is confirmed by those cases which list the fathers' occupational background; the fathers of 18 of the 57 girls resident in the Monastero di S. Maria e S. Niccolò in 1571 were involved in cloth production, including carders and weavers, reflecting employment opportunities in a city dominated by the woollen and silk cloth industry. However, a few occupations reflect the fact that the vast majority of girls came from the surrounding countryside, although this lack of information may simply indicate that less was known about the fathers of these girls.[98]

This brief discussion of these conservatories for girls has suggested that here at least one can see a very definite influence of the Counter-Reformation. While these foundations may have also reflected the sentiments of earlier north-east Italian movements such as that of Girolamo Miani and his Somaschi,[99] they were very much part of that later sixteenth-century concern for the vulnerability of both married and unmarried women, which also led to the creation of houses organised on almost conventual lines, such as that of the Malmaritate for unhappily married women.[100] Another expression of concern in this period for the vulnerability of unmarried women was the provision of dowries for the marriage of poor girls. Here the influence of the Grand Dukes was significant, especially from the 1590s.[101]

Charity and the Church

If the measures introduced by Cosimo de' Medici in the 1540s can be seen as an expression of his developing policy in the centralisation of his state, we cannot divorce the establishment of the Spedale dei Broccardi and the four female conservatories from the wider religious currents of the time. The preoccupation with the fate and education of orphaned children and the language in which these preoccupations are expressed clearly reflected the ideas of Catholic reform.[102]

Indeed despite strained relations with Popes Paul III and IV,[103] Cosimo made sure that he first obtained the consent and support of the Church before taking measures concerning charitable institutions and the poor. In the first place Cosimo stipulated that a senior member of the clergy should always be the president of the commission of the Buonomini; he was to be nominated by the Archbishop and in this way the Church, initially at least, retained control over those hospitals with a religious status.[104] The statutes which regulated the activities of the Buonomini were, moreover, given full approval in Rome, as can be seen from the brief of the Florentine Cardinal Penitenziere, Antonio Pucci, issued on 4 July 1542, followed by the approbation of the Archbishop in October 1542.[105] Finally, as we have seen, Paul III in his Bull of July 1543 authorised Cosimo to extend his control over all hospitals, whether under lay or ecclesiastical control, in order to help to finance the Abbandonati project.[106] This was an important and innovatory principle to have established, given the long history of conflict between local secular and ecclesiastical powers over control of the rights of visitation and taxation of charitable institutions.

Collaboration between the Medici regime and the Church remained an important element of the dukes' dealings with charitable institutions in the second half of the sixteenth century and made it easier for the Medici to exercise more control over the hospitals of the city and the provinces. This process was facilitated further when the Archbishop of Milan, Gian Angelo de' Medici, became Pope Pius IV in 1559. Although only a very distant relative, he clearly favoured the Tuscan dukes, reflected in the elevation of first Cosimo's 17-year-old son, Giovanni, to the cardinalate and then following his death in 1563 his brother Ferdinando, who was not yet 14. Ferdinando's connections in Rome furthermore stood him in good stead when he took over the reins of power and became Grand Duke in 1587.[107]

Although the relations between the Medici dukes and the church formed the background for the instigation of some of the grander initiatives in welfare policy, the broader influence of the Catholic reform movement can be seen to have been introduced rather through independent agencies than the ecclesiastical hierarchy. The most important of these agencies were the confraternity, often founded under the influence of individual religious, and the new Orders.

Confraternities

Perhaps most typical of the newer confraternities of the sixteenth century were the national networks of parochial sacramental companies and the Societies of Christian Doctrine. Although pre-dating Trent, they introduced the main elements of the message of Catholic reform to the local level. Between 1530 and the early seventeenth century twenty-four sacramental companies were founded in Florence.[108] In addition to their re-emphasis on the importance of the sacrament, religious education was an important element of these societies and reflects, as in the case of the hostels for boys and girls, the new perception of the necessity to educate children for their own moral improvement and for the good of society.

The new concentration on the role of the parish with the central importance of the sacrament stemmed directly from the influence of the Council of Trent; this was mediated through the local church and was a result of the joint collaboration between the Archbishop and the Medicean Dukes.[109] Thus the 1573 statutes of the provincial Synod of the Florentine Church encouraged the foundation of sacramental companies in each parish as well as Companies of Christian Doctrine.[110] At the centre of the rituals of many of these companies was the new devotion to the Quarantore, the Perpetual Devotion to the Blessed Sacrament.[111]

Many of these confraternities were established by prominent religious leaders in late sixteenth-century Florence, many of whom represented the ideals of the Counter-Reformation, but significantly were not themselves members of any of the new Orders.[112] Ippolito Galantini (d. 1619), for example, was principally concerned with the religious education of children and adults, particularly after the Council of Trent, and used for this the recently founded Compagnia di S. Salvatore in Ognissanti. The Dominican Alessandro Capocchi combined religious education with active charity towards the poor, using for this purpose three confraternities: the Compagnia di S. Benedetto Bianco, della Trinità and di S. Michele de' Ricci. But, as we have seen, he was also concerned with the fate of abandoned children, inspiring the foundation of the Monastero della Pietà for girls.[113] Another influential religious figure was Santi Cini (1524–70), who founded the important Compagnia di S. Tommaso Aquino, which met under the protection of both the Duke and the Medici Archbishop. The confraternity proved influential in promoting among its adherents, many of whom were from noble families, the message of Catholic reform. Many of these companies combined spiritual and charitable works, very much along the lines of the Oratory of Filippo Neri, a friend of Santi Cini. This underlines once again the way in which the early reformers made their influence felt, often without being directly involved, especially by using the confraternity as the vehicle through which their message and example was spread.[114]

It was, however, the earlier confraternities, and in particular that of the Misericordia and the Buonomini di S. Martino, which continued to provide the main source of confraternal charity in late sixteenth- and early seventeenth-century Florence. The Buonomini was largely responsible for direct subsidies in non-crisis years to the *poveri vergognosi*, or shame-faced poor, who included many textile workers. Then during epidemics the Misericordia came into its own, carrying the sick to Lazzaretti, burying the dead and generally fumigating the houses belonging to the *sospetti* and *infetti*.[115]

The new Orders and the poor

If confraternities and hospitals between them provided much of the charity in Florence, what, then, was the role of those new Orders, usually seen as closely associated with helping the poor and sick? The three major ones engaged in charitable works were all established in the city in the second half of the sixteenth century: that of S. Giovanni di Dio, the Camilliani, and the Frati Cappuccini. The Order of S. Giovanni di Dio, which had been founded in Spain by Giovanni Ciudadad, had rapidly spread throughout Europe; by 1588, when Ferdinando de' Medici granted them the Spedale di S. Maria dell' Umiltà in Florence, they had already founded seventy-nine hospitals and administered another twenty-nine in Catholic Europe.[116] The Fatebenfratelli, as they were popularly known, expanded the hospital of S. Maria della Umiltà, and dedicated themselves to looking after the sick poor.[117] The main areas of the hospital's activity appear to have been little different from those of other general hospitals. The ailments of many of their patients fell into the general category of 'fever', and treatment included the letting of blood, the extraction of teeth and the administration of various decoctions and infusions.[118]

The second new nursing Order were the Camilliani, whom we have already encountered working in the hospitals of Rome. Established officially in 1586, the Ministers of the Sick, as they were also known, arrived in Florence in 1599 when they immediately began to work as servants in the hospital of S. Maria Nuova. In the following year they established a seat in the house and church of S. Gregorio on Piazza de' Mozzi.[119] Next year San Camillo himself visited Florence and worked in the hospital where he is alleged to have miraculously cured a number of dying patients.[120]

The Frati Cappuccini, who were established in Florence in 1572 (although they had lived outside the city walls since 1535) at the invitation of Cosimo I, may not have had such miraculous powers.[121]

Nevertheless, in imitation of St Francis, they played an important part in looking after the sick. Furthermore, as successors to St Francis, they saw themselves as having an important role among the poor, hence their emphasis on the cheap cloth of their habits and, in contrast to the Jesuits, their preference for living in shabby rather than splendid surroundings. Instead of Francis' emphasis on lepers, they concentrated on those sick from those epidemic diseases most prevalent in the sixteenth century. As we have seen, they nursed those sick from the *Mal Francese* and other chronic diseases in the Incurabili hospitals, such as San Giacomo in Rome, and then worked among those sick from plague in the Lazzaretti of many of the cities of central and northern Italy. It was in particular for this work that they won dominion over the hearts, and therefore the purses, of the monied classes, who, despite the friars' aversion to all things of the world, in time came to accept subsidies to underwrite the cost of building their friaries and churches. Such was the case in Florence, where the Cappuccini made their home in the Convento di San Francesco next to the Benedictine abbey of San Miniato al Monte just outside the city walls. These buildings were taken over in September 1630 as the city's main Lazzaretto for plague victims during the epidemic that was to last until July the following year. The Frati inevitably became involved in looking after the *appestati* and some of them shared the fate of their charges.[122] However, it is significant of the reputation gained by the Camilliani since their arrival in Florence only thirty-one years before that the Grand Duke Ferdinando II chose Donato Bisogni, superior of the Padri Camilliani in Florence, to act as the director of the Lazzaretto.[123]

Conclusion

If we began this chapter with a crisis, the siege of Florence following on four years of epidemic disease and famine, we have ended 100 years later with another, the plague of 1630–1. How, though, did the influence of the Catholic Reformation change the way in which the Florentine authorities coped with either endemic or epidemic poverty? In the first place, it is evident that even though there was now a greater concentration on devotion to the sacrament at parish level – an effect of which could be seen as a more efficient system of social control of the poor [124] – the basic structure of charity and welfare remained largely as it had over the past 250 years. Thus the major hospitals, confraternities and orphanages continued to cope with the everyday poverty of the indigent and helpless members of society in the shape of widows, orphans and the sick, including unemployed textile workers. The New Orders made a valuable contribution to this system, providing personnel to tend to those sick from both endemic and epidemic disease.

But the Counter-Reformation did also lead to important innovations in the city's charitable system. This stemmed from what has been characterised as the 'redemptive charity' of the sixteenth century,[125] which sought to protect certain groups of society who were regarded as being more vulnerable to the evils of the downward spiral of poverty. Above all this policy was directed towards boys and girls. The former were, as we have seen, now taken off the streets into institutions where they lived and were taught to be good Christians and moral citizens, who would contribute usefully to society through exercising the profession in which they had been trained. Similar sentiments lay behind the establishment of the four conservatories for girls, through the added moral crusade underlying these institutions, namely the preservation of female honour.

It would be wrong, however, to attribute these moves as deriving exclusively from the Counter-Reformation, if this term implies the post-Tridentine church, because many of these initiatives had been begun before the Council met. The same was true of the second feature of sixteenth-century welfare policies, greater intolerance towards beggars. Even if these intolerant attitudes had already been present in the later Middle Ages, particularly in periods of epidemic poverty, it was the early sixteenth century which saw a closer association between poverty and disease, with the poor being seen increasingly as the cause of disease as much as its victims. The later sixteenth century saw a new movement, the greater forced institutionalisation of the poor in the Beggars' Hostels, the Spedali dei Mendicanti, which were founded in many major Italian cities from the late sixteenth century.[126] It could be argued that this was a response to the influence of Carlo Borromeo with his urging in 1565 to princes and magistrates to collect together beggars in the same place in order to ensure their maintenance. And behind this was the Church's more general interest in beggars because of their ignorance of Christianity. They were seen as sinners who needed to be saved and given religious education.[127]

If the regime in institutions for beggars may seem harsh, it should be remembered that many of them were set up during crises generated by severe dearth and disease, when measures to deal with the poor had traditionally been stronger and couched less in terms of charity and more in terms of social control. These sentiments and the actions which followed from them were characteristic of emergencies and should not be taken as necessarily representative of those taken in non-crisis years. Moreover, although the Medici dukes certainly now had a greater control over all these charitable and social institutions, the State's policies during periods of epidemic poverty caused by famines and plague were little different from those in the 1520s. They provided food for the starving and those who had been quarantined because they had come into contact with plague victims, and carried off the latter to isolation hospitals or Lazzaretti. No doubt the existence of these large institutions made it easier to enforce law and order and to prevent potentially disruptive behaviour, but we are still, even during periods of crisis, far from the absolutist state. Although the dukes may have gained greater control over the charitable system, the structure remained largely as it had over the previous 300 years. Hospitals and confraternities were still mainly run by the laity – though now with more guidance and help from religious – to provide both spiritual and material support. In the process, no doubt, the poorer sort were now provided with a more moral education, with greater emphasis on the institutionalisation of children and the preservation of female honour, thus reflecting the redemptive character of Counter-Reformation charity.

Notes

I am particularly grateful to Daniella Lombardi for her comments and suggestions on an earlier version of this chapter as well as to Philip Gavitt and Alessandro Pastore. Unless otherwise stated, all manuscripts cited are from the Archivio di Stato di Firenze (ASF).

1 See the collection of fundamental studies on the subject by Brian Pullan in: *Poverty and Charity: Europe, Italy, Venice, 1400–1700* (London, 1994), as well as G. Politi, M. Rosa, and F. della Peruta (eds), *Timore e carità. I poveri nell'Italia moderna* (Cremona, 1982).

2 See the surveys by M. Rosa, 'Chiesa, idee sui poteri e assistenza in Italia dal cinque al settecento', *Società e Storia*, 10 (1980), pp. 775–806; and A. Pastore, 'Strutture assistenziali fra chiesa e stati nell'Italia della contrariforma', in C. Chittolini and G. Miccoli (eds), *Storia d'Italia. Annali* 9, *La chiesa e il potere politico dal medioevo all'età contemporanea* (Turin, 1986), pp. 43–65; A. Pastore, 'Gli ospedali in Italia fra cinque e settecento: evoluzione, caratteri, problemi', in M.L. Betri and E. Bresson (eds), *Gli Ospedali in Area Padana fra Settecento e Novecento. (Atti del III Congresso Italiano di Storia Ospedaliera. Montecchio Emilia, 4–16 marzo 1990)*, (Milan, 1992), pp. 71–87.

3 Recent studies of the sixteenth-century economy have tended to modify the traditional picture of decline. See the discussion in J.C. Brown, 'Prosperity or hard times in Renaissance Italy?', *Renaissance Quarterly*,

xlii (1989), pp. 761–80. On Florence see: P. Malanima, *La Decadenza di un'Economia Cittadina. L'Industria di Firenze nei Secoli XVI-XVIII* (Bologna, 1982).

4 Cf. Pullan, 'Poveri, mendicanti e vagabondi (secoli XIV–XVII)', in Pullan, *Poverty and Charity*, Chapter IV, pp. 1008–20; P. Slack, *Poverty and Policy in Tudor and Stuart England* (London and New York, 1988), Chapter 5; R. Jütte, *Poverty and Deviance in Early Modern Europe* (Cambridge, 1994), pp. 42–50 and Chapter 9.

5 Cf. A. Carmichael, *Plague and the Poor in Renaissance Florence* (Cambridge, 1986), Chapter 5. See also B. Pullan, 'Plague and perceptions of the poor in early modern Italy', in Pullan, *Poverty and Charity*, Chapter 7.

6 On this see A. Foa, 'The New and the Old: the spread of syphilis (1494–1530)', in E. Muir and G. Ruggiero (eds), *Sex and Gender in Historical Perspective* (Baltimore and London, 1990), pp. 26–45; C. Quétel, *History of Syphilis* (Cambridge, 1990), Chapter 1; J. Arrizabalaga, J. Henderson and R. French, *The Great Pox. The French Disease in Renaissance Europe* (New Haven and London, 1997), Chapters 2 and 7.

7 Cited in D. Chambers and B. Pullan (eds), *Venice. A Documentary History* (Oxford, 1992), p. 309.

8 *Salvatoris Nostri Domini Jesu Christi*, 15 August 1515, in *Bullarium Romanum a B. Leone Magno usque a S.D.N. Clementem X*, ed. A.M. Cherubino, Lyon, 1892, i, pp. 567–71, especially p. 567; cited in P. De Angelis, *L'Arcispedale di San Giacomo in Augusta* (Rome, 1955), pp. 10–11.

9 Arrizabalaga, Henderson and French, *The Great Pox*, Chapters 2 and 7.

10 Pullan, 'Support and redeem', in *Poverty and Charity*, Chapter V, pp. 190–3.

11 B. Pullan, *Rich and Poor in Renaissance Venice. The social institutions of a Catholic State to 1620* (Oxford, 1971), pp. 264–5, and more generally P. Tacchi Venturi, *Storia della Compagnia di Gesù in Italia* (Rome, 1930), I.i, Chapters 18–19, and J. O'Malley, *The First Jesuits* (Cambridge, MA., and London, 1993), Chapter 5, especially pp. 171–3.

12 C. Cargnoni (ed.), *I Frati Cappuccini. Documenti e testimonianze del primo secolo* (Perugia, 1991), III.2, pp. 3411–46, especially pp. 3412–13 n. 6.

13 See P. Sannazzaro, *Storia dell'Ordine Camilliano* (1550–1699), (Turin, 1986), pp. 29–33.

14 Ibid., p. 50.

15 Ibid., pp. 47–8, 53–4, 57.

16 In general see C.F. Black, *Italian Confraternities in the Sixteenth Century* (Cambridge, 1989).

17 On Companies of Divine Love see: A. Bianconi, *L'Opera delle Compagnie del 'Divino Amore' nella Riforma Cattolica* (Città di Castello, 1914); and P. Paschini, 'Le compagnie del Divino Amore e la beneficenza pubblica nei primi decenni del cinquecento', in *Tre Ricerche sulla Storia della Chiesa nel Cinquecento* (Rome, 1945), pp. 11–32.

18 See the statutes of the Compagnia del Divino Amore in Genoa in Tacchi Venturi, *Storia della Compagnia di Gesù*, i, pp. 423–32, and

those of the Ridotto in Genoa: P. Cassiano da Langasco, *Gli Ospedali degli Incurabili* (Genoa, 1938), pp. 197–205.

19 On the development of the Incurabili hospitals in Italy see: Cassiano da Langasco, *Gli ospedali degli Incurabili*, and more recently: A. Malamani, 'Notizie sul mal francese e gli ospedali degli incurabili in età moderna', *Critica storica*, 15 (1978), pp. 193–216, and Arrizabalaga, Henderson and French, *The Great Pox*, Chapters 7 and 8.

20 On this hospital see: De Angelis, *L'Arcispedale di San Giacomo in Augusta*, and most recently A. Cavaterra, 'L'ospedalità a Roma nell'età moderna: il caso di San Giacomo (1585–1605)', *Sanità, Scienza e Storia*, 2 (1986), pp. 87–123, and Arrizabalaga, Henderson and French, *The Great Pox*, Chapter 8.

21 On this theme see Arrizabalaga, Henderson and French, *The Great Pox*, Chapters 7 and 8.

22 See S. Cohen, *The Evolution of Women's Asylums Since 1500. From Refuges for Ex-Prostitutes to Shelters for Battered Women*, Oxford, 1992; A. Camerano, 'Assistenza richiesta ed assistenza imposta: il Conservatorio di S. Caterina della Rosa di Roma', *Quaderni Storici*, xxviii, 1993, pp. 227–60.

23 Cf. B. Pullan, 'Per la difesa del corpo sociale: gli ospedali', in N.E. Vanzan Marchini (ed.), *De Natura* (Milan, forthcoming).

24 For a discussion of this whole subject see: A. D'Addario, *Aspetti della Contrariforma a Firenze* (Ministero dell' Interno, Pubblicazioni degli Archivi di Stato, LXXVII), (Rome, 1972).

25 B. Varchi, *Storia Fiorentina*, ed. L. Arbib (Florence, 1839–41), vol. 2, IX, pp. 100–01; his statistics may have been based on the 1527 census of the city of Florence in Biblioteca Nazionale Centrale di Firenze, NA 987.

26 Varchi, *Storia Fiorentina*, pp. 99–100, 118. On S. Maria della Croce al Tempio see: L. Passerini, *Storia degli Stabilmenti di Beneficenza e d'Istruzione Elementare della Città di Firenze* (Florence, 1853), pp. 482–96, and G.B. Uccelli, *Della Compagnia di S. Maria della Croce al Tempio* (Florence, 1864); for the Buonomini di S. Martino: A. Spicciani, 'The "Poveri Vergognosi" in fifteenth-century Florence: The first 30 years' activity of the Buonomini di S. Martino', in T. Riis (ed.), *Aspects of Poverty in Early Modern Europe* (Stuttgart, 1981), pp. 119–82, and 'Aspetti finanziari dell'assistenza e struttura cetuale dei poveri vergognosi fiorentini al tempo del Savonarola (1487–1498)', in *Studi di storia economica toscana nel medioevo e nel rinascimento: In memoria di Federigo Melis* (Biblioteca del Bollettino Storico Pisano, Collana Storica, 1987, 33), pp. 31–46; and for the role of the Misericordia see: C. Torricelli, M. Lópes Pegna, M. Danti and O. Checcucci (eds), *La Misericordia di Firenze Attraverso i Secoli. Note storiche*, (Florence, 1975), Chapter 3 and J. Henderson, 'Plague in Renaissance Florence: medical theory and government response', N. Bulst and R. Delort (eds), *Maladies et société (xii–xviiie siècles)*, (Paris, 1989), pp. 175–86.

27 On the Florentine Incurabili hospital see: ASF, Ospedale di SS Trinità degli Incurabili, and Passerini, *Storia*, pp. 203–16, and on the Lazzaretto: Carmichael, *Plague and the Poor*, pp. 102–3.

28 Passerini, *Storia*, pp. 206–10.

29 See F. Diaz, *Il Granducato di Toscana. I Medici* (Turin, 1976), Chapter II; A. D'Addario, 'Testimonianze archivistiche, cronistiche e bibliografiche', in: *La Comunità Cristiana Fiorentina e Toscana nella Dialettica Religiosa del Cinquecento* (Florence, 1980), pp. 165–6.
30 See Pullan, 'Support and redeem', pp. 190–3; Pastore, 'Strutture assistenziali', pp. 435–8.
31 On this period see: H.C. Butters, *Governors and Government in Early Sixteenth Century Florence*, 1502–1519 (Oxford, 1985), and J.N. Stephens, *The Fall of the Florentine Republic, 1512–1530* (Oxford, 1983).
32 Cf. Varchi, *Storia Fiorentina*, vol. 2, IX, p. 137; C. Roth, *The Last Florentine Republic* (London, 1925), pp. 197, 269–70. Another example is the Misericordia: *La Misericordia di Firenze*, p. 76.
33 Roth, *The Last Florentine Republic*, pp. 190–1.
34 Varchi, *Storia fiorentina*, vol. 3, XIII, pp. 30–1. Cf. also ASF, Magistrato Supremo 1, folio 52v.
35 Recorded in ASF, L'Ospedale di S. Maria Nuova (cited as SMN 4), folios 73v–74r: 21.iii.1533; ASF, Senato del Quarantotto 48, folios 56v–57v: 31.iii.1533 provided additional privileges to help their finances. Cf. Passerini, *Storia*, pp. 340–2 and D'Addario, *Aspetti*, pp. 81–82.
36 ASF, SMN 4, folio 73v: 21.iii.1533
37 ASF, SMN 4, folio 73v. Cf. Passserini, *Storia*, pp. 335–6.
38 ASF, Magistrato Supremo 1, folios 29v–30r; Senato dei Quarantotto 1, folios 56v–57r (also in SMN 4, folios 74v–75r).
39 ASF, Senato dei Quarantotto 5, folios 13v–15v: 19.iii.1542. Cf. Passerini, *Storia*, pp. 27–31, 799–800, and D'Addario, *Aspetti*, pp. 464–9, who discusses and publishes the final version of the document, dated 17.xi.1542. On this and subsequent developments see also: M. Sichi, *Un'Istituzione di Beneficenza Fiorentina: Il Bigallo* (Naples, 1927).
40 G. Parenti, *Prezzi e Mercato del Grano a Siena (1546–1765)*, (Florence, 1942), pp. 76–7; B. Licata, 'Il problema del grano e delle carestie', in G. Spini (ed.), *Architettura e Politica da Cosimo I a Ferdinando I* (Florence, 1976), p. 336.
41 Cf. D. Lombardi, 'Poveri a Firenze. Programmi e realizzazioni della politica assistenziale dei Medici tra cinque a seicento', in G. Politi, M. Rosa and F. della Peruta (eds), *Timore e Carità: I Poveri nell'Italia Moderna* (Annali della Biblioteca Statale e Libreria Civica di Cremona, xxvii–xxx, 1976–9), (Cremona, 1982) pp. 165–84, especially pp. 166–7.
42 ASF, Senato dei Quarantotto 5, folios 13v–5v: 19.iii.1542. Cf. Passerini, *Storia*, pp. 27–31, 799–800, and D'Addario, *Aspetti*, pp. 464–9. Confirmed by Pope Paul III: ASF, Diplomatico del Bigallo: under 4.vii.1543: Passerini, *Storia*, pp. 802–5.
43 The text of the Senate's deliberation is in ASF, Senato dei Quarantotto 5, folios 13v–15r: 17.xi.1542 and published by Passerini, *Storia*, pp. 807–9 and, with corrections, by D'Addario, *Aspetti*, pp. 465–67.
44 Ibid.
45 On the famine see Parenti, *Prezzi*, pp. 76–7.
46 See P. Gavitt, '"Perche non avea chi la ghovernasse", Cultural values,

family resources and abandonment in the Florence of Lorenzo de' Medici, 1467–85', in J. Henderson and R. Wall (eds), *Poor Women and Children in the European Past* (London, 1994), p. 84, and P. Gavitt 'Charity and state-building in Cinquecento Florence: Vincenzio Borghini as Administrator of the Ospedale degli Innocenti', *Journal of Modern History*, 69.2, 1997, pp. 230–70. I am grateful to Philip Gavitt for this suggestion.

47 Passerini, *Storia*, p. 799.

48 ASF, Senato dei Quarantotto 5, folio 13v; D'Addario, *Aspetti*, p. 465.

49 Passerini, *Storia*, pp. 807–9, discussed by D'Addario, *Aspetti*, pp. 89–90.

50 ASF, Diplomatico del Bigallo under 18.vii.1543; Passerini, *Storia*, pp. 810–12.

51 D'Addario, Aspetti, pp. 88–9; Lombardi, 'Poveri a Firenze', pp. 166–7.

52 Passerini, *Storia*, p. 31.

53 Passerini, *Storia*, pp. 802–5, and discussed on pp. 28–31. The two briefs of 1542 and the papal Bull of 1543 are in ASF, Bigallo 1669.4, folios 6r–10v, 14r–16r.

54 ASF, Bigallo 1669.2, folios 9r–25r, quoted by Lombardi, 'Poveri a Firenze', pp. 167–8.

55 The statutes as reflected in Cardinal Pucci's brief: Passerini, *Storia*, pp. 29–30, 802–5, on which the following discussion is based. In general on the problem of beggars see: D. Lombardi, 'L'ondata di pauperismo', in R. Romano (ed.), *Il XVII Secolo: la Dinamica di una Crisi,* in *Storia d'Italia*, ed. R. Romano (Milan, 1989), pp. 169–92.

56 Passerini, *Storia*, pp. 803–4.

57 Lincata, 'Il problema del grano', pp. 366–7.

58 Diaz, *Il Granducato*, pp. 130–2, and Licata, 'Il problema del grano'.

59 ASF, Practica Segreta 84, folio 64r, cited by Lombardi, 'Poveri a Firenze', p. 169.

60 Licata, 'Il problema del grano', pp. 333–71.

61 Discussed in J. Henderson, *Piety and Charity in Late Medieval Florence* (Oxford, 1994) for confraternities, and for hospitals: Passerini, *Storia.*

62 Passerini, *Storia*, pp. 308–10, and D'Addario, *Aspetti*, pp. 77–8. Cf. also ASF, SMN 10, folios 29v–30r. In 1561 the Portinari were elected as patrons of S. Maria Nuova again.

63 Passerini, *Storia*, pp. 810–12; D'Addario, *Aspetti*, pp. 89–90, and D. Lombardi, *Povertà Maschile, Povertà Femminile. L'Ospedale dei Mendicanti nella Firenze dei Medici* (Bologna, 1988), p. 71.

64 D'Addario, *Aspetti,* p. 78.

65 D'Addario, *Aspetti*, p. 75; cf. 'Uffici e Stato della città di Firenze': ASF, Archivio Mediceo del Principato 663; A. D'Addario, 'Burocrazia, economia e finanze dello Stato Fiorentino alla meta del Cinquecento, *Archivio Storico Italiano*, 121, (1963), pp. 385–456; '1561. Magistrati e ufizi della città di Firenze': ASF, Archivio della Guardaroba 50.

66 On S. Paolo see Passerini, *Storia*, 176–9; D'Addario, *Aspetti*, pp. 76–7; cf. also ASF, S. Paolo 912 on the reforms of the hospital in 1571.

67 Lombardi, 'Poveri a Firenze', p. 166 and n. 4.

68 D'Addario, *Aspetti*, p. 92, though it is not clear over what period these hospitals were surveyed.

69 ASF, Bigallo 154, folios 552 r-v: 13.i.1558: 'In decti spedali non solo non si serva hospitalità, ma si abandonava et si lassono ruinare et li spedalinghi in grave offesa de Dio et si grandissimo preiuditio et danno de' poveri . . . usurpono et appropriano e fructi di decti spedali'.
70 ASF, Bigallo 1237, folio 18r: 23.vii.1586: 'e vi informarete quello hanno d'entrata e di spesa accertandovene non solo per il detto loro e de' loro libri, ma in ogn'altro miglior modo che vi parrà convenirsi per ritrovarne il vero . . .'.
71 ASF, Bigallo 1237, folio 401v.
72 ASF, Bigallo 1237, folio 249r.
73 Passerini, *Storia*, p. 807.
74 Lombardi, 'Poveri a Firenze', pp. 169–72.
75 Lombardi, 'Poveri a Firenze', pp. 172–84, and in more detail: *Povertà Maschile, Povertà Femminile.*
76 D. Lombardi, *Povertà Maschile, Povertà Femminile*.
77 The Monastero di S. Maria e S. Niccolò was founded by Francesco di Giovanni Rosati.
78 D'Addario, *Aspetti*, p. 51.
79 Lombardi, 'Poveri a Firenze', pp. 167–8, 172; ASF, S. Maria Nuova, Monastero di Santa Caterina 7, folio 2r lists their names.
80 D'Addario, 'Testimonianze', pp. 135–6.
81 ASF, Monastero di S. Maria e S. Niccolò del Ceppo, 1 bis., folios 1r-v; ASF, Monastero di Santa Caterina 7, folio 1r.
82 D'Addario, *Aspetti*, pp. 51–2; cf. F. Marchi, *Vita di Alessandro Capocchi* (Florence, 1583).
83 ASF, Monastero di S. Maria e S. Niccolò del Ceppo, 1 bis., folio 1r; ASF, Monastero di Santa Caterina 7, folio 1r.
84 Diaz, *Il Granducato*, p. 134; B. Licata, 'Il problema del grano', pp. 333–71, especially p. 336.
85 ASF, Monastero di S. Maria e S. Niccolò del Ceppo, 1 bis., folio 12r. See also D'Addario, *Aspetti*, pp. 51–4; Lombardi, 'Poveri a Firenze', pp. 166–68.
86 ASF, Monastero di Santa Caterina 7, folios 6r–v.
87 Ibid., folios 14r ff: caps. vii–ix.
88 Ibid., folio 11v.
89 ASF, Monastero di S. Caterina, folio 4r.
90 ASF, Monastero di S. Caterina, folio 4r; Monastero di S. Maria e S. Niccolò del Ceppo, folio 11v.
91 ASF, Monastero di S. Caterina, folio 4r; cf. also Lombardi, 'Poveri a Firenze', p. 168.
92 ASF, Monastero di S. Caterina, folio 4r.
93 ASF, Corporazione Religiose Soppresse dal Governo Francese 112.78 (Spedale della Pietà), folios 1r–13r; ASF, Monastero di S. Maria e S. Niccolò del Ceppo 59, folios 105v–118v.
94 Lombardi, *Povertà, Maschile, Povertà Femminile*, pp. 85–6.
95 See above and A. Corradi, *Annali delle Occorse Epidemie in Italia, dalle Prime Memorie Fino al 1850* (Bologna, 1865–94, 1973 reprinted edn.), iv, pp. 506–521.
96 ASF, Bigallo 154, folio 52r; the story continued on folio 96r, a petition

to the Duke to allow the girl to become a nun of the Monastero di S. Domenico in Florence rather than simply a servant.

97 Passerini, *Storia*, p. 195.

98 ASF, Monastero di S. Maria e S. Niccolò del Ceppo 59, folios 105v–118v.

99 Cf. Pullan, *Rich and Poor*, pp. 259–62, 278–9.

100 See S. Cohen, *The Evolution of Women's Asylums*.

101 See M. Fubini Leuzzi, 'Appunti per lo studio delle doti granducali in Toscana', *Ricerche Storiche*, xx (1990), pp. 339–66, and 'Prescrizioni per la sposa. Il caso delle doti dei granduchi di Toscana tra teoria e prassi', *Atti e Memorie dell'Accademia Toscana di Scienze e Lettere. La Colombaia*, lxi, n.s. xlvii (1996), pp. 103–39.

102 Lombardi, 'Poveri a Firenze', p. 167.

103 G. Spini, *Cosimo I e l'Independenza del Principato Mediceo* (Florence, 1980), Chapter V; R. Cantagalli, *Cosimo I de' Medici Granduca di Toscana* (Milan, 1985), Chapter 5, especially pp. 237–8.

104 ASF, Bigallo 1669.4, folios 6r–10v, 14r–16r; cf. folios 26r–28v: 28.iii.1550.

105 Passerini, *Storia*, pp. 28–31, and document F: pp. 802–5; pp. 805–7: document G.

106 Passerini, *Storia*, pp. 810–12: document J.

107 Diaz, *Il Granducato di Toscana*, p. 186–8.

108 R.F.E. Weissman, *Ritual Brotherhood in Renaissance Florence* (New York and London, 1982), p. 206.

109 D'Addario, *Aspetti*, p. 195.

110 Weissman, *Ritual Brotherhood*, p. 223.

111 Weissman, *Ritual Brotherhood*, p. 229.

112 In general see: D'Addario, *Aspetti*, pp. 42–51.

113 D'Addario, *Aspetti*, p. 51; cf. F. Marchi, *Vita di Alessandro Capocchi* (Florence, 1583).

114 D'Addario, *Aspetti*, pp. 54–6. See also the contemporary life of Santi Cini in: S. Razzi, *Historia degli uomini illustri . . . del sacro ordine dei Predicatori* (Lucca, 1596), pp. 284–5ff. Cf. Passerini, *Storia*, pp. 516–18 for the charitable works of the company.

115 See *La Misericordia di Firenze*, and Henderson, 'Plague in Renaissance Florence', pp. 175–86.

116 L. Sandri (ed.), *L'Archivio dell'Ospedale di San Giovanni di Dio di Firenze (1604–1890)* (Milan, 1991), pp. 4–5. On the history of the Order see M. Francini, *Fatebene Fratelli. San Giovanni di Dio e i Suoi Seguaci in Italia* (Milan, 1985).

117 On the hospital in this period see Passerini, *Storia*, pp. 395–8, and 896–7 for the Grand Duke's letter dated 4.ii.1588 to the Buonomini del Bigallo concerning the Order taking over the hospital. Most recently see: L. Sandri (ed.), *I Fatebenefratelli a Firenze. San Giovanni di Dio da Borgognissanti alla Charité* (Florence, 1986) and L. Sandri (ed.), *L'Archivio*.

118 L. Sandri (ed.), *L'Archivio*, pp. 4–10.

119 Sanzio Cicatelli, *Vita del P. Camillo de Lellis*, ed. P. Sannazzaro (Rome, 1980), pp. 184–5, 356 n. 447.

120 Cicatelli, *Vita*, pp. 266–7.

121 E. Sisto da Pisa, *Storia dei Cappuccini Toscani con Prolegomeni sull'Ordine Francescano e le Sue Riforme* (Florence, 1906), i, pp. 145–50; D'Addario, 'Testimonianze', p. 130.

122 M.B. Ciofi, 'La peste del 1630 a Firenze con particolare riferimento ai provvedimenti igienico-sanitari e sociali', *Archivio Storico Italiano*, cxlii (1984), pp. 68–9. On this epidemic see also: D. Sardi Bucci, 'La peste del 1630 a Firenze', *Ricerche Storiche*, x (1980), pp. 49–92; G. Calvi, *Histories of a Plague Year. The Social and the Imaginary in Baroque Florence* (Berkeley and Los Angeles, 1989).

123 Sannazzaro, *Storia dell'Ordine Camilliano*, pp. 61, 67 (the Order was founded in Florence in 1599). On Padre Bisogni's role during the plague: pp. 132–3.

124 Black, *Italian Confraternities*, pp. 275–6.

125 Pullan, "Support and redeem": charity and poor relief in Italian cities from the fourteenth to the seventeenth century', in Pullan, *Poverty and Charity*, Chapter 5.

126 Lombardi, 'L'ondata di pauperismo'.

127 Pullan, 'Poveri, mendicanti e vagabondi', in Pullan, *Poverty and Charity*, Chapter IV, pp. 1017–18.

5

'AD UNA SANCTA PERFETTIONE': HEALTH CARE AND POOR RELIEF IN THE REPUBLIC OF VENICE IN THE ERA OF THE COUNTER-REFORMATION

Richard Palmer

'Finding a means to relieve beggars and the shamefaced poor in this city in their calamities, is not only laudable, pious and pleasing to our Lord God, but also honourable and healthy for our State because of the diseases which on many occasions have resulted.' In this typical preamble to legislation in 1545, the Great Council of Venice endorsed motivations for poor relief which were both secular and religious. Notaries were to remind testators of the needs of the poor, and to report bequests to the Provveditori alla Sanità, the magistrates responsible for public health.[1]

Famine and epidemic disease inspired the Venetian poor law of 1529, and the fear that plague might be imported into the city by wandering beggars ensured that poor relief in Venice was the responsibility of the Health Office, under the Provveditori alla Sanità. Later the association of mendicity with crime, especially theft and extortion by deceit, added a further spur to government action, as did the spectre of the armed beggar, which brought vagrancy dangerously close to brigandage. The less dramatic requirements of social order – the need, for instance, to protect honest citizens from importunate beggars who loitered around churches and disrupted services – also helped to merge poor relief and social control, and contributed to the establishment of hospitals for the confinement of beggars, in Venice and elsewhere in the Republic, at the close of the sixteenth century.

Christian charity provided a parallel motivation, not least because conspicuous State charity, along with the repression of heresy and vice, was a means of securing divine favour in a period when famine, plague and war were recurrent threats. Hospitals could for this reason be portrayed as 'bastions of the Republic'.[2] The Venetian patriciate also proved to be fertile ground for the piety and ideals of the Counter-Reformation, which became widely absorbed into the language of Venetian legislation. Before the end of the sixteenth century the Council of Ten was enforcing the regulation of prostitution on the grounds that the sins of the flesh not only brought disease to the body but infected the soul.[3] At the same time the Provveditori alla Sanità and the Provveditori sopra Ospedali were moving towards the confinement of vagrants, because of the sins committed by beggars at night in public places, and the fate of the poverty-stricken who died on streets without the sacraments of the Church.[4]

Well before the Council of Trent a 'new Catholicism' or 'new philanthropy' had taken firm root. Much of the spirit of this Catholic Reformation may be seen in the work of the Companies of Divine Love, which were introduced into the Republic in the 1520s by Gaetano Thiene of Vicenza and Bartolomeo Stella of Brescia, both of whom had been members of the Company in Rome.[5] These were societies of priests and laymen, bound together in a devotional life of prayer and frequent communion, whose aim was to express the love of Christ in service to the poor. Their prime concerns were the *poveri vergognosi*, the shamefaced poor, and the victims of the French Disease, whom they gathered together into new hospitals for incurables, the Incurabili. Closely linked to them, and active in hospitals in the Venetian Republic, were the new religious orders, the Theatines, founded in 1524 by Gaetano Thiene and Gian Pietro Carafa; the Barnabites, founded in 1530; and the Somaschi, founded in 1532 under the influence of a Venetian nobleman, Girolamo Miani. In 1537 Ignatius Loyola and his followers also made the hospitals of Venice a proving ground for ascetic self-sacrifice and self-mastery in nursing the sick poor, prior to the foundation of the Society of Jesus in 1540.

A further source of influence was the revival of the episcopate as a force for the moral and social reform of the diocese, prefigured in the De officio episcopi of the Venetian Gasparo Contarini, and actualised by Gian Matteo Giberti as Bishop of Verona from 1524 to 1543. Although Venice protected the lay status of hospitals, this did not prevent bishops from an involvement in the support and development of charities of all kinds, nor, after the Council of Trent, did it exempt hospitals from episcopal visitation. Giberti was active in numerous ways, in advancing Verona's hospital for incurables, the Misericordia, and in founding a Compagnia della Carità, a voluntary society for the outdoor relief of the respectable poor. Giberti proved to be a model for later Counter-Reformation bishops such as Carlo Borromeo in his Archdiocese of Milan (which included several Venetian dioceses) and Agostino Valier in Verona.[6] Valier, for example, was to introduce the Compagnie della Carità in Venetian Istria and Dalmatia during his Apostolic Visitation there in 1579.[7]

To the ideal of serving Christ in the sick poor and providing comfort in adversity, the Counter-Reformation added an urgent concern for the redemption of sinners and the salvation of souls.[8] Hospitals offered opportunities to minister to the spiritual needs of the poor, and frequently to attend at their deathbeds. The syphilitics of the Incurabili offered an obvious target for evangelical initiatives, and one which led on to other forms of moral welfare, in the care of repentant prostitutes and girls in moral danger. The protection and education of orphans, the need to keep them from lives of poverty, ignorance, idleness and crime also came to have a prominent place in the work of the Republic's hospitals, which could increasingly be seen as weapons in the Counter-Reformation battle against ignorance and sin. Inmates of hospitals were brought within the discipline and authority of an ordered Catholic society, a prospect which appealed to Church and State alike. This process influenced the character of the Republic's hospitals and the range of work which they undertook. Catholic reformers proved to be restlessly ambitious in piling up good works of different kinds one upon another, in their efforts to reach *una sancta perfettione*, a comprehensive system for the moral, spiritual and social needs of the poor. In this vision, medical care had a prominent place, but was by no means a priority amongst other forms of moral and social endeavour.

Long before the Counter-Reformation, all the provincial capitals on the Venetian mainland boasted substantial hospitals, amongst which care for the sick poor and for foundlings were standard elements amongst other social concerns. In the north-east the largest towns, Treviso and Udine, possessed hospitals deriving from the flagellant movement of the thirteenth century, Santa Maria dei Battuti at Treviso, Santa Maria della Misericordia dei Battuti at Udine. Management was in the hands of religious confraternities of laymen. At Udine responsibility lay with a Greater Council which came in the sixteenth century to have 300 members – an assembly larger than the town council – though a smaller committee dealt with day-to-day management.

On the other side of the Venetian mainland, in the west, the largest towns, Brescia and Bergamo, provide a different pattern. These shared in a widespread movement in the Archdiocese of Milan in the mid-fifteenth century which created centralised Ospedali Maggiori by the amalgamation of smaller institutions. The preaching of the Observant Franciscans was influential in their formation, though they also owed an explicit debt to the exemplary hospitals of Florence and Siena. Like the Ospedale Maggiore of Milan, these hospitals promoted the cross-wards of hospital architecture – four wards radiating from the intersection of a cross where an altar was placed. At Brescia the Ospedale Maggiore was again in the care of a lay confraternity with councils of 200 and 100, and a smaller executive committee. At Bergamo the situation was different, for the Ospedale Maggiore did not incorporate the town's great confraternity, the Misericordia, which played a systematic role in safeguarding the poor of the whole province in times of dearth. The hospital was managed by a small committee of fourteen governors elected by the town council with the co-operation of the cathedral chapter.

In the centre of the Venetian mainland charitable functions were more diffused amongst several institutions. At Padua, for instance, the hospital of S. Francesco, which became famous as the scene of clinical teaching by Giovanni Battista da Monte and his successors, was exceptional in its exclusive focus on the sick poor. Alongside it however was a separate foundling hospital, the Cà di Dio, and a major confraternity, the Fraglia della Carità, which was active in outdoor relief, feeding and clothing the urban poor, providing dowries for poor girls, and sustaining the poor of the countryside in times of dearth.

Venice imposed no central policy for medical care and poor relief on its dominions, and the character of hospitals and charities was often determined by local circumstances. The welfare system of Bergamo, for instance, responded to the town's notoriously infertile site, which was able to sustain its population for only part of the year.[9] Verona was also exceptional, in that the inherited patrimony of an unusually rich leper hospital, Santi Jacopo e Lazzaro alla Tomba, allowed the Town Council to finance the work of its Health Office, to build a huge *lazaretto*, to continue the idiosyncratic work of the hospital with regard to diseases 'tending to leprosy', and to engage in poor relief.[10]

Diverse as they were, each of these hospitals was exposed to the influence of the new Catholicism. Its impact may be seen for instance in the hospital of Santa Maria della Misericordia at Udine. There, in 1505, the hospital governors had pondered the success of their resident surgeon, one Maestro Angelo. He was attracting patients from far and wide seeking treatment for the French Disease, *morbo gallico*. Far from congratulating their surgeon, the governors sacked him, 'lest expenses in this place should be multiplied'.[11]

This hospital had grown out of the flagellant piety of the thirteenth century, and it continued to be managed by a fraternity 'of the beaten' (*dei Battuti*). But the fervour which had given rise to the hospital had passed, or, as one member of the fraternity put it in 1548, 'That first charity and brotherly love has grown not merely lukewarm, but stone cold and almost extinct'.[12] In place of its great flagellant processions, the fraternity could muster only a handful of paupers, in threadbare flagellant costume, hired for ceremonial occasions. This was a hospital with great civic importance and prestige. But its income, derived from its historic patrimony of land and property, was limited, and not always sufficient for the work of the hospital in caring for the sick poor and for children taken in from Udine's foundling hospital after weaning. Expenditure, as the prudent governors made clear in the case of Maestro Angelo, was not to exceed income. Long-term problems which went unresolved in consequence included the inadequacy of the hospital's infirmary. Situated on the ground floor, it was airless, very damp, and foul-smelling. According to reports in the 1540s, almost all the patients died. It was even said that if people in good health were housed in that room, they too fell incurably ill and met a wretched end.[13]

During the 1540s however the Hospital was repeatedly challenged to institute reforms and to adopt a true spirit of charity (*una vera carità*) towards God's poor (*i poveri de Dio*), on the model of other Italian hospitals. Meanness and faintheartedness in spending were now portrayed to the governors as the roots of all evil:

> In consequence we need not hesitate to spend money for the needs of the Hospital, not to spend recklessly, but for the great need of the sick even the chalices should be sold. For I have never seen a well-governed hospital ever in need, for when a well-governed hospital has a reputation for poverty, so much the sooner does it become rich, because God Almighty is its treasurer, and the blood of Jesus Christ crucified is converted into bread and wine, and other things

> necessary. And so by a reputation for good management the other hospitals of Italy have grown and increased, like the hospital of Florence which is worth 16,000 *scudi*, the hospital of Rome 20–25,000 *scudi* more or less, Naples 24,000, Palermo 12,000, Messina 8,000 and others in many parts of Italy. So the revenues of the hospital will be increased by a reputation for good administration, and not by meanness.'[14]

One of the aims of the reformers at Udine was to institute a 'truly Christian regime', through the revision of the hospital statutes on the example of those of other towns. Amongst the catalysts was the arrival in 1543 of a letter of advice from Verona. Its author is not named in the hospital records, but the respect which it commanded in Udine may indicate that it came from, or with the support of, Bishop Giberti. It occasioned an extraordinary meeting which brought together the inner council of hospital governors, the Venetian Luogotenente of the Patria of Friuli, a bishop, representatives of the town council and various 'lovers of the poor'. The letter set out model statutes for a Catholic Reformation hospital. There were to be twelve governors, the most spiritual to be found, motivated by the love of God. Each week two of them were to take direct control, managing expenditure, receiving the sick, and visiting the patients at least twice a day to see that they were well treated and to exhort them in the service of God. A priest was to hear confessions and give communion to patients and staff once a month. In addition patients were to confess on admission, and there was to be a daily mass. Every morning and evening there were to be litanies and prayers, with the patients giving the responses. During meals some devout Christian work was to be read aloud. The priest was to visit and console the sick daily, and especially those close to death. As the secretary who recorded the meeting put it, these were statutes 'for the regulation of the hospital and the religious instruction of the poor'.[15] The reformers were also in contact with the new avant-garde hospitals of the Incurabili and the Derelitti in Venice, to which they turned for a woman to reform the nursing of the sick, and to teach other staff.[16]

The city of Venice stood in remarkable contrast to its mainland dominions, for before 1500 the city boasted no substantial hospitals other than the Pietà, which was dedicated exclusively to foundlings. It had flirted momentarily in the late fifteenth century with the idea of creating an Ospedale Maggiore and had gone so far as to commission a model of the Milanese hospital from Donato Bramante, but with no significant result.[17] By 1600 however this situation had been transformed. Two major hospitals for the sick had been established – the Incurabili in 1522 for syphilis and other chronic diseases, and the Derelitti in 1527 for acute illnesses. The Venetian Health Office had also put into effect after 1545 the system of poor relief and medical care, based on the city's 72 parishes, which it had first envisaged in 1529. It had also fostered a fraternity for the care of the *poveri vergognosi*, covering the whole city, which had come into being in 1537. Finally from 1594 the Senate established the Mendicanti, a hospital designed to complete the Venetian edifice of charity by sweeping beggars from the streets.

Amongst these institutions the Incurabili, in Venice and elsewhere, deserve attention as a distinctive contribution of the Catholic Reformation to medical care. The terrifying physical effects of syphilis, and the abandonment and destitution which befell many of its victims, made them immediately attractive to the evangelical piety which sprang from the Companies of Divine Love. Verona's hospital for incurables, the Misericordia was inspired by the plight of sufferers dying like beasts on the street in extreme poverty, without confession and the rites of the Church – an offence to God, as the town's Council of Twelve and Fifty was reminded.[18] The work in Verona began with a group of devout laymen who took into their care two women suffering from *mal francioso*. The Council of Twelve and Fifty supported them by providing a house, one indeed with symbolic overtones since it was converted from a brothel near the Arena, so that 'where first there was a filthy public brothel, now there is a house of mercy . . .'[19]

In Brescia the Incurabili was promoted by Bartolomeo Stella, but founded by a decision of the town's General Council in 1521. The Incurabili of Venice, founded in 1522, began, as in Verona, when two noble women took into their care three women suffering from *mal franzoso*, an effort to which Gaetano Thiene soon lent his support. No founding decree was passed by the state, but the Patriarch of Venice and the Provveditori alla Sanità immediately supported it. The Provveditori were concerned that victims of *mal franzoso* and other ills were begging on the streets and public places 'with the greatest stench and contagion of their neighbours', a potential cause of disease which might be the ruin of the city. They were to be compelled to enter the new hospital or to be banished from Venice.[20]

The Incurabili of Venice, Verona and Brescia (by no means the only such foundations in the Republic) were all soon linked by Papal bulls to the Archhospital of S. Giacomo in Rome. This allowed them to share its indulgences and other privileges, emphasizing at the same time the common aims of these hospitals on the Roman model.[21]

In Venice the Incurabili immediately captured the public imagination, as the diaries of Marin Sanudo reveal. He records preaching at the hospital by the Bishop of Scardona which reduced the whole congregation to tears; the baptism of converted Jews; and the moving sight of the noble governors of the hospital, led by Vincenzo Grimani, son of the Doge, symbolically washing the feet of the patients. Most of all he was struck that a hospital with no secure income could yet attract huge sums in alms, allowing it to increase the number of its inmates from 80 in 1522 to 150 in 1525.[22]

Long before, in 1496, Sanudo had noted that syphilis was transmissible only through sexual intercourse, an association which blighted the character of its victims.[23] Called before the Venetian Holy Office in 1569 on the accusation of Lutheranism, a barber at the Incurabili argued that the witnesses against him were untrustworthy. 'Not many good people came to that place, but the dissolute and evil-doers.' As to his principal accuser, he was 'a man whom I believe has never done good in his life, because he has been in the hospital not once, but two or three times'.[24] Redemption was therefore an important aim, and by 1525 the Incurabili was also housing repentant prostitutes, and becoming a centre for a variety of other evangelical initiatives.

Syphilis, however, was not the only disease treated at the Incurabili. A ducale of 1520 in favour of the Misericordia of Verona described it as a hospital for 'the french disease and other incurable sores'.[25] In 1542 the Misericordia extended its work to include patients with phthisis,[26] and in 1580 it defined its scope as the treatment of 'french disease of all kinds, hectic fevers, dropsy and sores (*piaghe*)', a term which it subsequently understood to include incurable fistulas and cancers.[27] At Brescia however the definition and diagnosis of 'incurable' proved to be so problematic that from 1548 its Ospedale Maggiore and Incurabili simply distributed their patients by sex. Male patients, curable and incurable, went to the Ospedale Maggiore, and female patients to the Incurabili.[28]

Therapies for syphilis in these hospitals included not only the use of mercurial ointments, but also the *legno santo*, guaiac. Its seasonal administration in the Incurabili of Venice, as in that of Rome, brought large fluctuations in the size and nature of the hospital's inmates. At the same time its high cost and dubious effectiveness were common subjects for the agenda of hospital governors. At

Padua in the late sixteenth century the treatment was restricted to a limited number drawn by lot; each year a wretched few were disappointed in the ballot.[29]

Along with the Incurabili, the Compagnie della Carità may also be considered typical of the Catholic Reformation, although their roots were sometimes much older. These fraternities helped to undermine begging by bringing relief and medical aid to the poor in their homes, and especially to the *poveri vergognosi*, the shamefaced poor in reduced circumstances, whose calamity and despair exposed them to spiritual as well as bodily perils.

In Venice where a fraternity (later called the Fraterna Grande di Sant' Antonin) was founded in 1537, and in Verona, where the Compagnia emerged in the years 1538–39, these societies were supported by the joint action of Church and State. From Venice the Doge urged their establishment throughout the Republic, just as Gian Matteo Giberti promoted them throughout his diocese of Verona.[30]

Visitors of the Compagnie attended the sick poor in their allotted areas of the town, calling in doctors as necessary and obtaining medicines. In Venice the Fraterna developed its own pharmacy, which was able to supply medicines to the poor of the whole city during an epidemic of typhus in 1570.[31] Here, as at Verona in 1587, the society fulfilled a role in relation to a disease which did not call into action the draconian plague regulations, but which hospitals avoided for fear of contagion.[32]

The brothers of the Compagnia at Verona (according to the statutes which Giberti helped to draft) were to pray to God to inflame their souls with godly ardour.[33] These were spiritual brotherhoods, as at Vicenza, where the statutes of 1569 enjoined monthly communion and a weekly meeting for edification and religious direction. Their first concern was with the spiritual welfare and consolation of the sick, and visitors were also directed to keep an eye open for other needs, such as girls in moral danger.[34]

In Venice the work of the Fraterna Grande di Sant' Antonin ran in parallel with that of the parish fraternities which resulted from the poor law, which may have dealt with a wider spectrum of the urban poor. Conceived in 1529 as a civic response to epidemic disease, the parish fraternities only came into existence after 1545, in the era of the Council of Trent, and they proved to be deeply imbued with the spirit of the Counter-Reformation. The statutes of the parish fraternity of S. Canzian, compiled in 1577, required that members should be god-fearing, full of love, supported by frequent confession and communion, ready to visit the poor of Christ as instruments of the Lord. At the bedsides of the sick, visitors were to remind them that tribulations were sent by God for the good of their souls, and to urge them with contrition to turn to God through confession.[35] The similar statutes of the parish of SS. Apostoli of 1563 enjoined additionally that, before turning to the provision of doctors and medicines, visitors should remind parents to teach their children the Pater noster, Ave, Credo, Salve and other devotions, and to avoid swearing and dishonest words. If a patient was obstinate in obeying the orders of the Church, the Fraterna was to take no further care of him.[36] In the parish of S. Canzian, where visitors found boys wasting time in idleness, they might be sent to school, to learn a trade, or to sea. Girls in moral danger were to be lodged elsewhere, or sent to a hospital. In this way the parish fraternities served as one of the instruments through which Tridentine discipline was enforced at the local level.

The care and education of children represented a major initiative of the Catholic Reformation, expressed not only through the Schools of Christian Doctrine which sprang up from the 1530s, but through hospitals.[37] The care of foundlings was on a far larger scale than any other hospital activity in the Republic, with 1,200 children in the care of the Pietà of Venice in 1559, and up to a thousand in the smaller towns of Brescia and Bergamo later in the century. Typically, the multi-purpose Ospedale Maggiore of Bergamo which also dealt with acute and chronic illnesses could declare in 1572 that foundlings were its principal concern and source of expense.[38] Foundlings represented a long-term commitment. At Bergamo, where, in the late sixteenth century at least, the success of the Ospedale Maggiore in rearing children defies the Malthusian reputation of foundling hospitals for killing children at public expense, foundlings might remain with their wetnurses to the age of 10 or 12, when they returned to the hospital to learn a trade, perhaps weaving or silk manufacture, in the hospital workshops. The cost of dowries was a further burden on hospitals, especially as foundlings were generally assumed to be illegitimate, and might require larger-than-average dowries.

One of the long-standing aims of foundling hospitals was to prevent infanticide, and to save abandoned infants who might otherwise die without baptism. The Catholic Reformation added a concern for spiritual and moral education, and for the protection of children from idleness and vice. These aims also led hospitals towards the care of orphans. Through the work of Girolamo Miani orphanages were established in Venice in the Incurabili and in the Derelitti by 1531, and subsequently in the Incurabili of Brescia and at Bergamo. In Verona too the Misericordia decided in 1531 that the care of incurables was not enough; a true Christian could not please God by remaining as if asleep in one work alone, but must progress from virtue to virtue towards a holy perfection (*una sancta perfettione*). Therefore the hospital would take on the care of orphans in need, who would otherwise go to the bad.[39] Later, in 1572–73, the joint efforts of Bishop Valier and the Council of Twelve and Fifty added a further institution, the Veronese Derelitti, for the confinement of vagabond children. It was concerned with boys who were sometimes the victims of Fagin-like beggar-masters, often living lives of swearing and crime, and with girls whose conduct around the town day and night endangered their own souls and those with whom they mixed. It was a stage towards the Veronese Mendicanti, for vagabonds of all ages, which followed in 1590 to complete another civic network of charity.[40]

Like foundlings, orphans represented pressing needs, and Miani's orphanages grew like cuckoos in the hospital nests. Founded in 1527 for acute diseases, the Venetian Derelitti could declare by 1570 that the care of orphan girls was of greater importance than any other holy work which it performed.[41] At Verona the governors of the Misericordia decided in 1550 that funds for incurables and orphans should be pooled, since the separation of 'yours' and 'mine' was a dishonour to God; each should share the other's poverty or riches.[42] The needs of foundlings and orphans however could be more insistent, especially during the repeated shortages of the late sixteenth century, when the famished poor flocked into the towns in search of food. At such times there were crippling demands on hospitals and charities, not only to feed the poor, but to cope with huge increases in the number of infants abandoned, while the wages of wetnurses, often linked to official price indexes for grain, tended to soar. On nine occasions in the 1580s and 1590s the Ospedale Maggiore of Brescia was driven to alienate property on a large scale, worth a total of 104,000 lire.[43] Medical care in the hospitals was more of a constant, and could seem less glamorous than other objects of charity. At Udine the reform movement of the 1540s, which was initially concerned with desperate conditions in the infirmary, was soon diverted into the religious education of foundling children, and a school for boys from the town – an unhappy experiment, since the priest in charge proved so terrifying that nine of the boys went into epileptic fits at the very sound of his voice. The rebuilding of the infirmary waited until 1562.[44]

Although Ignatius Loyola and his disciples ventured briefly on to the wards at Venice, it was orphans and foundlings, rather than the sick poor, which mainly attracted the new religious orders to the hospitals, and which sometimes supplied the orders with new recruits. The Derelitti in Venice might equally arrange for a dozen of its boys to be trained for the priesthood, as it did in 1578, prompting the Patriarch of Venice to try to involve the hospital in founding a seminary.[45] Patients in hospital wards at this time were required to be obedient not only to the doctors but to the religious observance of the house, which began with confession on admission, and continued with daily mass. A patient might be dismissed, as at SS. Jacopo e Lazzaro at Verona 'for swearing as if she were in a brothel or an inn, without respect for the sacred altar where the most holy sacrament is celebrated'.[46] Orphanages came to have a discipline of incredible rigour, as may be seen from three successive versions of the statutes for the orphan girls at the Derelitti in Venice from 1570 to 1667. They reveal the development of a daily routine of almost constant religious observance, with the recital of the offices by the girls even as they toiled in the hospital workshops. Silence was otherwise to be almost complete, and no two girls were to speak to each other more than briefly, lest by the suggestion of the devil some sensual affection might develop. [47]

This chapter has examined the ways in which health care and poor relief developed in the Republic under the influence of the Counter-Reformation, and its role in defining the vision of what was to be done and the character of what was achieved. The restless advance from good work to good work went far by 1600 to realise a comprehensive system of charity, the 'holy perfection' conceived in outline in the decades before the Council of Trent. At the same time it brought with it an element of compulsion. From 1611 Venetian officials could earn 30 soldi for every beggar with sores or other lesions (*piaghe*) whom they arrested and consigned to the *Incurabili*.[48] Alongside the Venetian magistrates for the repression of heresy and swearing, the Health Office and the hospitals of the Republic were playing their part in the struggle for a disciplined and obedient Catholic society.

Notes

This chapter owes an overwhelming debt to Professor Brian Pullan, whose *Rich and Poor in Renaissance Venice* (Oxford, 1971) as well as numerous articles which have succeeded it, are fundamental to the subject.

1 Archivio di Stato, Venice (hereafter A.S.V.), *Provveditori alla Sanità*, Reg. 12, folios 103–04. The legislation extended existing provision for the shamefaced poor (*poveri vergognosi*), to cover beggars in general (*poveri mendicanti e vergognosi*).
2 A.S.V., Senato Terra, filza 90, 18 April 1584. The four hospitals named as *principalissimi bastioni* were the Derelitti, the Mendicanti, the Pietà and the Zitelle. Cf. Richard Palmer, 'L'assistenza medica nella Venezia cinquecentesca', in B. Aikema and D. Meijers, *Nel Regno dei Poveri. Arte e storia dei grandi ospedali veneziani* (Venice, 1989), pp. 35–42.
3 A.S.V., *Provveditori alla Sanità*, Reg. 2, folio 160, 28 March 1572.
4 A.S.V. *Provveditori alla Sanità*, Reg. 3, folios 92–93. This is a joint report of these Provveditori in March 1594. Cf. Pullan, *Rich and Poor*, p. 365.
5 Pio Paschini, *La Beneficenza in Italia e le 'Compagnie del Divino Amore'* (Rome, 1925).
6 Pullan, *Rich and Poor*, pp. 270–8, 328–9, 339. Cf. O.M.T. Logan 'The ideal of the bishop and the Venetian patriciate', *Journal of Ecclesiastical History*, vol. 29, 1978, pp. 415–450, and J.M. Headley and J.B. Tomaro, (eds) *San Carlo Borromeo* (Washington and London, 1988).
7 Giovanni Mantese, 'Il Card. Agostino Valier e l'origine delle Compagnie della Carità', *Archivio Veneto*, 5th series, vol. 90, 1972, pp. 5–26.
8 Brian Pullan, 'The Old Catholicism, the New Catholicism and the poor', in G. Politi, M. Rosa, F. Della Peruta (eds) *Timore e Carità. I Poveri nell' Italia moderna* (Cremona, 1982), pp. 13–25; Brian Pullan, "Support and redeem": charity and poor relief in Italian cities from the fourteenth to the seventeenth centuries', *Continuity and Change*, vol. 3, 1988, pp. 177–208.
9 *Origine, opere, leggi, et privilegi dell' Hospitale Grande di Bergamo* (Bergamo, 1580).
10 Vittorio Fainelli, *Storia degli ospedali di Verona* (Verona, 1962).
11 Udine, Seminario Arcivescovile, *Ospedale di S. Maria della Misericordia dei Battuti, Libro delle terminazioni 1483–1524*, folio 180r.
12 Ibid., *Libro delle terminazioni 1542–61*, folio 97v.
13 Ibid., folios 12r, 64v, 92v, 95v.
14 Ibid., especially folios 12–109, 1543–49. The petition quoted is at folios 108v–109r.
15 Ibid., folios 12–14. The extraordinary meeting was held on 26 March 1543. The bishop present is named only as '*Eligius episcopus*', with blank spaces in the text as if the secretary was uncertain of both his Christian name and his see.
16 Ibid., folio 16r.
17 Dulcia Meijers, 'L' architettura della nuova filantropia', in B. Aikema and D. Meijers, *Nel Regno dei Poveri*, pp. 43–69.
18 Archivio di Stato, Verona, *Santa Casa della Misericordia*, Reg. 8, folio 1, a decision of the Council of Twelve and Fifty, 18 April 1515.
19 Ibid., Reg. 1. A prelude to the statutes of the Misericordia, dating from the 1520s, includes an account of the foundation.
20 A.S.V., *Provveditori alla Sanità*, Reg. 2, folio 31r, 22 February 1521 m.v.
21 On S. Giacomo, see Alessandro Canezza, *Gli Arcispedali di Roma* (Rome, 1933), and Alessandra Cavaterra, 'L'ospedalità a Roma nell' età moderna: il caso di San Giacomo (1585–1605)', *Sanità, Scienza e Storia*, 1986, n. 2, pp. 87–123.

22 E.A. Cicogna, *Inscrizioni veneziane* (6 vols, Venice, 1824–53), vol. 5, pp. 305–09, brings together the diary entries relating to the Incurabili.
23 Marin Sanudo, *I diarii*, 58 vols (Venice, 1879–1903) vol. 1, cols. 233–4.
24 Palmer, 'L'assistenza medica', p. 40.
25 Archivio di Stato, Verona, Reg. 8, folio 2v. The *ducale* is dated 1 May 1520.
26 Ibid., Reg. 12, folio 23r., 5 February 1542.
27 Archivio di Stato, Verona, *Istituto Esposti*, Reg. 70, folio 59r, 21 October 1580. A much fuller interpretation is given in the statutes of 1633, *Capitoli et ordeni . . . delle venerabili case di Santa Misericordia e Santissima Trinità di Verona . . . MDCXXXIII* (Verona, 1669).
28 Archivio di Stato, Brescia, *Ospedale delle Donne (ex-Ospedale degli Incurabili)*, *Annali dell' Ospedale degli Incurabili*, vol. 1, pp. 16–18. A decision of the Ospedale Maggiore dated 11 January 1548, confirmed by the Consiglio Generale of the Incurabili 8 July 1548.
29 Archivio di Stato, Padua, *Ospedale di S. Francesco. Acta, 1553–1584*, folio 191v, 19 April 1582. Provision was made for 24 men and 24 women per annum, selected by lot.
30 Archivio di Stato, Verona, *Pia Opera di Carità*, Reg. 359, decisions of the Veronese Council of Twelve and Fifty, and *ducali* relating to the Carità.
31 Pullan, *Rich and Poor*, p. 373.
32 Archivio di Stato, Verona, *Istituto Esposti*, Reg. 70, folio 230r. An agreement by the Santa Casa di Pietà to supply medicines to the Compagnia della Carità for the emergency, 20 August 1581.
33 Ibid., *Pia Opera di Carità*, Reg. 359, folio 6r, 11 May 1539.
34 Giovanni Mantese, 'Il Card.', prints in an appendix the Statutes of the Compagnia della Carità of Vicenza of 1569.
35 A.S.V., *Fraterne Poveri, S. Canzian*, busta 9, Statutes dated 1 May 1577.
36 Ibid., *Fraterne Poveri, SS. Apostoli*, busta 1, folios 1–6, the Statutes of 1563.
37 On the Schools of Christian Doctrine, see Paul F. Grendler, 'Borromeo and the Schools of Christian Doctrine', in J.M. Headley and J.B. Tomaro, *San Carlo Borromeo*, pp. 158–71.
38 *Origine, opere, leggi*, (note 9). Published in 1580, this preserves the Hospital's Statutes of 1572.
39 Archivio di Stato, Verona, *Santa Casa della Misericordia*, Reg. 12, folio 1.
40 Alessandro Canobbio, *Discorso ai magnifici S. Presidenti della Carità di Verona, nel quale si dimostra l'importanza del provedere a' poveri mendicanti* (Padua, 1572); *Ordini e capitoli delli Derelitti instituito nella magnifica citta di Verona l'anno 1572* (Verona, 1573); Alessandro Canobbio, *Ordini con i quali si e introdotta nella città di Verona la santissima opera de Mendicanti* (Verona, 1590).
41 Venice, Archivio I.R.E., *Derelitti, Libro di Parti 1546–1604*, folio 51, 12 Feb. 1569 m.v.
42 Archivio di Stato, Verona, Santa Casa di Misericordia, Reg. 12, folio 42r.
43 Archivio di Stato, Brescia, *Ospedale Maggiore, Provvigioni*, Registri 12–15, 1576–1608. Decisions to alienate property were taken in 1584, 1586, 1587, 1588, 1589, 1590, 1592, 1598.

44 Udine, Seminario Arcivescovile, *Ospedale di S. Maria della Misericordia dei Battuti, Libro delle terminazioni 1542–61,* folios 17r, 33r, and *Libro delle terminazioni 1561–76*, folios 37v, 39v, 60r. The priest concerned was Giovanni Maria Savelli.

45 Venice, Archivio I.R.E., *Derelitti, Libro di parti 1546–1604*, folios 80r, 84r.

46 Archivio di Stato, Verona, *Ospedale di SS. Jacopo e Lazzaro alla Tomba*, Reg. 1490 (admissions and discharges, 1594), Anzola della Misericordia, admitted 25 Dec. 1594.

47 The Statutes of 1570 are in Venice, *Archivio IRE, Derelitti, Libro di parti 1546–1604*, folios 51v–52r, 12 Feb. 1569 m.v. The second version (undated, *circa* 1600) is in A. S. V., *Ospedali e luoghi pii diversi* , busta 910. The third, dated 1667, is substantially published in Istituto di Ricovero e di Educazione, *Arte e musica all' Ospedaletto* (Venice, 1978), pp. 141–53.

48 A.S.V., *Provveditori alla Sanità*, Reg. 738, folio 32r.

6

'A FOUNTAIN FOR THE THIRSTY' AND A BANK FOR THE POPE: CHARITY, CONFLICTS, AND MEDICAL CAREERS AT THE HOSPITAL OF SANTO SPIRITO IN SEVENTEENTH-CENTURY ROME

Silvia De Renzi

According to the 'confessionalisation thesis', strategies for imposing religious and social discipline are one of the most important changes in the making of Early-Modern European states, and one which cuts across confessional boundaries.[1] In Catholic countries, the Council of Trent was a watershed in this process and the Counter-Reformation can be defined as an ideological re-conquest involving the imposition of religious conformity as well as the reassertion of a social hierarchy. By focusing on the policy of coercion and control implemented by the state and by a state-controlled church, the confessionalisation thesis has emphasised the existence of a gap between the elite and popular culture and promoted a two-tier model of Early Modern society. Recently, the process of confessionalisation has been questioned, at least with regard to specific areas of the Catholic countries, and the need for a more flexible model has become clear.[2] Investigations have highlighted strategies of accommodation and compromise adopted by the Church towards popular devotion. The investment of unorthodox behaviour with accepted meanings was a much more common Church strategy than had previously been recognised. Moreover, in the lower strata of the clergy, the priests themselves often shared with their parishioners a relationship with the sacred which the higher hierarchy considered with suspicion. What was most often at stake in the clash of these different views was control over access to the sacred and over the boundaries between the natural, the supernatural and the diabolic. One of the areas where this issue had the strongest implications was healing. Recent research has made it clear that medicine in the Early Modern period was a pluralistic system, where various techniques and practitioners were available to different patients, not necessarily according to their social position.[3] Official medicine had a flexible strategy towards unofficial forms of healing; often, as long as a proper patent was issued and the boundaries of what was permitted were respected, midwives, barbers and even charlatans could carry out their activities.

The need for a more dynamic model of the relations between elite and popular culture, however, should not lead us to overlook the polarity between the powerful and the powerless that emerges from the sources, and the fact that conflicts did arise in the society of the ancient regime.[4] Healing techniques and the competence of practitioners remained controversial issues both for the Church and official medicine. Contempt for popular methods of healing like magic rituals, invocations, or the use of special herbs could turn into suspicion. Wise-women using herbs and rituals to cure, or snake handlers treating viper bites might be highly regarded among peasants, but they were also liable to inquisitorial investigation. As the historian Adriano Prosperi has recently shown, in Italy the Inquisition and episcopal courts were no less influential actors than the often complacent priests. While in the second half of the sixteenth century, the Roman Inquisition and a new emphasis on the sacrament of confession were used in the battle against the spread of heresy, later, as the danger of heresy subsided, they became the tools of a more specific control over morality and unorthodox forms of popular culture.[5] Simultaneously, sophisticated use of propaganda promoted a paternalistic model of society, which was based on the submissiveness and obedience of the lower social strata. In their writings and orations, theologians and preachers insisted on the enormous cultural differences between the learned and the vulgar, the rich and the poor, the city and the country.[6] The features of a political and cultural project emerge clearly from this literature. In this framework, policies of assistance and poor relief were one of the most important tools which civic and religious authorities developed to guarantee the social order while responding to new models of devotion.

In this chapter I intend to use some of the features of the Counter-

Reformation which I have outlined so far to examine some documents relating to the activities of the Hospital of Santo Spirito, which was one of the most important institutions for the care of the poor in seventeenth-century Rome. Rome stands out among other political entities in seventeenth-century Italy both for its political situation and for its extraordinarily rich network of charitable institutions. The Papal state was a unique example of a power which was both religious and secular, where the political elite overlapped almost entirely with the ecclesiastical hierarchy. Rome had long before lost its municipal identity and lacked the active urban elite which characterised other Italian cities. Though some independent administrative bodies and tribunals still had rights and jurisdiction over civic matters, the Papacy gradually increased its strict control over them.[7] Moreover, important and consistent reforms of the organisation of the state were introduced between the end of the sixteenth and the beginning of the seventeenth century as part of a dynamic politics of asserting the power of the Counter-Reformation church. New fiscal and criminal legislation led to an increasing presence of the State in spheres of social life which had traditionally been independent of the central political power. In this context, legislation concerning poor relief proved to be particularly useful both to reinforce the social order and to promote the new image of the triumphant Catholic Church.[8]

A key feature of poor relief was the medical assistance provided in hospitals.[9] The Hospital of Santo Spirito (see Figures 6.1, 6.2 and 6.3) was one of the oldest hospitals of the city and did not suffer from the oscillation of funds which affected other institutions for the relief of the poor. It had been established for the care of the sick and of abandoned children by Pope Innocenzo III in the twelth century, and since then had been run by the Order of the Santo Spirito. A network of hospitals run by the same order had quickly spread all over Europe as branches of the main centre in Rome. Subsequently, various Popes reinforced the fiscal privileges of the Hospital and helped it increase its power as a landowner. As a consequence, the hospital became one of the richest feudatories in the Papal state. The existence of a special link between the Order and the Pope is confirmed by the fact that he appointed its head (Commendatore) directly.[10] Its prominence makes the Santo Spirito an especially appealing case for which to unravel the ways in which the various actors in medical assistance – physicians, surgeons, governors of the hospital, as well as the recipients of the charity – related to it.[11] I shall argue that if medical practice was one of the most important terrains in the policy of poor assistance and at

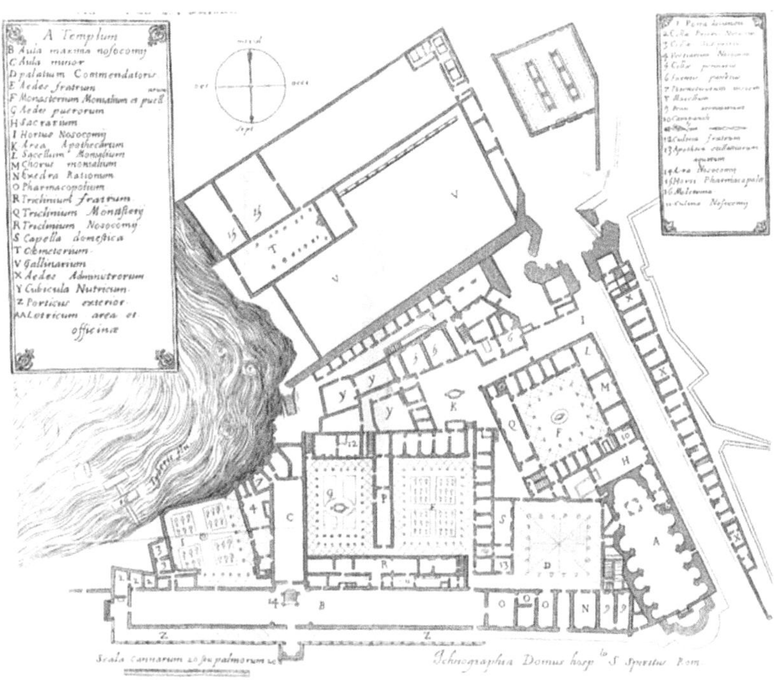

Figure 6.1 Hospital of Santo Spirito, Rome: plan. This, like all the following pictures of the Hospital of Santo Spirito, is taken from P. Saulnier, *De Capite Sacri Ordinis Sancti Spiritus Dissertatio*, Lyons; G. Barbier 1649
Source: Reproduced by permission of Wellcome Institute Library, London

the same time a highly controversial field in the relations between elite and popular culture, then a hospital offers an exceptionally powerful view of how the different perspectives of such actors intersected and sometimes clashed.[12]

I shall start by focusing on physicians, looking in the first section at the Hospital as an extremely active medical institution whose therapeutic and teaching function had expanded in the course of the sixteenth century. The hospital's strong links with the University and the papal court made it a key place in the making of a physician's career. Counter-Reformation Rome, with its huge court, hundreds of noble households and cardinals' families, as well as its network of charitable institutions, offered doctors excellent opportunities. By briefly analysing the cases of four eminent physicians, I shall show in the second section how their work at the Santo Spirito integrated with, and contributed to, other aspects of their careers.

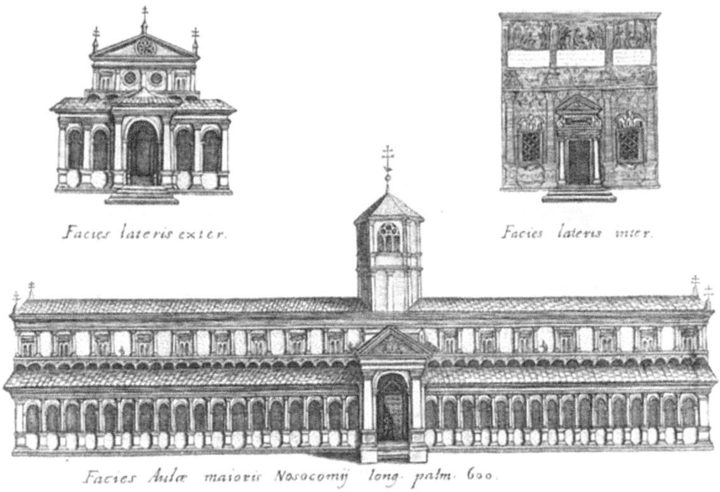

Figure 6.2 Hospital of Santo Spirito, Rome: elevation
Source: Reproduced by permission of Wellcome Institute Library, London

Although a special, separate ward was reserved for the nobility, the hospital was primarily intended to serve the poor. In the history of the Order of the Santo Spirito which Peter Saulnier published in 1649, he described the emblem of the centuries-old Order as a fountain which gathers water from various sources and showers it on to the 'thirsty poor of all ages'.[13] Research into the records of admission to institutions which mainly provided assistance to the poor has shown that the major recipients of care were members of artisans' families.[14] However, access to hospitals providing medical care was probably wider and, in a city like Rome, included beggars and people from the country. Given this variety of patients, the role played by hospitals in the pluralistic system of Early Modern medicine deserves further study. For instance more investigation is needed of the relations between the sets of practices and conventions of various groups active in a hospital – university-trained physicians, surgeons, apothecaries, members of confraternities, patients. In the third section, I shall discuss the case of a peasant who was admitted to the hospital and whose medical practice differed from, and somehow clashed with that carried out by the physicians. This will lead me briefly to highlight the issue of the production and circulation of drugs in institutions of medical care. While making certain types of expensive remedies available to the poor, hospitals became important

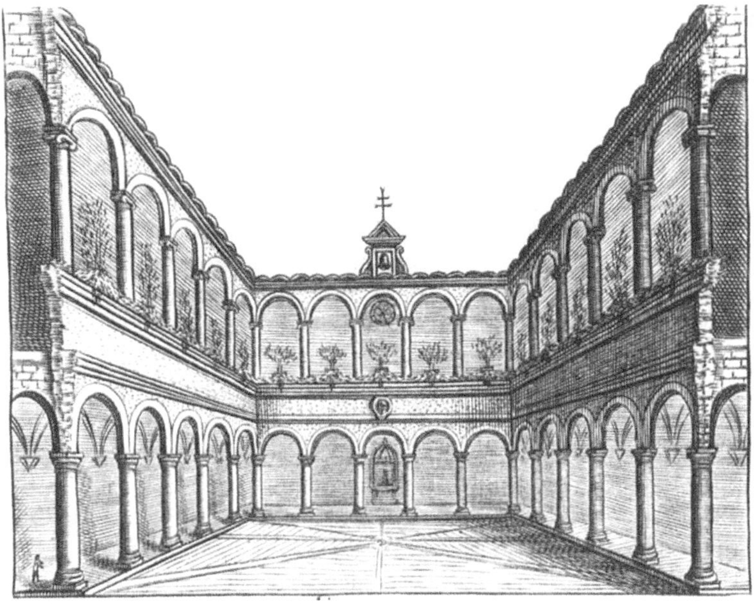

Figure 6.3 Hospital of Santo Spirito, Rome: the cloisters/courtyard
Source: Reproduced by permission of Wellcome Institute Library, London

actors in the business of producing and consuming drugs. Finally, in the last section I shall contrast two different ways in which the wealth of the Santo Spirito was used. I shall comment on the tricks which women devised to cheat the system of wetnurses arranged by the hospital; and I shall focus on the Santo Spirito as a fundamental source of papal finance. The foundation of a bank which used the enormous land properties of the Hospital as a guarantee to cover the budget deficit of the Papal state is also a part of its history.

Medical teaching and dissections at the Santo Spirito

The long commentary on the American fauna which the German physician Johannes Faber wrote for a book produced by the Accademia dei Lincei is a very rich, unusual and quite unexploited source for the history of medical activities in seventeenth-century Rome. Describing a specimen of an American bull, for instance, he recalls the huge number of oxen and buffaloes which were bred in the estates of the Hospital of Santo Spirito in order to supply food for the children and sick people of whom it took care. Faber remembers that in 1600, when he started his five-year training at the Hospital, more than 12,000 sick people received shelter, food and medication.[15] During his training, he learnt to dissect corpses; indeed, he writes repeatedly of the hundreds of bodies which he and his colleagues cut up together.[16] The profile of Roman medical teaching was in this period extremely high: students and young physicians would go to Rome to finish their medical education. The presence of Andrea Cesalpino, who was appointed in 1592 to teach *medicina pratica* at the Sapienza, certainly helped to increase the prestige of the teaching. Anatomical investigations had been flourishing since the 1540s and 1550s, with the teaching of Realdo Colombo and Bartolomeo Eustachi.[17] Public dissections were regularly performed not only at the Sapienza, but also in various hospitals of the city, like S. Maria della Consolazione and S. Giacomo. What emerges from Faber's remarks, however, is that anatomies were carried out at the Santo Spirito not just as ritual public events, but also as post mortems, and that this happened on a fairly regular basis.[18] This is an interesting addition to the fact that the Santo Spirito had a high reputation for medical training. Apart from Faber's testimony, we find confirmation of this in two other seventeenth-century sources, to which I shall be referring at length. One is the extraordinarily detailed description of the Hospital which the secretary of the Order of the Santo Spirito, Domenico Borgarucci, wrote in 1623.[19] It was the basis for Peter Saulnier's celebratory book on the Order, which I mentioned above, and is the second source to which I shall refer.[20]

Borgarucci recalls the very efficient rota which was established to guarantee assistance to the patients day and night. Seventy-two men, including laymen and members of the Order, were normally employed under the supervision of a prior and a sub-prior. Around twenty-four of them were young people who wanted to learn surgery; they had established a school (Accademia) within the Hospital and paid a surgery professor to teach them. This training led to a special licence; and the Pope himself, cardinals and Roman noblemen often took advantage of the expertise of those who had attended the Accademia at the Santo Spirito. Along with the surgeons, the hospital employed four principal physicians, each of whom had an assistant, a young doctor who wanted to learn medical practice.[21] This training too had a high reputation and, according to Borgarucci, allowed young physicians easily to find a job in the household of a Cardinal or of a powerful prince: to attend the lectures at the Santo Spirito put one on the road to a successful career.

What was this training like? From Saulnier we know that twice a week one of the four doctors and two surgeons had to lecture not just on the elements and foundations of medicine, but also on its secrets and, as it were, its tricks. His task was to train the young people of the hospital not only in the precepts which they found in their handbooks, but also by displaying things. For this reason, during winter time in the specially arranged theatre, he would describe the structure of the human body and display this marvellous thing 'by the art of anatomical dissection'.[22] If these anatomies were a good opportunity to learn the structure of the human body, the 'tricks' of the art were more likely taught during the daily rounds in the hospital. The Santo Spirito did not accept incurable patients; the most common diseases treated there were various types of fever and wounds. Twice a day, each doctor, accompanied by his assistant, by the person responsible for the care of the patients and by the assistant apothecary, would visit one of the four wards of the hospital, each of which had beds for twenty-five patients. He inspected and palpated the patients, questioned them about their symptoms, asked the assistant about the case, and looked for the signs which the *ars medica* would suggest.[23] Then he would scrutinise the blood which, after every blood-letting, was kept in a special niche near the bed, and he would prescribe the treatments (Figure 6.4).[24] Diets were noted in a special code on a little board at the head of the bed.

What emerges from this description is that at the Santo Spirito young doctors received a kind of bedside teaching, which was probably very similar to the practical teaching of the Hospital of S. Francesco in Padua.[25] Both Saulnier and Borgarucci regarded this highly organised system of teaching as evidence of the great concern the hospital had for its patients. The best physicians were available to them; even Papal doctors were employed to heal the poor: the charitable functions of the hospital were greatly enhanced by its good reputation as a medical institution.

But who were the doctors whom the Santo Spirito employed and how were they recruited?

Medical careers at the Santo Spirito

Between 1574 and 1664 seven of the twenty-one physicians of the Hospital were also professors at the Sapienza, while seven were

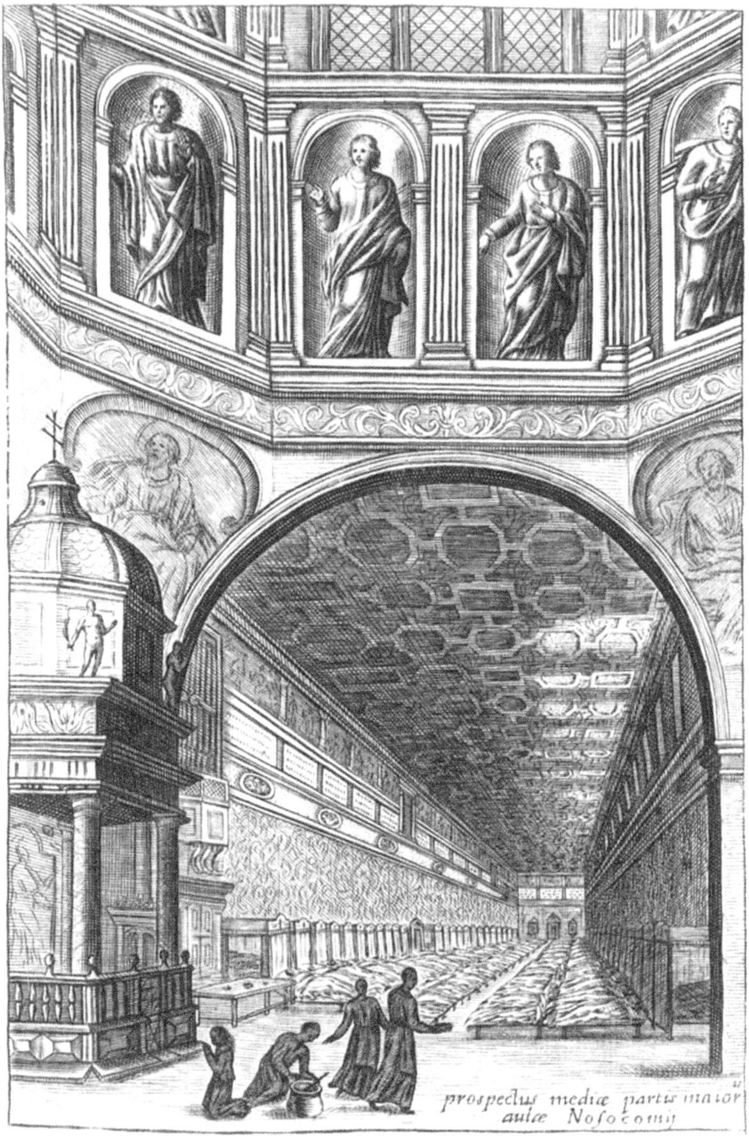

Figure 6.4 One of the four wards of the Santo Spirito
Source: Reproduced by permission of Wellcome Institute Library, London

registered in the payroll of the Hospital as '*scrittori*', which means that they had published some kind of medical work. We know that in 1595 the annual salary of the doctors was 100 scudi and that it did not increase much in the following century. Although the physicians could add bread, wine and barley produced in the Hospital's estate – and this could be equivalent to another 36 scudi – their remuneration remained low.[26] However, Saulnier claims, neither this nor the fact that dissections could be risky prevented the doctors from greatly enjoying their work and from actively looking for patronage in order to obtain a post there.[27]

To get a position at the Santo Spirito, physicians had to pass an exam, which was advertised both in and outside Rome.[28] According to Borgarucci, the fact that recruitment was on a non-local basis was among the clearest signs of the concern that the Hospital had for its patients. This rule was possibly designed to counter-balance the predominant system of patronage. To understand what induced physicians to apply to the Santo Spirito and what it meant for them to work there, I will briefly look at the careers of four physicians who were on the payroll at different periods during the seventeenth century: Giulio Mancini, Antonio Luciani, Giovanni Trullio and Paolo Zacchia.

Giulio Mancini was born in Siena of humble origins and studied medicine in Padua.[29] An extraordinary figure as a learned physician in Baroque Rome, he is now better known for his activities as an art collector and connoisseur. However, contemporaries praised him highly for his unbelievable skill in making quick prognoses of sick people just by looking at them. This was probably the basis on which, against heavy competition, he obtained a job at the Santo Spirito in 1595. Beyond being renowned for his interest in the highly controversial field of astrology and for his shaky faith, Mancini was also an expert in chemical investigations.[30] At the Santo Spirito, he became friends with the Commendatore of the Order of the Santo Spirito, Pietro Campori, who in 1616 was nominated Cardinal. His friendship probably greatly helped Mancini obtain the most prestigious position for a doctor in Rome, that of physician to the Pope, in 1623.[31] At this point he stopped work at the hospital and involved himself in the lively intellectual and social life at the court of the Barberini. We know that he took part in some controversial medical and philosophical discussions held at court.[32] Among his unpublished works, one offers a rational explanation of the ability of some people to forecast the future, while another is a defence of a woman charged with witchcraft. Mancini also maintained a public role, since in 1629 he was one of the three physicians appointed members of the Congregazione di sanità, which had been established by the Pope to co-ordinate action against the risk of a plague epidemic.[33]

Compared to Mancini, Marcantonio Luciani seems a colourless figure in the intellectual scene of Counter-Reformation Rome: as far as we know, he neither left intriguing manuscripts, nor was he a brilliant courtier. And yet he built for himself a successful career in the medical world of the city, holding some of its key positions at a time when the campaign for control over medical activities was particularly fierce. After his training at the Santo Spirito, he worked there for almost thirty years, but he also taught *medicina theorica* at the Sapienza. He was appointed Protomedico, that is the main authority of the College of Physicians, in 1625, when lively discussions about the drugs which should be listed in the *Antidotario romano* (the list of remedies used by Roman physicians) were taking place.[34] Related hot issues were the control over apothecaries, which the Protomedico had the right to visit on a regular basis, destroying drugs which he considered bad, and the fight against charlatans and all sorts of unauthorised drug sellers. In the same period, new rules to exert strict control over midwives were established.[35] Thus, for Luciani to work at the Santo Spirito was just a part of a very busy career, which included vigorous action in negotiating control over the available forms of healing.

In the case of Giovanni Trullio, a more specific connection with the care of the poor is apparent. Trullio had a valuable knack for treating kidney stones, and he was required to work in the infirmary of the Papal Palace. In 1636, Pope Urban VIII established a special fund to pay him, provided he remained in Rome and worked for 'public utility and benefit'. Thus, he started his surgical teaching at the Sapienza, but agreed also to treat the poor for free, and we know that he successfully cured a prostitute, called Brigida, who had a bad wound in her throat.[36] It was not until nine years later, however, that he became surgeon at the Santo Spirito: presumably he had previously offered his services to the poor in some other institutions or at home.[37] However, the appointment at the Santo Spirito was not at all a setback in his career. Trullio continued to be regarded as an outstanding surgeon and remained a member of the household of the *Cardinal Nipote* Francesco Barberini.[38] He specialised in dissecting and embalming rich and famous people – he embalmed Pope Urban VIII. There is evidence that he performed countless post mortems during the 1650s. Patients of the Santo Spirito offered him the opportunity to make medical observations, which were subsequently published.[39]

The work and career of Paolo Zacchia, the last doctor I shall look at, casts light on the growing authority of physicians in seventeenth-century Rome. In the 1630s he was Protomedico and in 1644 he became physician to the Pope Innocenzo X. We know from *Quaestiones medico-legales* that throughout his life Zacchia was consultant to the Tribunal of the Sacra Rota, a court the power of which had been expanded and strengthened after the Council of Trent. The cases debated by this court were published and clearly reveal that physicians were regularly appointed as expert witnesses.[40] It comes as no surprise to find that for more than ten years between 1648 and 1659 Zacchia worked at the Santo Spirito, which at this point we can regard both as an efficient stepping stone to, and as complementing, the careers of ambitious doctors.

We still lack both analytical investigations into, and synthetic accounts of, medical practice in seventeenth-century Rome. However, the cases of these four physicians show that boundaries between various sites of medical practice – noble households and the Papal court, hospitals, urban or state offices in public health policy – were very fluid. Physicians took full advantage of the process of centralising political power. They could complement their private medical practice with appointments in the public health system in periods of crisis, for example during epidemics. During more normal times, they reasserted the dominance of official medicine over other ways of healing through the activities of the College of Physicians. Finally, in the tribunals, they helped the papacy re-exert a strong grip on society, while strengthening their intellectual prestige and social authority. Far from being mutually exclusive, these tasks complemented each other in the construction of a physician's career. In such a network of sites and activities, offering medical assistance to the poor at the Santo Spirito did not ruin the respectability of a physician. On the contrary, thanks to the close links between the Santo Spirito and the Papacy, and to the high reputation of the medical training offered at the Hospital, the Santo Spirito was a good place for physicians to network, while offering wonderful opportunities to develop professional skills. Contemporary sources emphasised both the fierce competition for a position at the Santo Spirito, and the permeability of the hospital's borders. While surgeons and physicians trained at the Santo Spirito would easily find jobs in noble households, patients, regardless of their social position, would resort to the highly-regarded care provided at the hospital. At the same time, in stressing the long-standing and special links between the Order of the Santo Spirito and the Papacy, these authors recalled that the Commendatore of the Order was appointed directly by the Pope and chosen from the highest ranks of the ecclesiastical elite.[41] The chapter which Saulnier dedicates to praising the

Commendatori allows one to follow the progress of ecclesiastical careers. The prestige connected to the position of Commendatore could facilitate the move to higher positions. Between 1554 and 1616 three Commendatori of the Santo Spirito were nominated cardinals; more often a Commendatore would leave the Order after being appointed bishop, and it was not unusual for the Commendatore to have been head of another order and moved to the Order of the Santo Spirito before becoming Bishop.[42]

Thus, the fact that only in the case of Trullio do charitable motives seem quite clear, should not be surprising. Reasons to apply for a job at the Santo Spirito could be various: a somewhat difficult-to-detect religious and moral commitment, and the more evident search for a prestigious position were interwoven.

Drugs for the poor at the Santo Spirito

The biographical sketches I have provided above are a first attempt at exploring the uses of the Santo Spirito in its doctors' careers. By now turning again to the everyday organisation of the hospital, I aim to view it as a place where different perspectives on medical assistance and poor relief could meet and sometimes clash. By different perspectives, I mean on the one hand, the charitable projects which the establishment of the hospital, including the doctors, aimed at implementing, and the medical culture which shaped their activities; and on the other, the attitude towards this institution of the recipients of charity, who obviously went to the hospital with their own 'medical' experience and social views.

One matter which could easily become controversial was the treatment. According to Borgarucci, patients, regardless of their social status, could get the most expensive and precious drugs which the doctor prescribed.[43] Rome had a very rich network of apothecaries. And contemporary medical and pharmaceutical treatises throw light on the up-to-date treatments, including chemical drugs, available at its hospitals.[44] The apothecary of the Santo Spirito was certainly among the most famous and best supplied.[45] The chief apothecary, helped by five or more assistants, carried out an intense activity of distillation from plants and flowers.[46] In seventeenth-century Rome, distillation of drugs both from plants and metals, had become a fashionable pastime among the elite.[47] But, as I mentioned above when referring to the activities of the Protomedicato, the production and sale of drugs had increasingly become a matter of conflicts between physicians, apothecaries and charlatans.[48] I shall use one of the cases which involved

Faber during his training at the Santo Spirito to examine how different medical cultures and ways of healing could meet in a hospital.

At the end of June 1603, Faber wrote, a peasant was sent to the Santo Spirito after his hand had been bitten by a viper. Terrified, he had sucked his finger, with the result that his lips and tongue had swollen enormously. Then he had drunk an antidote which, Faber reported, was called Orvietanus after the charlatan who produced and sold it. According to Faber this antidote was 'very common among the people, much less effective than true theriaca, and for this reason much cheaper'.[49] The condition of the man was very bad, and Faber, concerned about his soul no less than about his body, ordered him to be confessed by a priest.[50] The medical image used by Faber to mean the purification of the soul through the expulsion of poisonous sins derives from the growing literature on confession, which was at that time a condition for admission to the hospital.[51] Then Faber prescribed the following treatment: a potion made by a dose of theriaca, a preparation of deer horn and a particular kind of water to be poured into the man's throat by a special silver cannula; lips, palate and chest to be constantly smeared with two different ointments made of theriaca. Meanwhile, the veins of his hand were incised, and later an ointment made of oil of scorpion, theriaca, vinegar, white of egg and bolo Armeniae was spread on hands and arms. By the end of the following day, after a blood letting, the peasant was in such good health that he could leave the hospital. Commenting on this episode, Faber proudly told the reader that he also possessed the recipe of a very good drug based on viper meat, which the famous cardinal Francesco Dal Monte gave him. It could be used, Faber added, not just by physicians who took care of the simple folk, but also by those who were in charge of the health of Princes.[52] Indeed, although its recipe was a secret, the Cardinal used to distribute the remedy free to both the rich and the poor. Clearly, Faber aimed to contrast Orvietanus, a cheap and nasty drug which country people bought at the market or prepared themselves, with better tested and official drugs with which generous noblemen and caring physicians could provide all the sick, regardless of their social condition. However, one can make sense of what Faber presented as disinterested care in a completely different way. In the first decades of the seventeenth century, Orvietanus was one of the most popular antidotes, based on a great number of herbs, and widely imitated.[53] Its recipe was jealously-kept secret for commercial reasons by its producers, charlatans who would sell it on market squares or at their shops. But it was the antidote of the poor. As Faber must have known very well, in 1613 the Protomedicato in Rome had licensed Gregorio Ferrante to sell Orvietanus in the city. Gregorio was the son of Girolamo Ferrante, a Neapolitan charlatan who may have invented the remedy and, for some reason, used the name of Orvietan (native of Orvieto). Apparently, provided a licence had been issued, Orvietanus was accepted by the medical authorities. And yet, controversies must have arisen, since more than once in the first half of the century the Protomedicato had to reinforce its strict regulation.[54] As is clear from Faber's remarks, Orvietanus was considered at best a completely useless drug, to be replaced by proper substances, which had been sanctioned by expert practitioners, though not necessarily physicians. Hospitals were appropriate places to carry out a campaign in which the boundaries between controls over popular remedies and their eradication were fluid. The episode reported by Faber provokes further reflections on the relationships between schemes of medical assistance and poor relief and the social implications of the preparation and consumption of drugs. Although practitioners of popular medicine often developed a scornful attitude towards the official medical establishment, one of the main reasons for the existence of a differentiated drug market was the price of the remedies.[55] Certain drugs were simply not available to a large majority of patients. How did this relate to the provision of medical care and what was the role of hospitals in this framework? While further research is needed on this issue, I would like to discuss a few cases which may throw some light on it.

Borgarucci stresses the generosity of the Santo Spirito in preparing and distributing expensive drugs, including precious stones, to all its patients, regardless of their social condition. The provision of drugs through hospitals was carried out in a variety of ways, including, for instance, appeals to the poor to go to the Hospital of San Giacomo for the distribution of the holy wood, which were hung in churches all over the city. People answered them, and apparently crowds gathered regularly in front of the Hospital's doors.[56] The holy wood (Guaiacum) became an extremely popular remedy and its provision one of the greatest expenses of the Hospital. The steady increase in the use of new substances and the replacement of older, more dangerous, but probably less expensive remedies like mercury, is part of the history of the commercialisation of the European economy.[57] It is well known that the Fugger family, the most powerful German banking-house, had a stake in the distribution of Guaiacum, since it had a monopoly on its trade to Europe.[58] Certainly this big business found an ally in the well-organised system for the diffusion of the drug among the poor and the incurable arranged at the S. Giacomo. In Rome, the Hospital had a monopoly on the holy wood, and other apothecaries of the city were supposed to obtain a special licence to sell it.[59] A similar case is that of the Peruvian bark (Cinchona spp.) against fevers, the distribution of which remained firmly in the hands of the Jesuits and their apothecaries.[60] Controversies about the efficacy and modes of use of the substance – wider or limited to specific types of fevers – were common, while resistance to the drug came both from the advocates of traditional treatments and the persistent diffusion of popular remedies. Links between medicine and economics in the spread of the powdered bark are apparent. While contemporary Catholic sources reported the generosity of the Jesuits in providing the powder to the poor without charge, other sources stressed that the Jesuits made huge profits by selling it at excessively high prices.[61] The economic implications of the distribution of the bark are proved even on a small-scale by the existence of an unofficial market: its free provision to poor patients was conditional on a statement of their illness and a promise not to sell the powder. And we know that other apothecaries complained about the increasing favour of the Jesuit apothecaries with their lay clientele. In this framework, the diffusion of the powder in hospitals, like the Santo Spirito in Rome or Pammatone in Genoa, were episodes of a well-orchestrated campaign.[62] Especially when the Jesuit Cardinal De Lugo was its director, the apothecary of the Santo Spirito became the main centre for the import, working and distribution of the bark. In addition, in Rome the Jesuits founded a special apothecary for shame-faced families. It was run by the Confraternity of the Twelve Apostoles and enjoyed the patronage of the *Cardinal Nipote* Francesco Barberini. Provided a person had a certificate of poverty from the parish priest and a prescription from a doctor, he or she could get drugs while avoiding the shame of a public hospice.[63] We know that Cardinal Barberini was very keen on having a well-equipped apothecary's dispensary, and we can assume that the new remedy introduced and marketed by the Jesuits was widely prescribed there.[64] In this framework of fierce competition for the monopoly of the production and sale of drugs, the provision of medical assistance to the poor can acquire a new meaning. If an efficient system was arranged, profit and generosity could go hand in hand. However, things could be more problematic. When the expense of providing free drugs to the poor became too high, as in Turin in the middle of the century, one of the exhortations made by the city to the doctors of the poor was to limit prescriptions to very urgent cases and to avoid expensive medicines.[65] On the other hand, officers of the Protomedicato of Bologna usually sent the bad drugs which they confiscated in the dispensaries of apothecaries to hospitals.[66] The way in which the economics and culture of medical practice intersected with, and affected, schemes of poor relief is particularly evident in times of emergency, such as during epidemics. During the plague of 1656, for instance, one of the commonest preservatives used by monks, priests and physicians in the *lazzaretti* in Rome was a very cheap toad-powder. Debates about its efficacy were very lively, but there was general agreement on the fact that it was a very cheap preservative, much more affordable than the incredibly expensive amulets made of precious stones, which were very popular among wealthy people.[67] Clearly, the drug market was highly differentiated, and along with other criteria, costs of drugs affected the range of choices of patients, physicians and governors.

Greedy women and the Papal finances

The request that the poor be proved sick and promise not to sell the powdered bark they received free bears witness to the widespread fear among governors of hospitals of being cheated by people faking illness. This case allows us to look at the different ways in which donors and recipients of charity related to it. Let us briefly consider another case where such contrasts were even clearer: the care of foundlings for which the Santo Spirito was so renowned. In his account, Saulnier wrote that the increasing number of children who were abandoned in the revolving box of the Hospital could not just be the fruits of illegitimate love; bad economic or health conditions, wrote Saulnier, often obliged God-fearing families to abandon their children. The distinction between deserving and undeserving children was a highly debated issue, and Saulnier thought that it was better to take care of the undeserving than to neglect the deserving ones.[68] What, however, the establishment of the Hospital considered unbearable were the tricks which women got up to in order to cheat the Hospital into taking care of their own children after they had abandoned them. While some of the children were kept in a special building inside the main area of the Hospital and fed by the fifteen wetnurses who lived there, many others were assigned to wetnurses outside the Hospital.[69] These were women who had just given birth. Before they received a baby to take care of, the Hospital would examine them by asking when their own baby had been born, if it was a boy or a girl, and whether he or she was alive or dead. All these questions aimed to prevent women 'blinded by greed', as Borgarucci put it, getting a salary from the Hospital for taking care of their own children, and thus damaging its finances.[70] Thus if a woman had had a boy, she would get a female baby to feed and vice versa. Furthermore, to avoid the replacement of a foundling who died by a child of the wetnurse, all the abandoned children were branded with ink put in a cut in their feet.[71] In Borgarucci's definition of these women as 'greedy' we find an echo of the image of the 'bad' poor which had already supplemented the more traditional notion of the poor of Christ. Usually, moralistic condemnations targeted the cunning of beggars who were able to feign all sorts of sickness to get alms. This time, however, the trick seems a cleverly devised strategy to take full advantage of a system of charity certainly not by desperate beggars – who could never apply for a job as wetnurses. Rather, we have to think of that big category of the families of artisans and peasants, whose means were constantly going above and below the level of subsistence. The care of abandoned children was, along with the distribution of dowries to poor women, one of the typical features of poor relief in the Early Modern period. Recent research has unravelled how strategies of distributing dowries and allocating foundlings to wetnurses fit into local economic and political networks.[72] Before being a matter of individual choice, charity responded to social models and rules. As E. Grendi has aptly put it, donors and receivers of charity shared a 'culture', a 'knowledge' of assistance: in a process of acculturation, people learnt how to conform to, and take advantage of, the system of charity.[73] This approach is very fruitful. However, the emphasis on the shared culture should not lead us to overlook those cases in which the recipients of charity appeared to break, or twist the rules. A source like Borgarucci's account involuntarily gives us a glimpse of such breaks. Sometimes they became open resistance, as in the case of the rebellion which broke out among the young women and the nuns of the Santo Spirito against the new policy implemented by the Commendatore Francesco Maria Febei in the 1670s.[74] But the cruel, preventive strategy of branding the babies and Borgarucci's moral censure of the women, have already shown that donors and recipients of charity sometimes had different views on what the latter should be allowed to obtain.

In discussing the fountain emblem, Saulnier represented the Popes as one of the major sources of the Hospital's wealth. So far, I have looked at the Santo Spirito as a medical and charitable organisation. I will conclude by focusing briefly on the other essential function which it acquired when in 1605 it became one of the Pope's most efficient financial tools. For my purposes here, it will be enough to recall briefly that after the Council of Trent the debit balance of the Papal State increased. While a variety of systems of borrowing, including venal offices and bond issues were devised, the problem of liquidity was never solved.[75] At the beginning of the seventeenth century even the finances of the Santo Spirito started to collapse. Though it was still one of the biggest estate owners in the State of the Church, due to a general reduction of income and probably to some irregularities in its management, the Hospital was in dire straits.[76] In 1605, Pope Paul V and the Commendatore of the Santo Spirito, Ottavio Tassoni, agreed to found a bank which would collect money from private creditors, using the countless properties of the Hospital as guarantee. According to the official documents the primary aim of this bank was to help small depositors avoid investing their money with unscrupulous bankers.[77] Behind this more charitable reason, however, the scheme aimed to convey fresh money to the coffers of the Hospital and through them to the Papal palace. Indeed, the bank was obliged to use the money for no other financial operations, but only to buy Papal bonds. Thus, while the Papacy could be partly rescued from the vice-like grip of private bankers, the interest from the bonds was used for the running of the Hospital. The bank was placed in the premises of the Hospital and members of the Order of the Santo Spirito were in charge of it. It was the first time anything like this had been arranged. In the beginning the bank operated a rather simple system and did not offer the sophisticated financial opportunities commonly provided by banks. But it worked quite well and soon the Papacy changed the rules, allowing lay personnel to be appointed to the management and removing some other restrictions. However, even when the bank had to move to bigger premises outside the Hospital, its administration remained firmly in the hands of the Commendatore of the Santo Spirito, whose position in the Papal bureaucracy was certainly enhanced as a result. Complaints about unfair competition started to be made.[78] In a few years the bank collected enough money to allow the papacy to undertake some important enterprises.[79]

While it is not surprising to find that a hospital was involved in financial activities to increase its income, it is worth stressing the peculiar partnership with the Papal State.[80] The main feature of political life in Rome after Trent was the attempt by the Papacy to increase its control over various aspects of public life and to centralise political authority. This process was particularly evident in the financial field. The thorough search for new solutions to its huge problems made the Papal state a sort of political laboratory in the making of the modern state. Within this framework the experiment of the bank of the Santo Spirito stands out even more clearly. One of the oldest charitable institutions became an essential element in the political and economic apparatus of the state. Somehow, however, this was perceived as clashing with the true vocation of the Hospital, and those who celebrated it played down the consequences of this financial operation.[81]

Conclusions

As contemporary devotional literature shows, concern for the poor and policies of poor relief were a good example of the ambivalent nature of the political and social project which we call the Counter-Reformation. On the one hand, appeals to new forms of charity became an important feature of post-Tridentine devotion. In Rome, which had to prove itself once again, though in a different way than previously, to be the centre of Christianity, this led to the establishment of hundreds of confraternities and institutions which devoted themselves to the assistance of the poor. On the other hand, images of the 'bad' poor were invested with new meanings, and as various, though abortive, attempts to enclose the poor show, the question was now to control and possibly hide throngs of vagrants and beggars.[82] At the same time, other tools for controlling non-disciplined forms of popular culture were created, including the new Roman Inquisition and the grip over consciences through confession. Within this broad framework, I have focused in this chapter on two main points.

First, by looking at the Santo Spirito I have shown how in Baroque Rome the institutions created to implement policies of poor relief and medical assistance became part of the intricate political system which revolved around the Papal court. I have looked at the efficient ways in which various actors involved in that policy took full advantage of the wealth and importance of the Santo Spirito to build their careers. In particular, I have examined how physicians exploited both the training and the opportunities for work which this extremely active medical institution provided. I have argued for a similar role played by the Hospital in boosting the careers of its ecclesiastical governors. Finally, I have looked at the Papal administration and showed how it benefited from the Hospital's properties. Each of these actors tells us one side of the multifaceted history of poor relief. In discussing the cases of the people selling drugs they had received for their own use, and of the children masquerading as foundlings I have argued that explorations into episodes of cheating and rules to prevent it will allow us to recapture the views of the recipients of charity, who usually did not leave records.[83]

My second point concerns the cultural and economic implications of the medical care provided by the hospitals. In the Early Modern period, medical practice was a pluralistic system where various techniques of healing were available. However, the competence of non-official practitioners was contested and certain types of healing were controversial and, especially in the framework of the political and cultural project of the Counter-Reformation, were subject to the control of both the Church and the official medical establishment. Furthermore, the production and consumption of drugs had huge economic implications. By analysing the case of the peasant admitted to the Santo Spirito after a snakebite, I have argued for the importance of reconstructing the economic and cultural role played by hospitals in contemporary medical debates and practices.

Acknowledgements

In addition to the comments which I received during the original conference, I have benefited from the criticisms of S. Cavallo. N. Hopwood and S. Cuomo have provided valuable help.

Notes

1 For a recent survey of the historiography of confessionalisation and the imposition of social discipline, see W. Reinhart, 'Disciplinamento sociale, confessionalizzazione, modernizzazione' in P. Prodi (ed.) *Disciplina dell'anima, disciplina del corpo e disciplina della società tra medio evo ed età moderna*, Bologna, Il Mulino, 1994, pp. 101–23; see also, W. Reinhart, 'Reformation, Counter-Reformation, and the Early Modern State: a Reassessment', *Catholic Historical Review*, 1989, vol. 75, pp. 383–404.

2 See M. Forster, *The Counter-Reformation in the Villages. Religion and Reform in the Bishopric of Speyer, 1560–1720*, Ithaca, NY/London, Cornell University Press, 1992; R. Scribner and T. Johnson (eds), *Popular Religion in Germany and Central Europe, 1400–1800*, Basingstoke and London, Macmillan, 1996.

3 For a description of the complex system of medical practices available in early modern Italy, see D. Gentilcore, *From Bishops to Witch. The System of the Sacred in Early Modern Terra d'Otranto*, Manchester, Manchester University Press, 1992.

4 See B. Scribner, 'Is a History of Popular Culture Possible?', *History of European Ideas*, 1989, vol. 10, pp. 175–91.

5 See A. Prosperi, *I tribunali della coscienza. Inquisitori, confessori, missionari*, Turin, Einaudi, 1996, especially Chapter 17.

6 For the paternalistic model, see A. Biondi, 'Aspetti della cultura cattolica post-tridentina' in C. Vivanti (ed.) *Storia d'Italia, Annali 4. Intellettuali e potere*, Turin, Einaudi, 1981, pp. 255–302. On the growing gap between high and low culture, see O. Niccoli, *Prophecy and People in Renaissance Italy*, Princeton, NJ, Princeton University Press, 1990, especially the 'Epilogue', pp. 189–96.

7 The historiographical debate over the Papal State in the Early Modern period is very lively and revolves around the extent to which the Popes implemented a consistent programme of building a modern state. Here I follow the view expressed by P. Prodi in his *Il Sovrano Pontefice. Un Corpo e Due Anime: la Monarchia Papale nella Prima Età Moderna*, Bologna, Il Mulino, 1982, especially Chapter 3; see also L. Nussdorfer, *Civic Politics in the Rome of Urban VIII*, Princeton, NJ, Princeton University Press, 1992.

8 See Prodi, *Il Sovrano Pontefice*, pp. 115–19. On the policy of poor relief in Rome between the 16th and the 17th centuries, see L. Fiorani (ed.), *Religione e Povertà. Il dibattito sul pauperismo a Roma tra '500 e '600*, (Ricerche per la storia religiosa di Roma, 3), Rome, Edizioni di Storia e Letteratura, 1979; P. Simoncelli, 'Origini e primi anni di vita dell'ospedale romano dei poveri Mendicanti', *Annuario dell'Istituto Storico Italiano per l'Età Moderna e Contemporanea*, 1973–74, vol. 25–6, pp. 121–72; P. Simoncelli, 'Note sul sistema assistenziale a Roma nel XVI secolo', in G. Politi, M. Rosa and F. Della Peruta (eds), *Timore e carità. I poveri nell'Italia moderna. Atti del convegno 'Pauperismo e assistenza negli antichi stati italiani', Cremona, 28–30 marzo 1980,* Cremona, Biblioteca statale e libreria civica di Cremona, 1982, pp. 137–56. For a 17th-century description of the incredibly rich network of charitable institutions in Rome, see C.B. Piazza, *Eusevologio romano, overo delle opere pie di Roma accresciuto & ampliato secondo lo stato presente. Con due trattati delle Accademie e Librerie celebri di Roma*, Rome, F. Cesaretti, Domenico Antonio Ercole, 1698 and C. Fanucci, *Trattato di tutte l'Opere pie dell'Alma Città di Roma*, Rome, L. Facius and S. Paolini, 1601.

9 By focusing on a hospital I do not mean to deny the vitality and variety of outdoor forms of medical care, like, for instance, the apothecary for the home assistance of the shame-faced poor, founded by the Confraternity of the Twelve Apostles. The Confraternity paid as many physicians as there were districts in Rome in order that they should visit the sick in their homes every day, prescribing drugs which could be obtained from the apothecary. See Piazza, *Eusevologio*, vol. 1, pp. 127–9.

10 On the history of the Hospital, see P. De Angelis, *L'Arciospedale di S. Spirito in Saxia nel passato e nel presente*, Rome (Collana di studi storici sull'Ospedale di S. Spirito in Saxia e sugli Ospedali romani), 1952; P. De Angelis, *L'Ospedale di Santo Spirito in Saxia*, Rome (Collana di studi storici sull'Ospedale di S. Spirito in Saxia e sugli Ospedali romani), 1960–62. On the Order of Santo Spirito, see the entry 'Ospitalieri di Santo Spirito' in G. Pelliccia and G. Rocca (eds), *Dizionario degli Istituti di Perfezione*, Rome, Edizioni Paoline, 1980, vol. VI, cols 994–1014.

11 In the Early Modern period hospitals had various functions: sometimes their therapeutic aims prevailed over the original task of assisting the poor; more often the two functions overlapped or alternated. But all hospitals tended to become centres of political power, which provided the elite with the opportunity to link devotion with political careers. See A. Pastore, 'Gli ospedali in Italia fra Cinque e Settecento: evoluzione, caratteri e problemi', *Sanità Scienza e Storia*, 1990/91, n. 2, pp. 71–87; A. Pastore, 'Strutture assistenziali fra Chiesa e Stati nell'Italia della Controriforma', in G. Chittolini and G. Miccoli (eds) *Storia d'Italia. Annali 9. La Chiesa e il potere politico dal medioevo all'Età contemporanea*, Turin, Einaudi, 1986, especially pp. 435–41.

12 In this chapter I will build a framework for further research in the archives of the Hospital. The main archive sources are in the Archivio di Stato in Rome. Documents relating to the apostolic visitation to the Hospital ordered by the Pope Urban VIII in 1625 are kept in the Archivio Segreto Vaticano. See S. Pagano, 'Le visite apostoliche a Roma nei secoli XVI–XIX' in *Ricerche per la Storia Religiosa di Roma. Studi, Documenti, Inventari, 4*, Rome, Edizioni di Storia e Letteratura, 1980, pp. 317–464.

13 P. Saulnier, *De capite sacri ordinis Sancti Spiritus Dissertatio*, Lyons, G. Barbier, 1649, p. 132. Peter Saulnier was a sub-prior of the Hospital in the 1640s. It is clear from the passage that Saulnier's '*Domus Sancti Spiriti emblema*' is more a mental image he himself devised than an image used by the Order.

14 For the various categories of the poor in early-modern Italy, see B. Pullan, 'Poveri, mendicanti e vagabondi (secoli XIV–XVII)', in C. Vivanti and R. Romano (eds), *Storia d'Italia, Annali 1 Dal feudalesimo al capitalismo*, Turin, Einaudi, 1978, especially pp. 981–1047, now in B. Pullan, *Poverty and Charity: Europe, Italy, Venice*, Aldershot, Variorum, 1994. A. Monticone argues that the main target of the policy of poor relief in Rome were families of artisans: assistance and distribution of money through dowries aimed at stabilising the highly unstable urban economy. See his 'Introduction' to L. Fiorani (ed.), *Religione e povertà*, pp. 19–24. For a similar pattern, see D. Lombardi, *Povertà maschile, Povertà femminile. L'Ospedale dei Mendicanti nella Firenze dei Medici*, Bologna, Il Mulino, 1988. But for a social analysis of the records of a hospital exclusively devoted to the cure of the sick, see J. Arrizabalaga, J. Henderson and R. French, *The Great Pox. The French Disease in Renaissance Europe*, New Haven, CT and London, Yale University Press, 1997, pp. 212ff.

15

> His enim in locis, in quibus celebre illud S. Spiritus Romanum Nosocomium non pauca oppidula possidet, Equorum ac Bubalorum ad amplificandam eorundem procreationem, centena aliquot vagantur & sustentantur eam quidem solam ob causam, ut Domui huic vere piae, plurimumque Charitatis operibus intentae uberius inde vectigal proveniat, ad tot millia aegrorum, puerorumque proiectitiorum alenda. Memini enim, nos toto Anni Secularis M.DC. curriculo, quo ibi mansi, ultra duodecim millia aegrorum suscepisse & necessaria alimentorum ac medicamentorum ope cunctis succurrisse

in Johannes Faber, *Rerum Medicarum Novae Hispaniae Thesaurus, seu Plantarum Animalium Mineralium Mexicanorum Historia* . . . Rome, Blasius Deversinus and Zanobius Masotti, 1651, pp. 593–4. On Faber's career, and especially his diplomatic activities, see S. De Renzi, 'Courts and Conversions: Intellectual Battles and Natural Knowledge in Counter-Reformation Rome', *Studies in History and Philosophy of Science*, 1996, vol. 27, pp. 429–49.

16 At the Santo Spirito, Faber built some of the strongest professional links of his twenty-year career as a physician and botanist at the Papal court. For the dissections performed by Faber at the Santo Spirito on 'hundreds of corpses', see Faber, *Rerum medicarum*, p. 493. In this text Faber repeatedly discusses the most amazing cases which he and his colleagues saw at the Hospital during their training.

17 For a survey of anatomical teaching and practice in Rome, see P. Capparoni, 'I Maestri di anatomia nell'Ateneo romano della Sapienza durante il secolo XVI', *Bollettino dell'Istituto Storico Italiano dell'Arte Sanitaria*, Sept.–Oct. 1926, pp. 194–227. See also E. Conte (ed.), *I Maestri della Sapienza di Roma dal 1514 al 1787: i Rotuli e altre fonti*, Rome, Nella sede dell'Istituto, 1991.

18 References to public, ritual dissections held in various hospitals of Rome are in 'Academografia. Trattato XII delle Accademie Romane del Secolo passato e presente', in Piazza, *Eusevologio*, vol. 2, pp. XXIII–XXVI. Further research on this topic may help revise the received view on the restrictions to dissections in sixteenth- and seventeenth-century Italy. See A. Carlino, *La Fabbrica del corpo. Libri e dissezioni nel Rinascimento*, Turin, Einaudi, 1994. For a revision of the 'myth' of the taboo surrounding dissections, see K. Park, 'The Criminal and the Saintly Body: Autopsy and dissection in Renaissance Italy', *Renaissance Quarterly*, 1994, vol. 47, pp. 1–33.

19 D. Borgarucci, 'Relatione del modo, che si tiene da religiosi di Santo Spirito in Sassia di Roma nel governo dell'archihospedale apostolico di Santo Spirito, et dell'ordine, che si osserva nella cura degl'infirmi, et esposti, scritta da Fra Domenico Borgarucci religioso, et secretario del medesimo Ordine'. It has recently been published by G. Reginald in '"Servizio dell'anima quanto del corpo" nell'Ospedale del Santo Spirito (1623)', in Fiorani (ed.), *Religione e Povertà*, pp. 221–54. The manuscript is held in the Vatican Library. A later copy of the manuscript is attached to the volume of Saulnier held at the Wellcome Institute Library in London. Borgarucci wrote his description at the request of a French nobleman who sought advice after having founded an institution for the care of the poor.

20 On Saulnier's account, see P. De Angelis, *L'insegnamento della medicina negli ospedali di Roma. Cenni storici*, Rome, Scuola Medica Ospitaliera di Roma, 1948.

21

> Li medici fisici principali, che attendono alla cura degl'infermi, sono quattro . . . Ciascuno delli suddetti medici principali dell'hospitale ha il suo pratico, o vogliamo dire assistente, che nell'atto del visitare gl'infermi assiste et osserva, poiche' con la pratica che fanno, acquistano anch'essi grandemente nella professione, et divengono celebri medici, come per Roma et fuori hoggidì si veggono al servitio de' cardinali et prencipi grandi.
>
> D. Borgarucci, 'Relatione', pp. 238–9.

It is likely that Faber worked in this position during the five years of his training, and from the extant book of payment of the Hospital we know that during his time there the four physicians were Fabio Moriconi, Giuseppe Venturini, the better-known Bernardino Castellani, who was also the doctor of Pope Gregory XV, and Giulio Mancini. I shall return later to Giulio Mancini's career. See P. Savio, 'Ricerche su medici e chirurghi dell'ospedale di Santo Spirito in Sassia sec. XVI–XVII', *Archivio Romano di Storia Patria*, III Series, 1971, vol. 25, pp. 145–68.

22 Lectori suus hic debetur locus, siquidem ex isto Medicorum collegio, vel certe ex Chirurgis Doctoribus deligitur semper unus, qui in Academia domestica manualis Medicinae binas habeat hebdomadis singulis praelectiones, illiusque non elementa tantum proponat, & principia, sed etiam recondita quaeque, & artis, ut sic dicam, strata-gemata. Exercet hic iuventutem Nosocomij, excolitque non praeceptionibus tantum quas commentariolis excipiunt, sed ipsa ostensione rerum; atque ita per aliquot hybernae tempestatis menses, excitato quotannis ad rem amphiteatro, audientibus spectantibusque non discipulis tantum sed externis etiam scientiae cupidis, humani corporis fabricam orationem describit, & anatomicae dissectionis arte spectandam exhibet.

Saulnier, *De capite*, p. 143

23 Bis diebus singulis a Medicis invisantur aegri, mane duabus circiter horis ante prandium: sero totidem ferme ante coenam: ubi apparent in valetudinario, Custodes illico Assistentem, Decurionem, & Pharmacopolam cuique deputatum advocant: ephemerides Medici sumunt in manus, Decurio et Pharmacopola diaria pariter sua in quae referant quae a Primario Medico decernuntur. Hic ergo per-spicit aegrum, tractat, percunctatur, audit tum ex eo, tum ex assistentibus si quis ei casus vel symptoma inciderit; indicia quae dictat ars aucupatur, tum si quid status aegri fert, dictat & ut pluri-mum scribit etiam ipse & Assistens.

Saulnier, *De capite*, p. 169

24 For the blood kept in a glass near the bed, see Borgarucci, 'Relatione', p. 243.

25 On the Hospital of S. Francesco, see J.J. Bylebyl, 'The School of Padua: Humanistic Medicine in the 16th century', in C. Webster (ed.), *Health, Medicine and Mortality in the Sixteenth Century*, Cambridge, Cambridge University Press, 1979, pp. 335–70; for a revision of the received view on S. Francesco, see G. Ongaro, 'L'insegnamento clinico di G.B. Da Monte (1489–1551): una revisione critica', *Physis*, 1994, vol. 31, pp. 357–70.

26 Savio, 'Ricerche', p. 153.

27 Cited in De Angelis, *L'Insegnamento*, p. 24. De Angelis quotes from an edition in Italian of Saulnier's work which I was unable to consult.

28 Li medici fisici . . . prima d'havere il luogo di medico principale si sottomettono al concorso con altri medici, et con rigoroso esame il qual'è indetto et pubblicato un mese avanti, dentro et fuori di Roma, acciò vi possino concorrere persone etiam lontane, e sperimentato il loro sapere, et trovatogli superiori a tutti gli concorrenti, sono admessi al servizio . . . dal che anco si può congetturare con quanta premura s'attenda alla salute di questi infermi.

D. Borgarucci, 'Relatione', p. 238

29 In his biography of Mancini, Eritraeus stresses both his humble origins (‘*honesto quidem sed humili loco natus*’) and his uncommon skills (‘*In praedictionibus longo multumque praestabant; ac, simul ac aegrum inviserat, statim quem exitum morbus ille esse habiturus, divinabat*’). See J. N. Erythraeus, *Pynacotheca Imaginum Illustrium . . . virorum*, Cologne, I. Kalcovius and Socii, 1645, pars altera, pp. 79–82. For further biographical details, see J. Hesse, ‘Note manciniane’, *Münchner Jahrbuch der bildenden Kunst*, 1968, Dritte Folge, vol. XIX, pp. 103–20. Recent research has focused on Mancini’s artistic expertise and on his work on painting, *Considerationi sulla Pittura*, first published by A. Marucchi with a commentary by L. Salerno, Rome, Accademia Nazionale dei Lincei. Fonti e Documenti per la storia dell’arte, 1956–1957. On his connoisseurship see M. Maccherini, ‘Caravaggio nel carteggio familiare oli Giulio Mancini’, *Prospettiva*, 1997, vol. 86, pp. 71–92, and Z. Wazbinski, *Il Cardinal Francesco Maria Del Monte, 1549–1626*, Florence, Olschki, 1994. Manuscripts of his works are in the Vatican Library. He died very rich and showed his commitment to poor relief by bequeathing his enormous wealth to the poor students of Siena.

30 See the description made by Gabriel Naudè: “Le Pape d’auiourd’ huy a eu un Medicine qui estoit moralement un fort bon homme, nommé Julio Mancini, grand Astrologue, fort sçavant dans les bonnes lettres et qui avoit des benefices, qui est ainsi mort à Rome, grand et perfait Athée . . .”, quoted in R. Pintard, *Le libertinage érudit dans la première moitie du XVIIe siècle*, Paris, Boivin et C.ie Éditeurs, 1943, pp. 261–262. For Mancini’s interest in chemistry, see Faber, *Rerum Medicarum*, p. 599.

31 See J. Hesse, ‘Note manciniane,’ p. 105.

32 For an example of such discussions, see Faber, *Rerum Medicarum*, p. 599.

33 See L. Duranti, ‘Le carte dell’Archivio della Congregazione di Sanità nell’Archivio di Stato di Roma’, in *Studi in Onore di L. Sandri*, Rome, Pubblicazioni degli Archivi di Stato, 1983, vol. 2, pp. 457–69.

34 For his teaching at the Sapienza, see E. Conte (ed.) *I Maestri della Sapienza*, in the index, under the name Marcus Antonius Lucianus Belfortensis. The payroll of the Santo Spirito lists Luciani from 1608 to 1636, see Savio, ‘Ricerche’, p. 153; in the regest of the archive of the College of the Physicians in Rome there is a gap in the list of the Protomedici between 1623 and 1626 and Luciani’s name does not appear. See F. Garofalo, *Quattro secoli di vita del Protomedicato e del Collegio dei Medici di Roma (Regesto dei documenti dal 1471 al 1870)*, Rome, Pubblicazioni dell’Istituto di storia della medicina dell’Università di Roma, 1951. However, Faber, after recalling that Luciani was his friend and colleague at the Santo Spirito, writes that he was appointed Protomedico in 1625. For this and for contemporary discussions about the Antidotario Romano, see J. Faber, *Rerum medicarum*, p. 577. For debates among physicians and apothecaries about the preparation and use of drugs in the 1620s see P. Castelli, *Epistolae medicinales*, Rome, Jacobus Mascardus, 1626.

35 See F. Garofalo, *Quattro secoli*, especially pp. 32–35; D. Gentilcore, ‘“All that Pertains to Medicine”: Protomedici and Protomedicati in Early Modern Italy’, *Medical History*, 1994, vol. 38, pp. 121–142.

36 On Trullio, see L. Belloni, ‘La dottrina della circolazione del sangue e la

Scuola Galileiana, 1636–1661', *Gesnerus*, 1971, vol. 28, pp. 7–35. Belloni quotes the document with which Urban VIII guaranteed a special salary to Trullio, provided he remained in Rome and treated the poor; see L. Belloni, 'La dottrina', p. 18. For Trullio's teaching at the Sapienza, see E. Conte (ed.), *I Maestri della Sapienza*, ad indicem, under the name Ioannes Trullius Romanus.

37 His appointment at the Santo Spirito is recorded in P. Savio, 'Ricerche', p. 165.

38 See M. Voelkel, 'L'Università romana ed i Barberini nella prima metà del XVII secolo', in P. Cherubini (ed.), *Roma e lo Studium Urbis: spazio urbano e cultura dal Quattro al Seicento: atti del convegno, Roma, 7–10 giugno*, Rome, Ministero per i beni culturali e ambientali, 1992, pp. 323–40.

39 Giovann Maria Lancisi recalls several post mortems performed by Trullio in his *De Subitaneis mortibus*, Rome, Franciscus Buagnus, 1707, p. 122; references to Trullio's observations on patients at the Santo Spirito are in the correspondence between T. Bartholin and H. van Moeinichen published by M. Lyser in *Culter anatomicus. Hoc est Methodus brevis facilis ac perspicua artificiose & compendiose humana incidendi cadavera* . . ., Copenhagen, M. Godicchenus, 1665, pp. 242 ff. Trullio was also appointed consultant to the important Tribunal of the Sacra Rota; see Belloni, 'La dottrina', p. 28.

40 P. Zacchia, *Quaestiones medico-legales. Liber primus [-secundus]*, Rome, A. Brugiotti and J. Mascardi, 1621–25. For the cases debated at the Sacra Rota, see for instance F. Blancus, *Elenchus sive Index Decisionum Sacrae Rotae Romanae in Libris impraessis per Dioceses extensarum* . . ., Rome, Nicolaus Angelus Tinassius, 1687.

41 See Borgarucci, 'Relatione', p. 236.

42 See in Saulnier, *De capite*, the section entitled '*Nomenclatio summorum Ordinis Magistrorum Romanae Domus, brevibus quamplurimum elogiis illustrata*', pp. 31–58.

43
> [. . .] il quale caporale di ciascun quartiere giontamente col speciale, scrive l'ordinatione del medico, che viene obedito in esse, ancorché fussero le cose che s'ordinano preciosissime, et di valore, essendo benissimo la speciaria predetta provista anche di gioie portabili, nel che non si guarda a conditione, ne a qualità dell'infermo; ma indifferentemente si danno a tutti conforme s'ordinano dal medico, a cui è data libertà d'ordinare senza alcuna riserva [. . .]
>
> Borgarucci, 'Relatione', p. 242

44 For the use of vitriol to cure lung diseases at the Hospital of S. Maria della Consolazione, see Castelli, *Epistolae medicinales*, p. 168.

45 On the apothecary of the Santo Spirito, see De Angelis, *La spezieria dell'Arciospedale di S. Spirito in Saxia e la lotta contro la malaria*, Rome, Collana di studi storici sull'Ospedale di S. Spirito in Saxia e sugli Ospedali romani, 1954; De Angelis, *L'Arciospedale di S. Spirito*, pp. 42 ff.

46 See Saulnier, *De capite*, p. 144.

47 In his *Epistolae medicinales*, Castelli refers to apothecaries engaged in the preparation of chemical drugs and working both in their shops and in various private households; for the chemical activities of virtuosi like the linceo Cassiano Dal Pozzo, see C. Dati, 'Delle lodi del Commendator

Cassiano Dal Pozzo' in *Raccolte di prose fiorentine raccolte dallo Smarrito Accademico della Crusca*, Venice, Dalla Stamperia Remondini, 1751, part 1, vol. III, pp. 77–96; for the pharmaceutical activites of Cardinal Dal Monte, see Wazbinski, *Il Cardinal Francesco Maria Del Monte*.

48 See, for instance, the animated discussions between the Protomedico Sebastiano Iozio and other physicians following the decision to allow apothecaries to sell vitriol. The main concern was to prevent incompetent charlatans from selling this kind of substance. See Castelli, *Epistolae medicinales*, pp. 174–185.

49

> Quare Orvietani antidoti portionem cum aceto hausit, sed nihilo melius inde valuit, nisi quod bis terve vitellinam bilem evomerit quam quidem confectionem plebei homines plerumque secum ferunt, a circulatore quodam huius nominis, sic appellatam, Theriaca longe inefficaciorem, vulgo tamen usitatiorem, ceu viliore pretio emptibilem.
>
> Faber, *Rerum medicarum*, p. 778

50

> Ego de ipsius animae salute, non minus quam de recuperanda corporis valetudine solicitus, peccata ipsum sua ceu perniciosa animae venena, si quae haberet, evomere prius iubeo, ob idque confessionem impero, quam Sacerdos ad nutum factam interrogando excepit.
>
> Faber, Rerum medicarum, p. 778

51 The procedure of admission at Santo Spirito was as follows: first an assistant physician 'on call' had to examine the patient to prevent people with incurable diseases or leper and scabies from being accepted; then a priest 'on call' would administer the sacrament of confession, and finally the patient would be taken to a bed; see Borgarucci, 'Relatione', p. 239. However, bitter discussions about compulsory confession arose among members of the widespread Confraternity of the Camilliani, who took care of the sick. See A. Prosperi's entry 'Camillo de Lellis', in *Dizionario Biografico degli Italiani*, Rome, Istituto della Enciclopedia Italiana, 1974, vol. 17 pp. 230–4.

52 J. Faber, *Rerum medicarum*, p. 778.

53 David Gentilcore has reconstructed the history of Orvietanus in his book, *Healers and Healing in Early Modern Italy*, Manchester University Press, 1998. I thank him very much for letting me read the manuscript version of the chapter.

54 Further controversies arose again in 1645 concerning who was allowed to sell Orvietanus; see Garofalo, *Quattro secoli*, p. 38.

55 Commenting on the work by Cosme de Aldana, *Discorso contro il volgo in cui con buone ragioni si reprovano molte sue false opinioni*, published in Florence in 1589, Niccoli recalls de Aldana's complaint about physicians being scorned by the common people, who heeded only the charlatans. See Niccoli, *Prophecy and People*, p. 194.

56 See Arrizabalaga *et al.*, *The Great Pox*, p. 189; and also A. Cavaterra, 'L'ospedalità a Roma nell'età moderna: il caso del San Giacomo (1585–1605), *Sanita' Scienza e Storia*, 1986, n. 2, pp. 87–123.

57 On the introduction into Europe of substances like tobacco, tea and coffee, and on the medical value soon attached to their use, see R. Matthee, 'Exotic Substances: The Introduction and Global Spread of

Tobacco, Coffee, Cocoa, Tea, and Distilled Liquor, Sixteenth to Eighteenth Centuries', in R. Porter and M. Teich (eds), *Drugs and Narcotics in History*, Cambridge, Cambridge University Press, 1995, pp. 24–51.

58 On lignum guaiacum, see R.S. Munger, 'Guaiacum, the Holy Wood from the New World', *Journal of the History of Medicine and Allied Sciences*, 4, 1949, pp. 196–229.

59 See Cavaterra, 'Ospitalità', p. 107.

60 S. Jarcho, *Quinine's Predecessor: Francesco Torti and the Early History of Cinchona*, Baltimore, Johns Hopkins University Press, 1993.

61 Ibid., p. 17 and 205.

62 For the Pammatone, see Jarcho, *Quinine's Predecessor*, p. 20. For the apothecary of Santo Spirito, see De Angelis, *L'Arciospedale di S. Spirito*, pp. 42–45, and De Angelis, *La Spezieria dell'Arciospedale*.

63 See Piazza, *Eusevologio*, vol. 1, pp. 127–9 and 373–7.

64 'E perchè molto rileva per benefizio de' Poveri, che la Spezieria per essi destinata, sia provista abbondantemente e puntualmente di quanto bisogna, perciò la Compagnia medesima sollecitamente vi invigila, visitando con la presenza di persone perite le Droghe, e robbe, che in essa si consumano, acciò i Poveri non siano defraudati della dovuta Carità [. . .]', ibid, p. 375. On the association of the Jesuits with a wide range of new remedies and exotic substances, and on the competing interests in the production of pharmaceuticals, see M. Baldwin, 'The snakestone experiments. An early modern medical debate', *Isis*, 1995, vol. 86, pp. 394–418. Baldwin stresses also the competition for the prestige connected to the monopoly of the production and sale of drugs like theriac in the early modern state.

65 See *Avvertimenti per la cura de' poveri infermi nella città di Torino*, Turin, 1680, quoted in S. Cavallo, *Charity and Power in Early Modern Italy. Benefactors and their Motives in Turin, 1541–1789*, Cambridge, Cambridge University Press, 1995, pp. 78–81.

66 See G. Pomata, *La promessa di guarigione. Malati e curatori in Antico Regime*, Rome-Bari, Laterza, 1994, p. 174.

67 See M. Baldwin, 'Toads and Plague: Amulet Therapy in Seventeenth-century Medicine', *Bulletin of the History of Medicine*, 1993, vol. 67, pp. 227–47.

68 P. Saulnier, *De capite*, p. 177–82. On the care of foundlings at the Santo Spirito, see C. Schiavoni, 'Gli infanti "esposti" del Santo Spirito in Saxia di Roma tra '500 e '800: numero, ricevimento, allevamento e destino', in *Enfance abandonnée et société en Europe, XIVe–XXe siècle. Actes du colloque international*, Rome, 30 et 31 January 1987, École française de Rome, Palais Farnèse, 1991, pp. 1017–64.

69 See Borgarucci, 'Relatione', pp. 250–1.

70 '[. . .] per prohibire alle madri, le quali accecate dal medesimo interesse di lucro, pongono le proprie [creature] in Santo Spirito con animo di rihaverle in mano, et far mercantia del proprio sangue in pregiuditio dell'hospitale.' ibid.

71 Officials would check that things went on as established. If mothers were sure to get their babies back, concluded Borgarucci, you would not find anybody taking care of their own children. Typical frauds

perpetrated by wetnurses included not reporting the death of a child or a pregnancy. See P. Gavitt, *Charity and Children in Renaissance Florence. The Ospedale degli Innocenti 1410–1536*, Ann Arbor, University of Michigan Press, 1990, pp. 230 ff.; C. Klapisch-Zuber, 'Blood Parents and Milk Parents: Wet Nursing in Florence 1300–1530', in her *Women, Family and Ritual in Renaissance Italy*, Chicago, University of Chicago Press, 1985, pp. 132–64.

72 See L. Ciammitti, 'Quanto costa essere normali. La dote nel Conservatorio femminile di S. Maria del Baraccano', *Quaderni storici*, 1983, vol. 53 (special issue 'Sistemi di carità. Esposti e internati nelle società di antico regime'), pp. 469–97; S. Cavallo, 'Strategie politiche e familiari intorno al baliatico. Il monopolio dei bambini abbandonati nel Canavese tra Sei e Settecento', ibid, pp. 391–420.

73 E. Grendi, 'Premessa', ibid, pp. 383–9.

74 This episode, on which more investigation is needed, is recalled by Schiavone in his 'Gli infanti "esposti" del Santo Spirito in Saxia', p. 1045.

75 See P. Partner, 'Papal financial policy in the Renaissance and Counter-Reformation', *Past and Present*, 1980, vol. 78, pp. 18–62, and M. Monaco, *Le finanze pontificie al tempo di Paolo V (1605–1621). La fondazione del primo banco pubblico in Roma (Banco di Santo Spirito)*, Lecce, Edizioni Milella, 1974. On the fiscal policy of the Papacy in relation to the building of the modern state, see Prodi, *Il sovrano pontefice*, pp. 122–4.

76 See Monaco, *Le finanze*, pp. 123–7.

77 Monaco discusses how contemporary sources boasted of charitable motives, while the more pragmatic ones remained covered; see pp. 134–5.

78 Ibid., p. 140.

79 Like for instance the building of a big waterworks, called Acqua Paola after the Pope. It may well be that this first outcome of the financial operation run by the Hospital is the reason why Saulnier used the emblem of a fountain to describe the Santo Spirito.

80 See Pastore, 'Gli ospedali in Italia', pp. 74–75.

81 Borgarucci does not even mention the foundation of the bank, while Saulnier recalls the main aim of liberating the people from the grip of usury and briefly mentions 'publicae rei magnam utilitatem, et aliquod etiam Domus commodum'; see P. Saulnier, *De capite*, p. 55.

82 See the 'Appello ai poveri di Gesú Cristo' with which C.B. Piazza opens his *Eusevologio*.

83 I am well aware that Confraternities, like the Confraternity of S. Camillo de' Lellis which was very active at Santo Spirito, stand out by their absence from my picture. However, here too, I would argue for a reconstruction of the controversies surrounding their activities. In particular, it is worth exploring what led to the marginalisation of Camillo, the founder of the Order of Camilliani, following fierce discussions about competing forms of the relief of sufferance in hospitals. See A. Prosperi, 'Camillo de Lellis', in *Dizionario Biografico degli Italiani* (see note 51).

7

'CRADLE OF SAINTS AND USEFUL INSTITUTIONS': HEALTH CARE AND POOR RELIEF IN THE KINGDOM OF NAPLES

David Gentilcore

As one of Europe's most populous cities cited throughout the Early Modern period, Naples had hospitals to match. The Casa Santa dell'Annunziata, for example, was Europe's richest. Built 'like a spacious castle', according to a seventeenth-century guide book, 'it maintained as their condition, age and health require, two thousand souls'. It took in many hundreds of children, 'between orphane and exposed infants as well as males as females', instructing them 'in letters and art, according to their inclination till they become great'.[1] It treated the sick of all kinds, dividing them up into wards. Each patient had, much to the amazement of an anonymous seventeenth-century English visitor, 'a clean bed, with all necessaries and attendance, as if he were at home in his own house, until he recovers, all gratis'.[2] What was more, 'every bed stood as in an alcove, and had a wall on both sides separating it from beds on both hands, and as much void space on both sides of the bed that the bed it self took up but half the room'.[3]

The Annunziata was but one of the city's many hospitals. Enrico Bacco's guide to the city, first published in 1616, lists eleven hospitals in operation, ten conservatories for women, eleven for girls, five for boys and one for the aged. Together, they assisted some 6,000 people every year.[4] The Annunziata and the Incurables' Hospital were by far the largest and most endowed. They were referred to as 'the two eyes of Naples, the two columns' supporting the city.[5] However, despite their imposing presence and the impression they made on visitors from abroad, their contributions to health care and poor relief in Naples were but part of a wide range of initiatives. Throughout the Early Modern period the kingdom lacked a coordinated programme of poor relief, depending instead on forms of charity that had their roots in the Middle Ages. The unification of smaller hospitals into one large 'Ospedale Maggiore' that took place in some other Italian cities during the second half of the fifteenth and first half of the sixteenth centuries did not occur in Naples. The study of poor relief and health care in Italy has tended to focus on the development of hospitals for beggars.[6] In Naples, this took place relatively late and was never very effective. This does not mean that poor relief was lacking, but that it was decentralised. As in other Italian states, forms of charity were extremely varied. And although the Counter-Reformation inspired a flowering in works of charity and devotion, most of this was *ad hoc* and sectorial, arising out of particular situations or in specific places and targeted at special groups. The Catholic Church, in the form of a strengthened episcopacy, did seek to exercise increased control over hospitals, as it did over confraternities and other 'pious works'. Yet this went in the face of ever-increasing politicisation of hospitals, more closely linked to civic and state authorities. These are the features of health care and poor relief during this period.

Hospitals and religious renewal: the Incurables Hospital

It was the sixteenth century that witnessed the greatest expansion in the city's hospital structure, beginning with the Casa degli Incurabili, the Incurables Hospital, in 1519. Hospitals for 'incurables' were a response to a new plague which had been spreading through Europe since the closing years of the previous century: the 'French pox' or syphilis. It first appeared on the European scene in Naples, explaining why the French called it the *mal de Naples.* The response to the disease is best seen in a devotional context, in the religious renewal that was taking place throughout Europe and would lead to both the Protestant and Catholic Reformations. Syphilitics were generally treated with compassion, the disease being seen as the result of the general sins of humanity. The Incurables Hospital in Naples was founded by the Catalan noble and widow Maria Laurenzia Lonc, through the assistance and inspiration of the Genoese Ettore Vernazza. The latter had set up the pious association known as the Oratory of the Divine Love, first in Genoa and then in Rome. The Oratory had a close relationship with hospitals for incurables: in

Genoa it would run S. Maria del Ridotto, and it founded other hospitals elsewhere.

The project to build such a hospital in Naples attracted substantial donations and bequests, and within three years it had moved to new, larger quarters at S. Maria del Popolo. Lonc was indefatigable and chose to live in the hospital. By 1525 it was taking in all sorts of sick, especially the poor.[7] In fact, like many of its counterparts elsewhere on the peninsula, initial specialisation in the care of syphilitics did not mean a shift to an exclusively therapeutic function.[8] The hospital was unusual in being founded and run by a woman. In 1535 Lonc retired to a strict enclosed Capuchin convent, which she herself had founded. She was succeeded by her assistant and confidante, Maria Ayerbe d'Aragona, the Duchess of Termoli. Ayerbe was likewise a pious noblewoman and widow, a source of inspiration to the hospital staff. At the same time, the hospital was acquiring a more regular bureaucratic structure, with the viceroy, Pedro de Toledo, seeking some sort of control over the institution. As of 1539 the appointment of governors had to meet with the approval of the civil authorities, according to the hospital's statutes of that year, recognised by the viceroy. The statutes suggest that Ayerbe's role was increasingly spiritual and hint at possible tensions between her and the governors. They concluded with a reminder to all members of the governing body 'to show all possible reverence and respect, as befits her Ladyship's services, and involve her in all the affairs of the hospital'.[9]

Links between the Incurables Hospital and the viceregal administration expanded over the course of the century. The formation of its governing body went far beyond purely municipal dynamics. One of its governors had to be designated from amongst the ranks of the kingdom's Collateral Council, another had to be a titled nobleman, another a knight of the city's noble *seggi*, another a Spanish member of the great central tribunals, two were to come from the Seggio del Popolo and one was from the representatives of the foreigners in the kingdom.[10] This did not mean that the Hospital was somehow secularised, but it did ensure that serving on its governing body became a mark of prestige for those holding important administrative offices.

Hospitals and the Counter-Reformation

If there is no real dividing line separating hospitals founded before Trent and those founded after it, there is no doubting the great impulse that the Counter-Reformation gave to hospital charity. It is worth emphasising in this context that we must resist the temptation to see hospitals as existing in a medical or welfare sphere that is outside the religious. This is especially true after Trent when, with their increased powers, bishops sought to exercise jurisdiction over them. For contemporaries, hospitals were pious institutes, sacred places, in the same category as churches, monasteries, convents and chapels. Communities of religious lived in the hospitals, along with other pious individuals who dedicated themselves to serving them. This is why they are so often the theatre of religious devotions, the nature of which changes as the religious climate at large changes. At the same time, and not always harmoniously, they were also sources of political power, as we have seen. It is only in the latter decades of the eighteenth century that hospitals become the focus of medical learning (competing with the universities) and treatment (competing with home visits by practitioners). But even in the 1780s the Incurables Hospital had more ecclesiastics than medical practitioners and nursing staff combined.[11]

The Annunziata too had the ability to adapt to the changing climate ushered in by Trent. Even before the Council had ended in 1563 the hospital had become a renewed focus of spirituality and charity. In 1556 the Hospital's governor, Alfonso Piscicelli, downplayed its activities in an attempt to involve the nascent Society of Jesus. He told St Ignatius that the Hospital was only working to half its capacity: caring for bodies most splendidly, but ignoring people's souls. This opinion was not shared by other Jesuits in the city. In the same year Cristoforo Mendoza informed Ignatius that 'if there is any piety in Naples, it is all at the Annunziata'.[12]

The Hospital's liturgical and spiritual activities came to be performed by a well-prepared clergy, resident at the hospital. The clerical body consisted of sixty priests and thirty deacons. In 1575, after the Jesuits had declined to become directly involved, it even established its own seminary, training twenty-five priests. The Hospital's superior, the *sagrista*, was usually a bishop, and was an important figure in the life of the city. The Hospital's church became a centre for preaching the Tridentine message, including such preachers as the Jesuit Salmeron. The splendour of its ceremonies was well known: one thousand ducats a year was spent on music alone.

The Annunziata's wealth was the result of centuries of bequests. But the fame of the Annunziata also rested on the fact that the money was spent, and spent charitably. It maintained some 8,000 foundlings a year, many of whom were sent out to its 2,500 wet-nurses. Whatever the infants' places of origin – and many foundlings were sent in from other nearby towns – they were considered Neapolitan-born, acquiring the right to Neapolitan citizenship.[13] At the age of 8, boys were entered into a trade, via the city guilds, or into a family. Occasionally, they became clerics. Girls could remain in the hospital until the age of 18, where they were taught 'feminine activities and skills' by the Hospital's several hundred teachers.[14] Each year seventy girls were awarded dowries of 90 ducats.

Although the abandonment of infants was a regular practice, the Tridentine Church did not attempt to eliminate it. Rather it insisted that infants only be abandoned out of dire necessity, and only once they had been properly baptised. Infants were to be left with a note around their neck bearing their name. And they were to be left only at hospitals and other places prepared to take them. The phenomenon seems to become worse during the second half of the seventeenth century with the decline in living standards. In some areas parents temporarily left children at foundlings' homes, as part of an economic strategy to cope with lean times.[15] The effects were particularly acute for those living from day to day on temporary work. It may explain the constant increase in the number of foundlings taken in by the Annunziata. Despite an only gradually increasing population throughout the Kingdom, the annual average intake of the hospital climbs from around 600 foundlings in the 1680s to around 1,100 in the 1730s.[16]

The Annunziata was also a hospital for the sick, divided into several separate wards: infirmary, fever sufferers, curable sores and convalescents. It also supported charitable activities outside its walls. Its five *maestri* had a list compiled of deserving or shamefaced poor, to whom was destined a sum of 100 ducats a month. For the more common poor the Hospital could spend up to 30 ducats a day, plus 1,000 ducats every Saturday. In addition to dowries for its own foundlings, it provided 100 poor girls from the city and surrounding countryside with dowries of 60 ducats and contributed to the dowries of the less poor to the tune of 12 ducats each. Every year it made 2,000 ducats available for priests and religious institutions fallen on hard times, as well as providing some convents and monasteries with medicines. It supported the city's smaller hospitals and contributed one complete meal to the inmates of each of the city's ten prisons once a week.[17] It even responded to private requests for assistance, providing help to take up a trade or pay the rent.[18] Such was the Annunziata's place in the heart of Neapolitans that when a fire destroyed part of it in 1574, donations poured in from all sides, including 2,000 ducats from the Incurables Hospital.

Although private charity in Naples continued to revolve around the Incurables and the Annunziata, individuals did establish their own, smaller hospitals. This was a continuation of traditional models of charity, where institutions were set up to meet a specific need. Such was the conservatory and hospital of S. Onofrio, for the aged, founded by Ottavio Cassano in 1607, the conservatory 'for blind youths', founded by Aniello de Mano the following year, and the hospital 'for poor cripples' founded by Tiberio Melfi in 1655.[19] The inspiration behind such foundations was primarily devotional and charitable, but practical considerations had an important role in governing them, dependent as they were on private funds for their continued survival.

Lay confraternities

Private citizens could contribute in other ways: both the Annunziata and the Incurables Hospital were assisted in their operations by members of the city's numerous confraternities. The obligation for confrères to perform acts of charity was not new by any means, but the Tridentine emphasis on the performing of good works as a means to salvation was formally written in to the statutes of the many confraternities founded or renewed after Trent. The 1562 statutes of the Santa Croce confraternity asserted that 'since visiting the sick is so important, the Lord himself having clearly indicated that by visiting the sick He himself is visited . . . all our brothers must visit the sick of the hospitals of this city; that is, for each hospital three brothers of our company . . . must visit the said poor sick, giving them that comfort and consolation that God inspires in them'. The emphasis was on spiritual assistance, ensuring that sufferers died without 'any hate or obstinacy'.[20] The confrères reserved *physical* aid for one another.

The statutes of the Santissimo Crocifisso confraternity, founded in 1553, noted that 'Naples [is] extolled as the garden of Italy, not just for its pleasant hills, but indeed because [it is] a land rich in talented people and lively intellects, cradle of saints and useful institutions'.[21] The large number of confraternities active at the city's hospitals causes us to wonder whether their efforts were in any way coordinated, either by the confraternities themselves or by the hospitals' governing bodies. Or did they all target the same types of sick in the same hospital, aiming for the most visible impact? It is almost impossible to gauge actual practice. One account does praise Camillo de Lellis (on whom more below) for being the one to rationalise the confraternities' visits at the Incurables. This suggests that such was not the case up until then. The confraternities were to take turns, coming on different days of the week, providing meals for the hospital's sick amongst other services.[22]

As an extension of service in hospitals, confraternities occasionally contributed to the upkeep of a certain number of beds, presumably assuming the right to nominate who would occupy them. It may also have been a form of investment, attracting interest, as in Turin.[23] The hospitals came to depend on such outside support. The charitable functions of confraternities were generally administered by *monti*, special funds or banks, which they set up for the purpose. A typical example is the confraternity of knights who set up the Monte dei Poveri Vergognosi in 1614 for the benefit of the 'shamefaced poor'. It supported twenty-nine beds at the Incurables Hospital, as well as feeding a certain number of the hospital's sick every Tuesday. It also assisted the poor in prison, supplied twenty poor girls with dowries each year and contributed to the dowries of poor girls of noble families wishing to enter a convent.[24]

Congregations were also set up with the specific intent of founding and running a hospital. This was especially the case with large communities of *forastieri* (outsiders) present in the capital. As soon as numbers and economic fortunes permitted, they sought to establish their own confraternity, church and simple hospice caring for the sick and poor of their community. Religious devotion mixed with notions of national prestige. Due to the Kingdom's status as a Spanish dominion, there were large numbers of Spanish nobility, administrators and military personnel concentrated in Naples. This led to the creation of a brotherhood '*pro pauperibus Hispanae nationes*'. With the support of the viceroy it received Papal approval in 1532. This permitted them to build a hospital dedicated to S. Giacomo, complete with church, cemetery, apartments and offices. What resulted was no ordinary hospice, however. In 1583 and 1585 Papal bulls exempted the church and hospital from local episcopal jurisdiction, putting them under the direct authority of the Holy See.[25]

The wealthier and larger Neapolitan confraternities could afford to found their own hospitals. The 900-strong confraternity of S. Trinità dei Pellegrini founded the hospital of the same name in 1579, which specialised in taking in vagabonds, for three nights at a time, and convalescents from the other hospitals. Most of the kingdom's confraternities could not aspire to such great works of charity and prestige. Instead they were dependent on the alms they collected in order to carry out their visits to hospitals and prisons. In practice, hospital visits by confrères were not as consistent as implied by the rousing words of the confraternity statutes. The Santa Croce confraternity statutes were mentioned above; but the subject of hospital visits never came up at any of the confraternity's meetings or featured in its registers over the centuries.[26] This is to say nothing of those confraternities which functioned sporadically, were underfunded or otherwise fell into decline. The impressions of English visitors notwithstanding, there was a lack of basic provision for the sick in hospitals of the time. Constant nursing care was virtually non-existent. The situation was that much worse in hospitals operating on a shoestring, in debt or governed by officials more concerned with their own careers. Ecclesiastical visitations, which frequently provide descriptions of the conditions – physical and otherwise – of a diocese's hospitals, remind us that lists of charitable institutions in a given locality tell us only part of the story.

The Ministers of the Sick

It was to provide continuing, reliable care, both spiritual and physical, that the Abruzzese Camillo de Lellis set up his male nursing order, the Ministers of the Sick, in 1586. It was to be a congregation of priests, along the lines of other 'clerks regular' like the Jesuits, Theatines and Oratorians. This arrangement, typical of the Counter-Reformation, gave individual members and houses a certain degree of freedom to adapt to differing pastoral situations. According to its statutes, members of the order were to tend the sick according to physicians' wishes, informing physicians of any changes in the patients' conditions. They were to help the sick to eat, wash them, make their beds and help them to die a 'good death'. There were very few conditions put on what was referred to as 'complete service' in hospitals: they were not to undertake porterage, kitchen work, pharmacy or care of the insane. Sensing possible sources of conflict with hospital administrations, de Lellis stressed that they were to resist the temptation to become 'syndic or controller' of the hospitals in which they served.

Tentative beginnings were made at Milan's Ospedale Maggiore in 1594. Ten years later they were firmly established in Naples, under de Lellis' direct supervision. Twenty-four Camillians were serving at the Annunziata, fourteen at the Incurables Hospital and six at S.

Giacomo degli Spagnoli.[27] What, exactly, they did is not easy to say. We know little of their actual day-to-day routine. At the introductory hearing into de Lellis' canonisation, held in Naples, it was said that 'he conferred with physicians on the things necessary for the health of the sick, of which he had made a list'. This could include fairly specific nursing tasks. He would make the rounds of the sick, 'carrying a box with four or five jars of various kinds of water, according to the needs of the sick, to refresh them, wiping their tongues and rinsing their mouths'. In addition, he 'carried a chamber pot at his belt for the use of the sick, even bearing the necessary pots for them'.[28] Members of the order, like medical practitioners of the time, also visited the sick at home. They were recognisable because of the small red cross on their habits, for which they were soon popularly known as 'Padri della crocella'. Once their founder acquired a reputation of saintliness, the priests would bring along a relic of his on their visits, if requested.[29] Given the belief in the powers of relics to bring about a saint's miraculous intercession to heal disease, they form another aspect of the charity offered to the sick. While the focus of this study is on the *supply* or provision of poor relief and health care, this example suggests how historians might also benefit from looking at the other side of the coin. That is, shifting the focus of study to the *demand:* the use people made of what was available and the strategies shaping their decisions.[30]

Just as it is difficult to ascertain the practical role of confraternal assistance and how it fit into the day-to-day management of a hospital, the same can be said of the contribution made by the Ministers of the Sick. The fact that they were allowed into institutions like the Annunziata on a full-time basis suggests a need and desire for what they offered. There is no doubting the difficult and sacrificial nature of their work. From the start the Camillians were given the most thankless tasks. When Spanish galleys were quarantined at Pozzuoli, outside Naples, in 1589 because of an epidemic of petecchial typhus on board, the viceroy turned to the Camillians to give succour to the sick and minister to the dying.[31] Their commitment was tested to the full during epidemics. During the plague of 1656 three Camillians entered into service at the S. Gennaro pesthouse. The archbishop – from the relative safety of the mountain-top monastery of S. Martino – sent others to the parishes of S. Maria della Scala and S. Arcangelo agli Armeni to assist plague victims. Others alternated between day- and night-time duty in various places in the city. While the epidemic raged through the city some Camillians had to be withdrawn from active service to tend the increasing numbers of Camillians who were themselves becoming plague victims.

In all, forty-three Camillians died of plague in Naples, almost all as a result of tending plague victims throughout the city.[32] The plague was a disaster of unprecedented proportions for Naples (to say nothing of the kingdom as as whole). For the Camillians it resulted in the suspension of regular service at the city's hospitals. The provincial superior was amongst the victims, as were the prefects of each of the order's three Neapolitan houses. Complete service to the Annunziata was restored only in 1678, along with only weekly visits to the Incurables Hospital.

The *monti*: types and functions

Mention of the *monti* as a form of charity has already been made. The first Neapolitan Monte di Pietà was founded in 1539, though the period of greatest development was in the closing years of the century. Between 1587, the establishment of a bank at the Annunziata, and 1602, the founding of the Monte delle Misericordia, five additional banks were founded. They were associated with charitable institutions: the Incurables, S. Giacomo, S. Eligio, S. Spirito and the Monte dei Poveri. These were the kingdom's largest banks throughout the Early Modern period and many trade guilds and confraternities invested the funds of their own smaller *monti* in these banks.

One of the largest was the Monte della Misericordia. Founded in 1602 by a small group of Neapolitan noblemen who had already been meeting regularly at the Incurables Hospital, it went on the become the city's wealthiest. As early as 1607 it had enough funds to pay Caravaggio the enormous sum of 400 ducats for his painting entitled Our Lady of Mercy, depicting the seven acts of mercy. In 1658 it began work on its own palace and church and by the eighteenth century had an annual income of some 60,000 ducats. It supported forty-five beds at the Incurables Hospital, and provided lunch for the hospital's sick every Friday. The latter activity alone cost the Monte 2,000 ducats a year, more than the income of most town hospitals. In addition, the Monte ran a hospice on the island of Ischia for the mineral baths, to which it organised two trips a year of some 200 people, including accompanying clergy. It provided 206 girls with dowries each year.[33]

Smaller-scale *monti* were a typical Counter-Reformation response to the threat of hardship, mingling piety with practical concerns.

This was true for any sort of group of people sharing similar interests: national communities, trade guilds, family lineages, a town's peasants. In fact, notions of poverty and poor relief were dominated by ideas about the group. It was considered the business of the group and helped to define it. The kingdom can be seen as a network of *monti*, which existed in even the smallest towns. The dominance of the group in providing various forms of charity, from dowries to health care, helps explain the relative absence of state involvement in poor relief in the kingdom.

For the kingdom's guilds and artisanal confraternities *monti* were the most common form of mutual assistance. While many of these trade corporation-cum-religious brotherhoods had been in existence since the Middle Ages, many more had sprung up after Trent. Piety overlapped with trade protection, even attempts at wage control. In 1599 the archbishop was prompted to remark that, in Naples, 'the number of confraternities and congregations claiming to have charitable purposes has multiplied greatly'.[34] A guild's *monte* was administered by the guild itself, by appointed governors, either to assist guild members or to undertake a variety of welfare schemes. The members of the guilds would contribute either a monthly quota or a percentage of the trade's total output. When a guild member fell sick a guild representative would visit him to ascertain his condition. A visit from a physician would be arranged if necessary. The physician might then issue a medical certificate stating the nature of the illness, which would determine the financial recompense due the guild member. The amount was usually around one or two *carlini* a day for the the first month; then half that rate the second month. If the invalidity lasted a third month the governors of the *monte* would meet to decide on eventual further payment. In the case of a guild member who could no longer practise his trade because of disability, the governors were to use their discretion to decide on a monthly allowance, 'so that he does not go begging'.[35] Allowances were also issued when old age or imprisonment (as long as the cause was 'honourable') prohibited a member from earning a living. And widows might receive a pension to permit them to live an 'honourable life', though the sum was a relatively low three or four *carlini* a week.

Reasons of mutual support also propelled another type of social grouping to form *monti* – family lineages. The creation of family or clan *monti* was a particular kind of interested charity, set up primarily to fund dowries. Their expansion during the sixteenth and seventeenth centuries is less a result of religious fervour and charity towards the poor, than an increasing tendency to exclude women from inheritance, providing them only with a dowry. To this we must add notions of honour that the old Neapolitan noble families possessed, resulting in the requirement to provide ever-larger dowries for the daughters. The dowries of noble girls were often measured in the tens of thousands of ducats.[36] It must be said that poverty only becomes a criterion at a very late date: benefactors sought to assist all their marriageable descendants, rich or poor, helping the entire group. Only when and if the number of endowable female descendants increased excessively was poverty introduced into the equation. As for piety, there is usually no 'moral' limitation in the conditions of access: no mention of the need to be a 'good Christian' or an 'honourable' girl (words that are ubiquitous in the Early Modern period). But one could argue that such conditions were assumed, built in to being a family member.[37]

Another type of fund was that set by municipalities to counter the worst effects of poverty among its own inhabitants. They varied a great deal from place to place. The most basic and specialised were the grain banks, *monti frumentari,* which made seed corn available for the next year's planting. They sought to protect peasants from unscrupulous landlords who made loans which forced the peasants into lifelong debt. But during years of dearth their loans of grain were more likely to end up in the stomachs of famished peasants than be planted in the soil. Many towns also set up more generalised funds for the poor, known as *monti dei poveri*, but little research has been done to ascertain their actual impact.

Community physicians and surgeons

The setting up of *monti* was not the only sort of charitable initiative that towns could take. Feudal structures put great demands on the kingdom's towns, but they were able to show some vitality nevertheless. In terms of medical provision, most towns would seek to bring in a community physician (*medico condotto*) and surgeon (*chirurgo condotto*), or at least the latter. The arrangements were usually for a fixed period, during which the *condotto* was to reside in the community and treat the poor gratis. Factors like the town's size and the amount its budget could permit would affect the nature of the contract. No systematic study has yet been carried out for the kingdom, along the lines of Carlo Cipolla's research on parts of the Tuscan grand duchy, so we must rely on occasional data. In the 1590s the municipal officials of the town of Trani, despite a deficit, salaried two community physicians and one community surgeon as part of the town's budget.[38] Even small, hill-top towns like Atena and Brienza in the province of Principato Citra were, according to baronial assessments of the time, able to attract physicians to serve their communities.[39]

The decision to hire a *condotto* was usually taken with reference to the necessity of providing for the community's needy poor. But it was not just the poor who stood to benefit from their presence. Small towns had special reasons for attracting *condotti:* they would provide a private medical service to all classes of the local population in areas which could not otherwise generate sufficient well-off clientele to support a physician. Those sections of the population able to afford his services hoped that the *condotto* would set up a private practice and stay on. This was especially the case where other possible areas of patronage – local noble households and religious institutions – lacked sufficient resources or were too small in number to set up a contractual relationship with a physician and surgeon. It is questionable whether many of the inhabitants would have been able to afford the remedies prescribed by the physician, even if his visits came free. Testimony to this, and one possible solution, come from an unexpected source: the canonisation processes. To counter the problem of expensive remedies, the bishop of Bovino, Antonio Lucci, set up a *monte* for the sick poor of the town. According to devotees, the bishop gave a sum of money in trust to a local merchant. This was made available to the sick on the basis of chits signed by the town's physicians, corresponding to the cost of the medicines required. Witnesses interrogated at the ecclesiastical investigation into Lucci's life viewed this charity as being so exceptional that they used it as an example of his undoubted saintliness.[40]

The hiring of community physicians was not restricted to small towns. In Naples the urban territory was divided into twenty-nine districts, or *ottine*, each of which had a physician salaried by the city. Their duties were to treat the poor and distribute medicines free of charge. In order to qualify, paupers were issued with a certificate by the Maestri della Carità. The authority for such decisions belonged ultimately to the Tribunal of S. Lorenzo, the city government. The Tribunal was run by six elected officials (*Eletti)* from each of the five noble assemblies (*seggi nobili)* and from the popular assembly (Seggio del Popolo). Amongst other things, the Eletti controlled the import of grain and were responsible for the city's food provisioning measures.[41]

The Tribunal of S. Lorenzo was also responsible for the city's public health board, the Deputazione della Salute, set up in response to the plague of 1656. During the epidemic the deputees rounded up fifty-three physicians to serve the city's twenty-nine districts (*ottine*), a figure that represents only a fraction of the physicians then resident in the city.[42] Each was assigned to a particular area in their *ottina*. They were not to refuse treatment to any sick person, especially when requested by the deputees of the *ottine*, and they were to wear a cross of red cloth of at least a palm's length pinned to their chests so they could be recognised. Fifty-four surgeons and sixty-seven barbers were to serve the populace in the same way. Plague epidemics had a double-barrelled impact, especially on the poor. First of all, they tended to be the first and most numerous victims of the disease, given the conditions in which they lived. And, they were the most affected by the stoppage in all economic activity that resulted as government edicts were put into force, having least in the way of reserves.

Poverty, public order and the state

The thousands of migrants arriving from the provinces of the kingdom each year in search of work or food made it a national issue. This was a problem faced by capitals of all the Italian states. Naples' large size and its economic relationship with the rest of the kingdom made it particularly acute. Years of dearth exacerbated the problem, as in the 1580s when, according to an anonymous account, it was 'impossible to walk the streets, such was the number of poor people'.[43] Even in normal years, beggars and vagrants were said to form one-tenth of the city's population.

It was concern with beggars that occasioned the only concerted activities by the state with regard to poor relief. Not that the government's response ever formed part of a coherent policy or strategy. The Spanish viceroys never sought to institute a magistracy for the poor, for instance. In this they differed from other Italian states. Even Spanish Sicily had its Ufficio della Carità from 1555. On the plus side, this relative inaction meant that no serious attempts were made forcibly to enclose or segregate the poor. In any case, the reasons for this lie in part with the presence of separate organs of government, which dealt with problems as they arose, on an *ad hoc* basis. In serious cases, the viceroy intervened directly. Viceregal pragmatics were issued from time to time to forbid begging and oblige all beggars from outside to leave the Kingdom. But nothing substantial was done. Given the large numbers of people pouring into the capital each year, any policy outlawing vagrants would have been impossible to enforce. Early Modern governance remained the art of the possible. In 1638 the government set itself more realistic objectives, targeting outsiders (*forastieri*) staying in private houses, inns and hospices. Those responsible for taking them in were obliged to report them to the authorities within a day of their arrival.[44]

The only appreciable government initiative before the founding of the Albergo dei Poveri in 1751 consisted of turning the city's plague hospital into a hospice for the poor. This was done under instructions from the viceroy, Pedro Antonio de Cardona, in 1667, creating the 'Real Hospizio di SS. Pietro e Gennaro extra moenia'. It was not the first time that a viceroy had involved himself in the founding of a charitable institution. In 1616 the Duke of Osuna founded the conservatory of S. Maria di Costantinopoli for girls and in 1649, Iñigo-Velez de Guevara founded the conservatory of S. Nicola a Nilo for children orphaned in the 1647 revolt. But the 1667 initiative was on a much larger scale, in line with initiatives taken elsewhere in Italy. As early as 1581 Genoa had converted its former pesthouse to take in beggars, used as such until the next plague epidemic, of 1648. The analogy between plague sufferers and beggars – both threats to social order and public health – is clear.[45] So on 14 February of 1667 all the Naples beggars were ordered to present themselves at the Hospice within eight days. Eight hundred would be distributed into its five divisions or *quartieri:* for young girls, women, boys, married and unmarried men. In December the viceroy announced that the city's ministers, noblemen, knights, citizens and guilds would be taxed to support the nascent hospice. So too would all of the kingdom's municipalities, once it had been discovered that one-tenth of its inmates were from outside Naples.[46]

In line with responses typical of Catholic Europe, the Hospice mixed the provision of charity with repressive measures. Its seven governors had numerous duties, which included touring the city to identify and punish beggars who had not presented themselves, helping boys into a trade, finding places for girls as servants in 'honourable houses' and ensuring that the alms that were collected were deposited in public banks to make the best use of the money. But despite all these provisions the Hospice was a failure. Three years after opening, it was already in deficit. Most of the inmates had managed to distance themselves from it and an edict of 1671 was unsuccessful in obliging them to return. In fact most such institutions in the Italian states fell far short of their original ambitions to eliminate begging. This was due in part to inadequate funding and misplaced goals of being able to support themselves on the labour of their inmates. They were unable to keep inmates from coming and going, and economic realities soon forced them to restrict entry to certain categories.[47]

The example of the Kingdom of Naples brings together many of the themes discussed throughout this book. The Kingdom's mixed geopolitical condition as both an Italian state and a prized Spanish dominion makes it an interesting test case for models of Early Modern charity. Yet the sheer size of its capital, and its overbearing presence on the rest of the country, makes its experience *sui generis*.

When it came to medical organisation, in terms of the functioning of its Protomedicato, the Kingdom closely resembled the modest and loosely structured Aragonese Protomedicato, rather than the highly centralised and powerful Castilian tribunal.[48] Along the same lines, the Kingdom of Naples' charitable structures remained *ad hoc* and haphazard. Spanish viceroys lacked the power to affect great changes, and were satisfied with minor contributions and adjustments. In this sense at least the Neapolitan experience is in sharp contrast to that of other Spanish kingdoms whose hospitals were centralised early on: under Ferdinand and Isabella, in the case of Barcelona, Saragossa and Valencia, and under Philip II in the case of Castile. In this, Naples was also unlike other Italian cities, which saw the early amalgamation of several smaller hospitals into large general hospitals.

It could be argued, however, that the city already had a general hospital in the Annunziata, given both its vast size, wealth and the multiplicity of functions it performed. And, if the state was absent, the Church certainly was not. Especially in the years following the Council of Trent, it claimed jurisdiction over charitable institutions. Though some, especially the larger foundations, were exempt, the Church's presence did ensure that they were at least inspected and reported on from time to time, though the emphasis of the visitations was, of course, pastoral. To this we must add the devotional impulse and charitable zeal of innumerable individuals, imbued with the spirit of the Counter-Reformation.

Notes

1 Edmund Warcupp, *Italy, in its original glory, ruine and revival,* London, 1660, pp. 264–5; cited in Edward Chaney, 'Giudizi inglesi su ospedali italiani, 1545–1789', in G. Politi, M. Rosa, F. della Peruta (eds), *Timore e carità: I poveri nell'Italia moderna,* Cremona, Biblioteca statale e libreria civica di Cremona, 1982, pp. 77–101, at p. 96; Chaney's article is available in English as 'Philanthropy in Italy: English observations on

Italian hospitals: 1545–1789', in T. Riis (ed.), *Aspects of Poverty in Early Modern Europe,* Stuttgart, Alphen aan den Rijn Sijthoff, 1981.

2 J. Malham (ed.), *The Harleian Miscellany,* London, 1808–11, vol. xii, pp. 118–19; cited in Chaney, 'Giudizi inglesi', p. 95.

3 Gilbert Burnet, *Some letters containing an account of what seemed most remarkeble in Switzerland, Italy, etc.,* Rotterdam, 1686, p. 193; cited in Chaney, 'Giudizi inglesi', p. 95.

4 Enrico Bacco, *Descrittione del Regno di Napoli,* Naples, 1671. Available in English as *Naples: an Early Guide,* translated and edited by E. Gardiner, New York, Italica, 1991, p. 55.

5 Cornelio Musso in a sermon of 7 March 1570, cited in Romeo De Maio, 'L'Ospedale dell'Annunziata: "il megliore e più segnalato di tutta Italia"', in his *Riforme e miti nella Chiesa del Cinquecento,* Naples, Guida, 1973, p. 246.

6 See discussion in Brian Pullan, '"Support and redeem": charity and poor relief in Italian cities from the fourteenth to the seventeenth century', *Continuity and Change,* iii (1988), pp. 177–208, especially pp. 197–9.

7 A Papal brief of that years refers to the '*innumerabiles fere pauperes languentes infirmi . . . plagarumque et diversarum infirmitatum miseria oppressi*' being taken in. Francesco Saverio da Brusciano, 'Maria Lorenza Longo e l'Opera del Divino Amore a Napoli', *Collectanea Franciscana,* xxiii (1953), p. 45, note 54.

8 Alessandro Pastore, 'Gli ospedali in Italia fra Cinque e Seicento: evoluzione, caratteri, problemi', in M. L. Betri and E. Bressan (eds), *Gli Ospedali in Area Padana fra Settecento e Novecento (Atti del III Congresso Italiano di Storia Ospedaliera. Montecchio Emilia, 4–6 Marzo 1990),* Milan, Franco Angeli, 1992, 71–87, at p. 78.

9 '*Capitoli et ordinationi da osservarsi per li ecc.ti et mag.ci S.ri governatori et maestri del venerabile hospitale dell'Incurabili*', transcribed in Giuliana Vitale, 'Ricerche sulla vita religiosa e caritativa a Napoli tra medioevo ed età moderna', *Archivio storico per le province napoletane,* lxxxv-lxxxvi (1968–9), pp. 207–91, at p. 264.

10 Piero Ventura, 'Le ambiguità di un privilegio: la cittadinanza napoletana tra Cinque e Seicento', *Quaderni Storici,* xxx (1995), pp. 385–416, at p. 403.

11 According to Galanti there were sixty-eight clerics (including priests, chaplains, confessors and 'assistants to the dying'), plus five nuns, to the forty-five physicians and surgeons, and twenty cleaning and nursing staff (of whom just six were 'assigned to the washing of the sick'). Giuseppe Maria Galanti, *Nuova descrizione storica e geografica delle Sicilie,* Naples, Gabinetto Letterario, 1786–90, vol. iii, p. 142.

12 *Epistolae Mixtae, ex variis Europae locis ab anno 1537 ad 1556 scriptae,* Madrid, 1901, vol. v, p. 402; cit. in De Maio, 'L'Ospedale', pp. 245, 252.

13 This was just one of the Annunziata's jurisdictional and fiscal privileges, Ventura, 'Ambiguità', p. 402.

14 Francesco Imperato, *Discorsi intorno all'origine, regimento e stato della gran Casa della Santissima Annuntiata di Napoli,* Naples: Egidio Longo, 1629, p. 41.

15 Brian Pullan, 'Poveri, mendicanti e vagabondi (secoli XIV-XVII)', in C.

Vivanti and R. Romano (eds), *Storia d'Italia. Annali 1: Dal feudalesimo al capitalismo,* Turin: Einaudi, 1978, pp. 981–1047, at p. 1025.

16 Giovanni Battista D'Addosio, *Origine, vicende storiche e progressi della S. Casa dell'Annunziata di Napoli,* Naples, 1883, p. 527; cited in Ruggiero Romano, *Napoli: dal Viceregno al Regno,* Turin, Einaudi, 1976, p. 59.

17 De Maio, 'L'Ospedale', pp. 249–50.

18 Archivio della Casa Santa dell'Annunziata, *Appuntamenti,* viii; cited in Ventura, 'Ambiguità', p. 414, note 76.

19 Giovanni Muto, 'Forme e contenuti economici dell'assistenza nel Mezzogiorno moderno: il caso di Napoli', in Politi *et al., Timore e carità,* pp. 237–58, at p. 254. Available in English as, 'The form and content of poor relief in early modern Naples' , in A. Calabria and J. Marino (eds), *Good Government in Spanish Naples,* New York: Peter Lang, 1990, pp. 205–36.

20 Archivio Storico Diocesano, Naples, *Santa Visite,* vii, fol. 609v.; in Appendix to Silvana Musella, 'Dimensione sociale e prassi associativa di una confraternita napoletana nell'età della Controriforma', in G. Galasso and C. Russo (eds), *Per la storia sociale e religiosa del Mezzogiorno d'Italia,* Naples, Guida, 1980, vol. I, pp. 341–438.

21 'Regola del Venerabile Oratorio del SS. Crocifisso dei Cavalieri', in Maria Gabriella Rienzo, 'Nobili e attività caritativa a Napoli nell'età moderna. L'esempio dell'Oratorio del SS. Crocifisso dei Cavalieri in S. Paolo Maggiore', in ibid., vol II, Galasso and Russo *Per la storia sociale,* 1982, pp. 251–89, at pp. 254–5.

22 Teresa Filangieri Ravaschieri Fieschi, *Storia della carità napoletana,* Naples, Giannini, 1875, pp. 245–9.

23 Pastore, 'Ospedali in Italia', p. 74; Sandra Cavallo, *Charity and Power in Early Modern Italy. Benefactors and their Motives in Turin, 1541–1789,* Cambridge, Cambridge University Press, pp. 141–3.

24 Galanti, *Nuova descrizione,* vol. iii, p. 187.

25 Maria Gabriella Rienzo, 'Inventario sommario dell'Archivio della Confraternita del S.mo Sacramento dei nobili spagnoli di S. Giacomo in Napoli', in Assoc. degli ex-allievi (eds), *Le chiavi della memoria: Miscellanea in occasione del I centenario della Scuola Vaticana di Paleografia Diplomatica e Archivistica,* Vatican City, 1984, pp. 461–90, at pp. 461–4.

26 The requirement to visit hospitals disappears altogether from the Santa Croce's statutes of 1779. Musella, 'Dimensione sociale', p. 375.

27 Piero Sannazzaro, *Storia dell'Ordine Camilliano (1550–1699),* Turin, Edizioni Camilliane, 1986, p. 67.

28 Archivio Segreto del Vaticano, *Congregazione dei Riti,* no. 2631, folios 41v–42r.

29 Ibid., folio 129v.

30 I discuss this in my study, *Healers and Healing in Early Modern Italy,* Manchester, Manchester University Press, 1998.

31 Sanzio Cicatelli, 'Vita di P. Camillo de Lellis Fondatore della Religione de Chierici Ministri dell'Infermi', 1608, Ms., Archivio Generale dell'Ordine dei Ministri degli Infermi, Rome. Edited by R. Corghi and G. Martignoni, *Un uomo venuto per servire: Camillo de Lellis nell'antica cronaca di un testimone oculare,* Milan, Rusconi, 1984, pp. 79–81.

32 Sannazzaro, *Ordine Camilliano,* p. 179. Jean Delumeau gives the number of victims as ninety-six, out of 100 members in Naples; in his *La peur en Occident (XIVe-XVIIIe siècles). Une cité assiégée.* Paris: Fayard, 1978, p. 128.
33 Galanti, *Nuova descrizione,* vol. iii, pp. 188–9.
34 Archivio Segreto del Vaticano, *Relationes ad limina,* Archbishop Alfonso Gesualdo, Naples 1599; cited in Rosario Villari, *The Revolt of Naples,* translated by J. Newell, Cambridge, Polity Press, 1993, p. 219, note 57.
35 As the statutes of the salt-dealers' guild put it. Archivio di Stato di Napoli, *Capellano Maggiore: statuti e coporazioni,* b. 1182, 58; cited in Muto, 'Forme e contenuti', p. 245.
36 Maria Antonietta Visceglia, *Il bisogno di eternità: i comportamenti aristocratici a Napoli in età moderna,* Naples, Guida, 1988, pp. 81–93.
37 Gérard Delille, 'Un esempio di assistenza privata: I Monti di maritaggio nel Regno di Napoli (secoli XVI-XVIII)', in Politi *et al.*, *Timore e Carità,* pp. 275–82, at pp. 277–8.
38 N. J. Faraglia, 'Il censimento della popolazione di Napoli fatto negli anni 1591, 1593, 1595', *Archivio storico delle Province Napoletane,* xxii (1898), p. 379.
39 Tommaso Astarita, *The Continuity of Feudal Power: the Caracciolo di Brienza in Spanish Naples*, Cambridge, Cambridge University Press, 1992, pp. 141–3.
40 From the testimony of Dr Tommaso Rossomandi, in ASV, *Riti,* n. 279, folio 89. The Franciscan Antonio Lucci was bishop of Bovino from 1729 until his death in 1752.
41 Muto, 'Forme e contenuti', pp. 240–1.
42 'Bannum Deputatorum Salutis', 30 May 1656, *Pragmatica, edicta, decreta, regiaque sanctiones Regni Neapolitani...collocatis per...Blasium Altimarum,* Naples, Jacobi Raillard, 1682–95, vol. iii, pp. 1287–1302. The city's population was between 400,000 and 450,000.
43 N. J. Faraglia (ed.), 'Il tumulto napoletano dell'anno 1585', *Archivio Storico per le Province Napoletane,* x (1886), no pp.; cited in Villari, *Revolt of Naples*, p. 219, note 55.
44 'De Officio Magistratus Politiae in urbe et regno', in Lorenzo Giustiniani (ed.), *Nuova Collezione delle Prammatiche del Regno di Napoli,* Naples, Stamperia Simoniana, 1805, vol. x, pp. 20–2.
45 Alessandro Pastore, 'Strutture assistenziali fra Chiesa e Stati nell'Italia della Controriforma', in G. Chittolini and G. Miccoli, (eds) *Storia d'Italia. Annali 9: La Chiesa e il potere politico dal Medioevo all'Età Contemporanea,* Turin, Einaudi, 1986, pp. 433–65, at pp. 445–6.
46 G. Pandolfi, *La povertà arricchita o vero l'Hospitio de' poveri mendicanti fondato dall'eccellentissimo signor Don Pietro Antonio Raymondo Folch de Cardona,* Naples, 1671, p. 16; cited in Muto, 'Forme e contenuti', p. 257.
47 Pullan, 'Support and redeem', p. 197.
48 David Gentilcore, 'Il Regio Protomedicato nella Napoli spagnola', *Dynamis* (1996), in press.

8

POOR RELIEF IN COUNTER-REFORMATION CASTILE: AN OVERVIEW

Jon Arrizabalaga

Aitari, esker onez

Introduction

Until the 1970s most studies on health care provision and poor relief in Counter-Reformation Europe were locked between the apologias of Catholic-minded historians and the accusations of 'Whig', 'Weberian' and, in general, Protestant-minded ones. The former used to praise the charitable works for social welfare provision promoted by the complex institutional network making up the Roman Catholic Church, on the assumption that for any Catholic country poor relief and social assistance were synonymous with Christian charity unless that country stopped being Catholic. On the contrary, the latter claimed that poor relief in Catholic countries was – I quote Linda Martz's words – 'disorganized and haphazard, controlled by an over-indulgent church that sought to preserve a class of paupers so the rich would have ample opportunity to exercise their charitable obligations', in contrast to a supposed 'new form of rational, discriminating relief, directed by secular authorities' provided by Protestantism.[1]

Since Brian Pullan's and Jean-Pierre Gutton's seminal works twenty-eight years ago,[2] these Manichean views have been gradually dismantled by showing that fear of the poor and vagrant was shared by Catholic and Protestant city authorities, and that social welfare policies and services employed to cope with this problem were carried out by the authorities of Early Modern Catholic cities and states as efficiently as on the Protestant side, irrespective of the different reasons to which poverty was attributed, and of the different ways it was coped with.

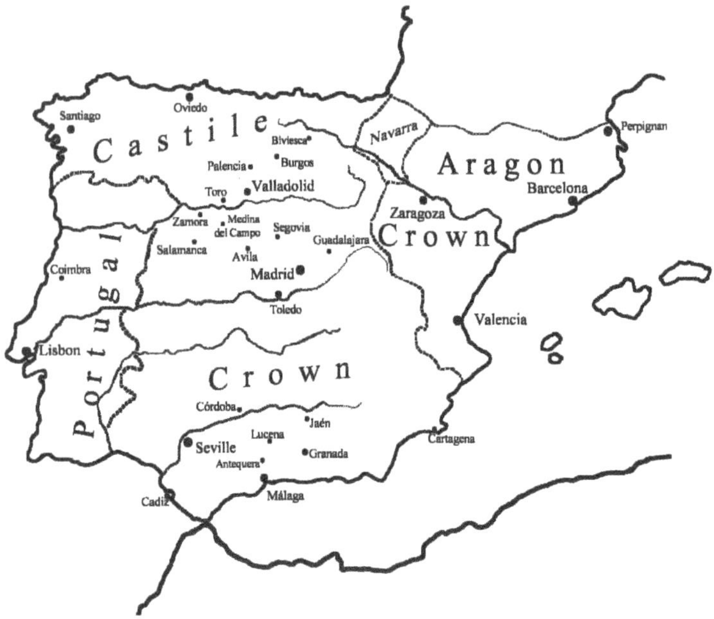

Figure 8.1 The Crown of Castile in the sixteenth and seventeenth centuries

From the Christian conquest of Granada in 1492 to the accession to the Spanish throne of the Bourbon dynasty in the early eighteenth century, the Crown of Castile included all the peninsular territories which did not belong to Aragón, Navarra or Portugal (Figure 8.1). As the leader of the imperial expansion which made the Spanish monarchy become the hegemonic power in Europe during the sixteenth and the first half of the seventeenth centuries (until the Peace of Westfalia in 1648), the Crown of Castile was also the titular head of all the American territories under the Spanish monarchy. This expansion was accompanied by an unparalleled development of the state bureaucracy to administer the territories under the rule of the Spanish monarchy all over the world. During the reign of Philip II (1556–98), the Spanish empire reached its zenith, although from the late 1560s a series of economic, social and political circumstances periodically created many difficulties for the monarch. These difficulties gradually increased during the reigns of Philip III (1598–1621) and Philip IV (1621–65), and in the long term brought about its final decline in the face of the new emerging powers in Europe. Among these troubles it is worth mentioning the chronic financial problems of the monarchy, the increasing attempts to prevent social unrest in the vast territories under its rule, and the widely varying demands of its foreign politics.[3]

The history of social welfare provision in Counter-Reformation Castile has not yet been thoroughly investigated. Apart from the classical work that Hernández Iglesias wrote more than 120 years ago, two overviews on the history of this topic throughout Spain up to and including the Enlightenment were published during the two central decades of this century, coinciding with the post-Civil-War national debate on the setting-up of a social security system for industrial workers.[4] From the 1970s a number of historians have explored the debates and developments in poor relief which took place in Early Modern Castile (and Spain). Except for some more general works,[5] studies have mostly focused upon the history of institutions,[6] the lives and works of outstanding 'reformers';[7] and the publishing of proposals for social reform.[8] Additionally, historians of the Spanish picaresque novel have paid some attention to poverty and the poor in Early Modern Spain.[9] Finally, some historical studies on Habsburg Spain have included chapters or sections dealing with the dispossessed and with poor relief.[10] To the best of my knowledge, only three works focusing at length upon significant case-studies of poor relief in Early Modern Castile have been published, namely that by Linda Martz on the imperial city of Toledo in the late sixteenth and early seventeenth centuries, that by Alberto Marcos Martín on the city and region of Palencia between 1500 and 1814, and that by Maureen Flynn on the city of Zamora.[11]

The present chapter attempts to review the development of poor relief in the Crown of Castile during the Counter-Reformation, with particular emphasis on the second half of the sixteenth and the early seventeenth centuries. Despite its being part of the Crown of Castile, the interesting case of Spanish America will remain outside the scope of this study, which is focused on Europe. Indeed, America represented for the Spanish Crown a sort of laboratory where the kings could develop their poor relief projects (including health care) without the obstacles they had to cope with in Castile; and the Crown wisely exploited this resource in the New World as a tool to Christianize the Indians just as the Spanish kings had used hospitals as a way to persuade the Moors to convert during the Christian conquest.[12]

Dealing with this general topic calls for specific attention to be paid to the powerful religious determinants which operated in Counter-Reformation Castile, particularly in the reign of Philip II. His full identification with the Counter-Reformation doctrinal and pastoral programme that the Roman Catholic hierarchy promoted after the Council of Trent (1545–63) made Philip II the champion in defending the Papal authority against heretics and infidels. It was because of this that he exerted a rigid vigilance over Catholic orthodoxy throughout the Spanish Empire; that he supported the Catholic party in the face of the Calvinist challenge in France; and that he promoted wars inside and outside his huge dominions, among them the repression of the Morisco revolt of 1568, the battle of Lepanto against the Turks (1571), the naval expedition of the Armada to England (1588), and the repression of continuous revolts against the Spanish monarchy in the Low Countries. In the course of this chapter we will attempt to see to what extent the religious circumstances influenced the development of a system for poor relief (including health care provision) in Early Modern Castile.

A new perception of poverty in sixteenth-century Castile

As with other European countries,[13] the difficulties of quantifying and qualifying poverty in the Crown of Castile during the Early Modern period are notorious. Robert Jütte's claim that 'poverty is a rather relative and variable concept because its definition is governed by the patterns of needs and values which exist in a given society'[14] applies fully to Castile. In terms of type, the triad of poor–beggar–vagabond – typical of poverty in *ancien régime* Europe – is, in principle, applicable to contemporary Castile, too. In fact, the corresponding words *pobre–mendigo–vagabundo* (or *vagamundo*) seem to have been widely used in Castile and were even recorded in the most significant contemporary dictionaries of the Castilian (i.e. Spanish) language.[15] But within permanent poverty, the three major categories which are more usual and practical to characterise it in Counter-Reformation Castile, are the 'deserving poor', or 'those unable to maintain themselves by labour'; the 'undeserving poor' or 'those who are physically able but preferred not to labour'; and the '*envergonzantes*', or 'those people in need of relief who do not beg publicly'. If the former two were universal in Europe, the latter were typical of the Catholic countries.[16]

An additional source of difficulties in measuring poverty in Castile is the fact that there are very few quantitative studies of it in its main setting, the cities, and none which allows us to estimate its overall level during the sixteenth and seventeenth centuries. However, all the signs indicate that the poor represented a high proportion of the Castilian population at the time, and that their numbers did not stop growing during the period.[17] In 1533, for example, 55.9 per cent of the residents at the city of Palencia fell into this group, and the numbers had risen up to 60.4 per cent fifteen years later (1548). For the following decades the precise numbers of the poor are not known but, at all events, they continued growing during the long Castilian crisis which lasted from the 1580s to the 1660s.[18]

In the Crown of Castile, repression of vagrancy was usual at least from the mid-fourteenth century, as can be shown from the successive laws promulgated by different Castilian kings at the Courts of Toro (1369), Burgos (1379), Briviesca (1387) and Valladolid-Madrid (1435).[19] Yet, until the late fifteenth century legal measures against idleness were sporadic; these were not intended to eliminate begging, and the fact of their repetition makes their practical ineffectiveness clear.[20]

Only during the sixteenth century, and particularly from the 1520s, did the question of begging and vagrancy each become in Castile – as in the rest of Europe – socially relevant.[21] In the complex economical, social and cultural transition from feudalism to capitalism, a new perception of the poor as a social problem and a threat to public order and health was promoted in the urban areas, where poverty manifested itself most dramatically, in contrast with a perception, more traditional in medieval Christendom, of the poor as individuals who were materially and spiritually complementary to the rich and therefore helped make up the balance of the whole social structure.[22]

As a result of all these new circumstances a growing number of initiatives, of various kinds, to cope with poverty are detectable in Castile from the early sixteenth century, both 'from below' (e.g., petitions by the courts and individual reports by public servants, priests, lawyers, physicians and others addressing the monarch with proposals for social reform), and 'from above' (mostly, legal dispositions by royal, municipal and religious authorities). Generally speaking, most of these initiatives were aimed at relieving the effects of poverty, keeping begging under control, and/or repressing vagrancy. In the course of the sixteenth century a tendency can be detected towards an increasing coerciveness, including compulsory seclusion of the poor in institutions allegedly established for their social rehabilitation; and towards a greater involvement of the monarchs in these measures, resulting in their becoming increasingly centralised. Yet, from the early seventeenth until the mid-eighteenth century this tendency seems to have declined as a result of the gradual collapse of the Spanish imperial state and of the predominance of the involvement of centrifugal forces in poor relief.

Let us overview the most pertinent proposals, debates and legislative measures on poor relief which took place in sixteenth- and early seventeenth-century Castile, before focusing upon the contemporary institutional achievements.

Poor laws and proposals on poor relief

The occurence of poverty among the poor in Castile in the early sixteenth century caused a great wave of beggars and vagrants. This increase of poverty lay behind not only the reiterated provisions on poverty promulgated by the Emperor Charles V at the request of the Castilian Courts at Valladolid (1518, 1523), Toledo (1525), and Madrid (1528, 1534),[23] but also behind the poor laws which the municipal authorities of important cities like Zamora, Toledo, Salamanca, and Valladolid adopted in the early 1540s.[24] None of these legislative measures sought the elimination of begging, but instead sought the control of this alarming phenomenon by means of certificates which allowed the poor to beg inside the cities and towns they were natives of or residents in, as well as by means of expulsion orders for the vagrants.[25]

The serious social situation created by the 1539 drought and subsequent disastrous grain crop was the main reason behind the poor law (*Real Cédula*) that Charles V promulgated in 1540. Issued by Cardinal Tavera, the Primate of Toledo (1534–45), as a regent in the absence of the Emperor, the 1540 poor law established a licensed begging system according to which only the 'deserving poor' natives of, or residents in, any city or town were allowed to beg, although begging by the sick poor, students and blind, or during famines and pestilences would be allowed as an exception. Additionally, this poor law recommended the designation of one person by each municipality to supervise its execution, and encouraged the ecclesiastical and civil authorities to make sure that the *envergonzantes* in any city or town were adequately provided with relief.

Yet its concluding paragraph suggested that public begging might not be considered the best way of providing poor relief (although it was not actually prohibited), and instructed the religious and civil authorities to ensure that hospital rents and any others designated for charitable purposes in the cities and towns were actually spent on healing and feeding the poor.[26] Martz has emphasised the confused and contradictory state of this law, and interpreted it as a way for the crown 'to avoid criticism by stating its policy of social welfare reform mildly, almost as an afterthought tacked on the main body of the law'. She believes that the Emperor 'did not force upon Castile the policies he had adopted in the Netherlands; rather he let the Castilians work out their own means of solving the problem'.[27]

Despite its mildness, the 1540 poor law, which was only published in 1544, promoted a paper controversy which was very influential in further debates on poor relief in Counter-Reformation Castile. It was held between the Dominican friar Domingo de Soto (1494–1570) and the Benedictine monk Juan de Robles (or de Medina) (1492–1572), both of them resident in Salamanca, where their respective works on the topic were also published in 1545.[28]

Domingo de Soto, the Dominican prior and professor of theology at Salamanca, fired the opening shot by attacking this law as being contrary to Christian charity, and defending the freedom to beg and beggars' freedom of movement as sacred rights established in the Christian religion. He resisted the idea of distinguishing between deserving and undeserving poor, was opposed to incarceration of the poor in hospitals, and rejected any attempt to assign social welfare provision to civil authorities.[29]

To the Benedictine abbot Juan de Robles, however, poverty could be treated as a social problem in the same way as disease or crime, that is by coping with it as diseases were treated or criminals were put into prison. Obviously influenced by Juan Luis Vives' views, Robles defended, by contrast, the spirit of the 1540 poor law and rejected the views of those supporting an unconditional freedom for beggars, by claiming that begging should be regulated. He stated that after their proper identification, the deserving poor should be provided with relief, and the *envergonzantes* should be attended at home, while vagrants should only benefit by virtue of working. Robles also claimed that foreign poor should not be excluded from alms and from being cured if they were sick, that social welfare provision should be assigned to the civil authorities, and that alms administration should be entrusted to lay people (albeit under the supervision of the bishops).[30]

The difficult economic situation in Castile during the central decades of the sixteenth century explains the repeated requests by the Castilian courts to the monarchs to enact complementary measures to the 1540 poor law such as creating a 'Father of the Poor' in every town, to be in charge of looking for a paid job for all those who lacked one.[31] But the political tension during this period – which coincides with the end of the reign of Charles V and the beginning of Philip II's – made this law (actually in force until 1565) and any complementary measure, in practice nothing more than mere words. In fact, in its role as a 'fortress of the militant Counter-Reformation' the Hispanic monarchy was then leading the Catholic struggle against Protestantism with the support of the religious orders (particularly the Dominicans), and reaffirming its most intransigent orthodoxy in the face of any spiritual renewal movement. In 1555, for instance, Erasmists went from being tolerated to being openly persecuted by the Inquisition. The doctrinal 'rigorism' and the religious intransigency of the sections of the Catholic Church then prevailing were reinforced during the third and last period (1562–63) and the years immediately subsequent to the Council of Trent (1545–63). The revival of the medieval ideal of charity, questioning any measure to regulate begging (along Soto's lines), prevented Robles' proposals from having any relevant social impact during this period. The new dominant religious atmosphere in the lands of the Hispanic monarchy is plainly illustrated by the strong invective against Vives' *De subventione pauperum* (Bruges, 1526) which the Spanish Augustine preacher and secret agent of Philip II in the Netherlands, Lorenzo de Villavicencio (died in 1583), included in his reply (1564) to Gilles Wijts' explanatory work on Vives' proposals (1562) on the occasion of a new attempt at social reform in Bruges.[32]

In 1565, in the context of an alarming spread of pauperism over the Hispanic kingdoms, Philip II promulgated another poor law in Castile.[33] After having recognised the failure of the 1540 poor law, the new royal *Pragmática* voiced very similar concerns, all of them apparently in accord with the re-Christianising spirit of the new, post-Tridentine times. First of all, it maintained the requirement for begging licences, although they were not restricted to natives of a place. Second, it gave to parish priests the duty of designating 'two good persons' (*dos buenas personas*) to be in charge of gathering information about the poor in their district, and of issuing the relevant begging licences, although these licences had to be endorsed later by the municipality in order to be valid. And third, the references at the end of the 1540 poor law to an eventual prohibition of mendicity and to the confining of beggars within closed institutions were suppressed.

The economic problems of the Spanish monarchy grew dramatically during the last third of the sixteenth century, leading to a long general crisis from the 1580s to 1660.[34] In the context of an enormous increase of poverty the question of poor relief was repeatedly considered in the Castilian Courts from the mid 1570s. Between then and the beginning of the seventeenth century, two major proposals to cope with poverty emerged in the Crown of Castile, namely the projects of social reform by the canon Miquel Giginta and by the royal physician Cristóbal Pérez de Herrera. Both of them relied upon the establishment of closed institutions as the best way to deal with poverty, an idea already outlined in a brief anonymous manuscript dated Madrid 1560, which additionally claimed that each state and city should be in charge of maintaining their poor.[35]

The 'new hospitality' of Miquel Giginta

In 1576 the Roussillon canon Miquel Giginta (*c.* 1534–*c.* 1588)[36] submitted to the Courts of Castile assembled at Madrid a report on poverty entitled *Representación para que se remedien los pobres*. The 'new hospitality' (*nueva hospitalidad*) he proposed was a new poor relief scheme closely inspired by a programme devised by the Portuguese Camara for the Lisbon confraternity of the Misericórdia. This scheme which was to be maintained by means of an 'ordered charity' (*caridad ordenada*), required the construction of a network of beggars' hospitals throughout the Hispanic kingdoms. While these common houses for the poor had been called 'Houses of Mercy' (Casas de Misericordia) in the Aragon Crown, in Castile they came to be named General Hospitals of Beggars.[37]

Thanks to the support of the powerful bishop of Segovia, Diego de Covarrubias, who was the president of the Castilian Courts and Royal Council, Giginta's reform proposals were approved and their practical aspects passed on to be studied by an *ad hoc* commission. Three years later he published this work under the title *Tratado de remedio de pobres* (Coimbra, 1579), dedicating it to Antonio Mauriño de Pazos, bishop of Ávila and successor to Covarrubias in the presidency of the Royal Council. His tireless campaigning for poor relief in Castile, Portugal and Aragon was reflected in three more publications between 1583 and 1587, the one he published in 1584 being dedicated to another prominent person, Gaspar de Quiroga, the cardinal-archbishop of Toledo and a member of the Royal Council as a result of his charge of General Inquisitor.[38] These two influential addressees of his works were the firmest supporters of his reform in Castile. Little wonder, since in addition to them being close mutual friends, they had spent many years of their lives in Italy, the place where the new beggars' hospitals promoted by the Catholic Church after the Council of Trent had been first founded in the 1560s.[39] Giginta's projects were also given support by the Jesuits, whose presence behind the foundation of many beggars' hospitals in Counter-Reformation Europe hardly needs emphasising here. His biographical traces vanish after his two last interventions before the Castilian Courts in July 1588 at Madrid, urging them to extend to the whole kingdom his proposals for reform of the hospital system.

Giginta argued[40] that the poor begged because they had no alternative way to maintain themselves. If their basic needs were provided for by adequate institutions where they could be lodged and fed, only vagrants and other undeserving poor would continue to beg. In such an ingenious way Giginta managed to avoid Soto's serious theological objections to any restrictive measure on the freedom of public begging.

By the time of Giginta's proposals the idea of hospital consolidation had been circulating for some time in the Crown of Castile, although it had not yet been carried out there – in contrast to the Crown of Aragón, where it had been completed by the early sixteenth century.[41] Giginta claimed that all the hospitals of any city or town should be consolidated into two different institutions, one for the sick poor and another for beggars. Giginta was mainly concerned with the latter and claimed that any important city in the Crown of Castile should have its own beggars' hospital.

To maintain these beggars' hospitals Giginta called not only on the traditional sources of charity funds (alms collections, bequests and donations by the well-to-do), but also on novel sources like charitable raffles and charges to visit a sort of museum called 'wards of wonders' (*cuadras de maravillas*), as well as taxes upon admissions to comedies. Additionally, he tried to engage bourgeois collaboration by proposing a more 'rational' and rigorous administration of the funds and properties resulting from the hospital consolidation, by encouraging saving, and by claiming that those products manufactured by the poor lodged in the hospitals should be sold in the market.

This latter feature leads us to emphasise that according to Giginta's views the beggars' hospitals were not closed institutions where the recipients should be merely confined – a term which Giginta carefully avoided as being suggestive of Protestant-minded repression of the poor – but active centres where the poor were taken in, trained in a craft (particularly children, the brightest of whom should even be taught to read, write and count), and set to manufacture products (the profit from this work was to contribute not only to maintain these establishments, but also to pay the workers). Therefore, he combined a utilitarian pedagogy with the idea of labour as a means of self-improvement. Giginta was never very clear about the kind of administration he conceived for his beggars' hospitals, but he appears to have intended a model of management under municipal control, although it is thought that he was respectful of the Tridentine decrees in accepting the subordination of the managers to the bishop's deputy.

In his *Atalaya de caridad*, his last work, which he published in 1587, Giginta advocated introducing the Montes de Piedad in all the major towns. This charitable institution of Franciscan inspiration had arisen in fifteenth-century Italy with the aim of providing loans in kind or in cash against collateral guarantees and under beneficient conditions as to repayment time and interest rate. Although institutions rather similar to the Italian Monti di Pietà, such as the 'Granaries' and 'Boxes of Mercy' (Pósitos and Arcas de Misericórdia), were active in Castile from the fifteenth century, and the Council of Trent explicitly recognised the Montes as charitable works, the plans to establish them were very controversial in late sixteenth- and early seventeenth-century Castile, where they developed only from the second half of the eighteenth century.[42]

The 'General Reformation' of Pérez de Herrera

The project of general social reform by Philip II's court physician Cristóbal Pérez de Herrera (1558–1620)[43] should be seen in the context of the catastrophic *fin-de-siècle* crisis in Castile, when hunger and plague were added to a serious economic recession caused by the price revolution, by the collapse of trading and by the decay of manufacturing activities. The cities were the main setting of the crisis, on this occasion particularly those of Southern Castile like Madrid and Seville, which had experienced a population explosion during the second half of the sixteenth century after manufacturing enterprises had collapsed in Northern Castile.

After having studied medicine at the University of Salamanca (1573–77), Pérez de Herrera was examiner of the Castilian Protomedicato (1577–80) and galley *protomédico* of the Spanish army (1580–92). From 1592 to his death about 1618 he was court physician, close to the monarchs Philip II and Philip III. This more comfortable position allowed Pérez de Herrera to publish widely on medicine, on poor relief and on general policy. These latter activities made Pérez de Herrera one of the *arbitristas*, a mixed group of people (army men, public servants, priests, traders, lawyers, doctors), who offered the kings and the ruling elites proposals for solving the misfortunes of 'the republic' in seventeenth-century Spain.[44]

In 1592 – the same year as the Castilian Courts initiated in a new series of sessions in Madrid, lasting until 1598 – Pérez de Herrera was allegedly commissioned by Philip II to write on poverty and poor relief. His hard work during the following years under these favourable circumstances allowed him to successively publish up to ten discourses on the topic between 1595 and 1598, all of them addressed to this king. They were eventually collected together and re-published under the title *Discursos del amparo de los legítimos pobres y reducción de los fingidos; y de la fundación y principio de los albergues destos reinos, y amparo de la milicia dellos* (Madrid, 1598).[45]

In these discourses Pérez de Herrera proposed to immediately set in motion a 'general reformation' (*reformación general*) of poor relief in every city or town of the Crown of Castile in order to prevent beggars escaping these social measures – as had been the case with Giginta's proposals – by moving to other places. For the same reasons he proposed that the reforms should be extended to the remaining kingdoms under the Hispanic monarchy and even to the whole Catholic world.[46]

His proposals for social reform were based on setting up 'shelters' (*albergues*) in all the major Castilian towns (about fifty), the purpose of which was merely to serve as 'parishes and dormitories'. Since the indigent were supposed to receive only spiritual attention and night accommodation in these *albergues*, a substantial saving of expenses was to be expected, these aims being more limited than those of Giginta's beggars' hospitals. Like the latter, however, the *albergues* were intended to provide assistance only for the healthy poor – in contrast to other contemporary poor relief institutions like the hospitals of the Order of Saint John-of-God which looked after both healthy and sick poor all together.

The administration of the *albergues* was intended to be in the charge of four people: a priest administrator, the city *corregidor* who would exert judicial control, and two delegates (a canon and a town councillor) elected each year. In the event of a stalemate between ecclesiastical and civil authorities, the priests were to intervene in the management, but they were to play a secondary role in the introduction and control of the reform, the supreme direction of which was expected to be kept in the monarchy's hands. In fact, Pérez de Herrera claimed that the reforms should be directed by a 'General Protector of the Poor' (Protector General de los Pobres) and a 'General Commissioner of the Shelters' (Comisario General de los Albergues). For these posts he proposed the president and one member of the Royal Council, respectively. He also proposed the creation of a body of 'censors' (*censores*) who should look after the fulfilment of the royal laws and watch over beggars' behaviour. This body should be headed by the 'General Solicitor of the Shelters' (Procurador General de los Albergues) who should also act as their 'General Administrator' (Administrador General).

At the core of Pérez de Herrera's reform plans was a distinction between the deserving poor, and those undeserving and vagrants. To establish this distinction, he proposed that all the poor, should be registered irrespective of their place of birth; otherwise they would be considered as offenders and therefore punished along the lines of the 1565 poor law. According to the expected procedure, the poor would be examined by the administrator of the shelter and by the representive of both the cathedral chapter and the city council in the presence of a physician or a surgeon. When someone was identified as a deserving poor person, he or she would be granted a renewable licence to beg in that city for one year. In contrast to Giginta's proposals, most of the deserving poor were expected to beg each day and to pay for their meals from the collected alms which were also to cover their accommodation. Only the less physically able deserving poor were expected to work within the shelters.

As to the 'undeserving poor', whose introduction to work was actually the main target of Pérez de Herrera's plans of reform, he assumed that they would feel sufficiently persuaded to work on crafts useful for the republic once they were under the control of the shelter registration system. In order to avoid them claiming a lack of work so they could remain idle, he proposed the election in each town of a 'Father of the Workers' (Padre de los Trabajadores) to be in charge of providing work for them.

Pérez de Herrera's plans of reform paid specific attention to female poverty – responsible for the increase of prostitution in the urban centres – to foundlings and to the army. He argued for the setting-up of 'Workhouses' (*Casas del trabajo y labor*) in the major Castilian cities, where prostitutes should be confined and sentenced to compulsory work for a variable time (from one year to a life sentence) in order to rehabilitate them. On the other hand, Pérez de Herrera recommended distributing most foundlings among wealthy families and welcoming the rest into the 'Houses of Foundlings' (Casas de Expósitos) and shelters until they were 7 years old. At this age they were supposed to enter schools to learn a craft, and the brightest ones to be trained as architects, engineers and artillerymen. Finally, Pérez de Herrera proposed the institution of a 'House of Relief for the Militia' (Casa de Amparo de la Milicia) under the control of the War Council, to relieve those members of the Army and Navy disabled as a result of wars.

Pérez de Herrera conceived the funding of his general social reform through alms, bequests from those who died without making a will, taxes on the income of permanent theatres, and donations from the Catholic Church, aristocracy and high public servants. For this purpose he successfully called on the support of King Philip II. The fact that his reforms began to be implemented in Madrid, Sevilla, Valladolid and Toledo, implies that his projects were by no means perceived as Utopian at the time. Yet, after Philip II's death, Pérez de Herrera's proposals met with the new king's lack of concern for them, and resulted in a total failure. Only in the mid-eighteenth century did similar proposals emerge with any chance.

Poor relief institutions

In Counter-Reformation Castile, as in other regions of Catholic and Protestant Europe, hospitals were the most representative institutions of poor relief. In the Middle Ages most hospitals had played the role of asylums and could indiscriminately take in every sort of healthy, sick or disabled poor person, physically or mentally ill, male and female, children (foundlings and orphans) and the aged, beggars, vagabonds and pilgrims. From the fifteenth century on, many of these small, widespread, and rather unspecific institutions of poor relief were consolidated into a much more limited number of larger hospitals. This resulted from a process usually prompted by the political powers both civic and ecclesiastical, by means of which their rents and services were optimised. These new institutions were intended to care for more specific groups of poor people and/or to provide a more 'specialised' care for their needs. Thereafter, hospitals became more and more medicalised institutions, with their traditional purposes of social control increasingly combined with new medical ones. Similarly, from the late fifteenth century new hospitals to care for the poor suffering from specific diseases were erected, and poor relief was effectively reorganised all over Catholic Europe into new institutions both closed and open, particularly after the Council of Trent.

As María Luz López Terrada has emphasised,[47] the consolidation of the numerous small medieval infirmaries existing in most Castilian cities into one or two great hospitals only began in the late sixteenth century, in contrast with the Crown of Aragón where this process had been completed in the most important cities (Barcelona [1401], Zaragoza [1425], Valencia [1512]) during the fifteenth and the early sixteenth centuries. This delay occurred in Castile in spite of the steady support given to the idea by the Catholic kings, who even founded several new hospitals e.g., Santiago (1499), Granada (1504), which, because of their size, appeared to be destined to play such a role.[48] The delay occurred despite even the repeated petitions of the Castilian Courts [Segovia (1532), Valladolid (1548, 1555), Madrid (1563) and Córdoba (1570)] to the Spanish kings;[49] and of Charles V's apparent order of 1540 to reduce the number of hospitals in Castile to one per town.[50]

Irrespective of all the difficult circumstances which the Crown of Castile passed through in the mid-sixteenth century, the reasons why there was no successful process of hospital consolidation before the 1580s, seem to have been mainly political and financial. The political included the strong opposition by the old hospitals' administrators and owners, mostly religious confraternities and brotherhoods. It also included disputes over respective competences, and conflicts among the partners to control and to lead the processions. The financial included lack of capital to cope with this kind of project. Nor did the climate of religious rigorism then pervading Castile – including the revival of an unselfish and medievalised view of charity – help to overcome these difficulties.

The activities of the Order of Saint John-of-God splendidly illustrate the pattern of poor relief institutions which were promoted in this religious atmosphere.[51] In 1537 John-of-God (1485–1550), a Castilianised Portuguese adventurer, had a Pauline 'conversion' as a result of the preachings of the influential priest John of Ávila (1499/1500–1569). For the rest of his life he devoted himself to charity by taking the poor into the house he had established in Granada in 1537, and by collecting alms among the wealthy people to maintain his foundation. In his hospital John-of-God admitted every kind of poor person (beggars, vagrants, pilgrims, travellers, children, prostitutes, the aged), whether healthy, sick (lepers, insane, epileptics, sufferers from the French Disease) or disabled (cripples, one-handed, dumb, blind, and so on), but he also aimed to cope with the needs of widows, young girls, pilgrims and *envergonzantes*. Through successive endorsements by different popes between the 1570s and the 1610s, his followers eventually became recognised as the Order of the Hospitallers of Saint John-of-God, which was explicitly devoted to the care of the poor.

By 1570 this religious community had already founded, among others, hospitals in Madrid (1552), Lucena (1565) and Córdoba (1570). In 1608 the order was divided into two congregations, namely the Italian and the Spanish. The Italian extended over the Catholic countries of Europe, included the religious provinces of Italy, France, Germany and Poland, and eventually reached a total of 165 hospitals. The Spanish congregation included Spain, Portugal and the dominions of both imperial powers, and encompassed nine provinces and 172 hospitals.[52] Among the earliest hospitals held by this order in the New World were those settled or re-founded at La Habana (1603), Santiago de Chile (1617), Santo Tomé de la Guayana (Venezuela) (1625), Mérida de Nueva Granada (Venezuela) (1630), Santiago de la Vega (Jamaica) (1630), and Tarija (Bolivia) (1632).[53]

Soon after the death of John-of-God his followers began to be criticised as parasitic on charity, as people who collected alms to enrich a excess staff and to construct ostentatious buildings where indigents were indiscriminately packed in with no attention paid to their needs nor any activity offered to them other than mendicity: 'Walls of marble and bellies of wind', according to the expressive phrase of the anonymous author of the *Viaje de Turquía* (*c.* 1557/8).[54] But from the formidable spread of this hospital order over the world and the proliferation of other religious orders and brotherhoods with similar aims in sixteenth- and seventeenth-century Castile,[55] it is obvious that the impact of these criticisms among the political elites, both civic and ecclesiastical, was very limited.

Only in the 1580s – a decade during which Philip II ordered no less than four royal provisions in favour of hospital consolidation in the Crown of Castile (1581, 1583, 1586, and 1589) – were the steady royal attempts over the previous two decades in favour of this aim able to break down the strong resistance to it.[56] As Linda Martz has emphasised, hospital consolidation in Castile, like most poor relief reforms, was mainly a project of the crown, although Philip II's actions 'were tempered by certain conditions and limitations, innate to a ruler of a sixteenth-century Catholic state' and, in the end, this process was 'sponsored, supported and executed by the combined forces of church and crown'.[57] In fact, for this achievement Philip II relied, on the one hand, on the support of those bishops favourable to this reform once the Council of Trent had assigned to the bishops the actual control over hospital administration and activities, and, on the other hand, on Pope Pius V's two letters (1566 and 1567) sanctioning the consolidation of any hospital whose serious financial difficulties made it unable to fulfil its duties, and reaffirming that any process of this kind should be under the control of the bishop of each diocese.[58]

Among the cities of the Crown of Castile where hospital consolidation was completed during the late sixteenth century are

Salamanca, Madrid, Seville, Medina del Campo, Jaén, Toro, Antequera, Segovia and Valladolid.[59] The cases of the first four of these are enough to illustrate the whole process.

In September 1581 the bishop of Salamanca consolidated nineteen local hospitals into two, namely the Hospital de Santa María La Blanca and the Hospital General de la Santísima Trinidad, the latter being for pilgrims (who could stay there up to three nights) and for every sort of injured and poor sick person, both male and female, except those suffering from buboes and contagious diseases (who were taken care of at the Hospital de Santa María). The Hospital del Estudio in the possession of the University of Salamanca from 1413 to provide care for the 'ill students and their servants', and which from the second half of the sixteenth century was used for practical teaching by its medical faculty, remained out of this consolidation, and survived independently until 1810.[60]

In January 1587, the cardinal-archbishop of Toledo ordered the reduction in numbers of the hospitals of Madrid, the seat of the court, from fifteen to five. This implied the preservation of four existing ones, namely the Hospital de la Corte (which used to move with the Castilian court and looked after the courtiers), the Hospital de los Italianos (which attended to the needs of the Italian community in the Castilian court), the Hospital de La Latina (a wealthy private hospital founded in 1534), and the Hospital de Santa Catalina de los Donados; and the consolidation of the remaining eleven into the Hospital General. This new institution was originally conceived as being divided into two separate houses (albeit with a single administration and direction), namely one for those poor people suffering from contagious and incurable diseases, and another for the remaining poor who were either healthy or suffering from non-contagious diseases. The former were lodged in the premises of one of the hospitals affected by the consolidation, the Hospital de Antón Martín (founded in 1552 by this follower of St John-of-God); women of the latter were housed at another of the affected hospitals, La Pasión, while from 1589 to 1596, men were gradually lodged in the buildings of the old beggars' hospital, founded in 1581 under the influence of Giginta. These premises were soon perceived to be unhealthy and insufficient for all of their functions and so, in 1603, Hospital General men were transferred from these lodgings to the more spacious premises of the new paupers' *albergue*, built according to Pérez de Herrera's plans between 1596 and 1600.

Although all of these institutions, including the largest one, the

Hospital General, were administered by religious congregations or brotherhoods, a Junta de Hospitales whose members represented the crown, the church and the city council provided overall supervision of the system. In the event this consolidation of Madrid hospitals was not rigorously enforced and a number of 'suppressed' hospitals were still active a century later.[61]

Also in 1587, after a century of failed attempts (1488, 1507, 1522), the seventy-four hospitals of Seville were consolidated into two, namely the Hospital del Amor de Dios and a new, recently-built hospital of Saint John-of-God which was named the Espíritu Santo. The local cardinal-archbishop Rodrigo de Castro played a key role in this consolidation from which five other hospitals were excluded.[62] While the hospital of the Amor de Dios was dedicated to poor males suffering from non-contagious fevers, that of the Espíritu Santo was intended for male and female poor suffering from buboes, sores, contagious diseases and pains, and incurable diseases including venereal disease. Both centres included a number of administrative, religious and health care positions, staff for which were appointed by the archbishop of Seville.[63]

In the same year, after having made continuous attempts to achieve this aim from the late 1570s, the abbot, the *corregidor* and two town councillors of Medina del Campo ordered the consolidation of all the hospitals in the city except two (no less than eleven) into a single General Hospital (Hospital General) as well as the union of all their goods and incomes to build and finance it. Yet, as a result of administrative and financial difficulties the Hospital General only commenced construction after 1591, when the city council of Medina secured funds for this purpose and also for the further maintenance of the new hospital, thanks to the generous contribution of the rich banker Simón Ruiz. The building was not completed until 1619.[64]

Hospital consolidation was neither generally nor permanently completed in the Crown of Castile. In cities like Zamora the serious obstacles created by the administrators of the small hospitals to the plans of centralisation made the authorities cease trying to unify them, and the Zamora hospital system continued to be decentralised until the mid-eighteenth century.[65] Furthermore, as Maureen Flynn has emphasised, the general crisis of the 1590s soon made the 'cities with centralised relief agencies and those with traditional private forms of welfare' confront 'the real test – the test of the comparable effectiveness of their respective systems'. By 1592 the Castilian Courts considered the results of the hospital consolidation as unsatisfactory, and representatives of the three states were asking for a return of consolidated hospitals to their previous condition, and promoting the private foundation of new hospitals.[66]

As already said, discussions at the Castilian Courts around Miquel Giginta's projects of poor relief coincided with, and to some extent were reactivated by, the process of hospital consolidation. Giginta's reformist proposals were approved in 1576, although the earliest of his beggars' hospitals was only opened in early 1581 at Toledo thanks to the unconditional support of the influential cardinal-archbishop of Toledo, Gaspar de Quiroga. One year later (1582), two more beggars' hospitals were established in Madrid and Granada, and in 1583 in Barcelona, but other attempts like those of Jaén, Seville, Burgos, Valladolid, Oviedo and Santiago de Compostela failed, mostly as a result of local opposition from the city rulers.[67]

Finally, the 'General Reformation' promoted during the general crisis of the 1590s by Pérez de Herrera under the steady support of King Philip II led to the building of a number of shelters in different Castilian towns. In September 1596 the shelter of Madrid (*Hospitium pauperum*) commenced construction. In 1597 fifty major Castilian towns were urged by the Royal Council to complete Pérez de Herrera's reform. By the summer of 1598 the shelters of several other towns were being built, and the beggars of Madrid, Seville, Valladolid and Toledo had already been registered.

Following the death of Philip II in 1598, Pérez de Herrera's reform projects gradually stagnated as a result of the growing financial difficulties of the Crown and of the new king's lack of interest. The case of the Madrid shelter illustrates this point well.[68] In 1599 it was already being used as a plague hospital, and, as previously stated, in 1603 the General Hospital was transferred to its premises, which by 1608 also housed 'The Galley' (La Galera) – a closed institution intended for vagrant women and prostitutes.[69]

Only from the mid-eighteenth century were Pérez de Herrera's ambitious schemes taken up. Yet his ideas may have been behind some projects of poor relief developed during the seventeenth century. This seems to have been the case with the already mentioned *galeras*, which may have been partly inspired by Pérez de Herrera's workhouses project (*Casas del trabajo y labor*), although the new name rightly emphasised their greater punitive nature. Among the earliest Castilian *galeras* were, apart from that of Madrid, those of Granada, Salamanca and Valladolid, all of them founded during the early seventeenth century, while others like those of Cádiz and Málaga were only completed in the last quarter of the century.[70]

Conclusions

Although a comprehensive history of social welfare provision in Counter-Reformation Castile is still to be written, some general conclusions may be pointed out – at least tentatively.

It is extremely difficult to give a direct answer to the core question of how the Counter-Reformation affected health care provision and poor relief in Castile. The religious forces in action in Counter-Reformation Castile were extremely powerful but they were not always pushing in the same direction. In the face of the medievalising and centrifugal patterns of charity practised by most religious confraternities and brotherhoods, as well as by some of the religious orders that apparently were favoured during the later stages of, and soon after, the Council of Trent, the Tridentine resolutions tended to stimulate centralisation, reinforced the absolute power of the pope and of the bishops in the Catholic Church, and made the care of beggars into a cornerstone of the Catholic Reformation. In the context of a Europe divided along religious lines, where Catholic and Protestant sides rivalled each other for social and economic development, post-Tridentine Popes and King Philip II seem to have agreed not only that poverty was a serious social problem to be coped with, but also that the Catholic world – and the Hispanic Crown at its head – should show its alleged moral superiority over the Protestants by organising the systems of social welfare provision in a more Christian and efficient way.

In this context, the projects for poor relief (including health care) that were completed during Philip II's reign seem to have been as ambitious (if not more so) as other contemporary ones on the Catholic as well as on the Protestant side. In fact, during the last three decades of the sixteenth century the Spanish monarchy, in conjunction with a number of influential bishops, vigorously supported and enforced (at least, partly) the important proposals of centralised social reform put forward by Miquel Giginta and Cristóbal Pérez de Herrera.

That most of these reforms collapsed in the early seventeenth century was due to political and economic reasons rather than to religious ones. After Philip II's death the vigorous royal impulse vanished as the subsequent Habsburg kings of Spain took no interest at all in these projects. For over a century the demands posed by other formidable pressures, mostly the management of a huge empire in the context of growing financial difficulties, prevented the Spanish Crown from being actively involved in promoting poor relief. Only from the 1730s, once the new Bourbon dynasty succeeded in consolidating its presence on the Spanish throne, and particularly during the Enlightenment, did the royal impulse toward poor relief become perceptible, although it never appears to have been absolutely decisive in *ancien régime* Spain.

The structural weakness of Castilian municipalities after their defeat by the royal power in the War of the Castilian Communities (1520–22) also limited very seriously the range of the measures instigated by the municipal powers, and prevented them from playing the same active role as the municipalities of the Aragon Crown cities did during the same period.[71]

In these circumstances, it is no wonder that in contrast with other Early Modern Catholic states where the monarchy and/or the municipalities took poor relief under their control earlier, a decentralised system of social welfare was dominant in Castile until well into the nineteenth century.[72] This system whose resources, just for the period between 1500 and 1800, have been estimated at no less than 5,000 new foundations (among them about 2,000 for hospitals, 500 for *Casas de Misericordia* and shelters, 2,500 for dowries and scholarships, and 600 for alms), was mostly in the charge of religious orders, confraternities and brotherhoods.[73]

Acknowledgements

To María Luz López Terrada for generously offering me her expertise and guidance on this topic; to José Pardo Tomás for his helpful advice, criticism and encouragement; and to Alfonso Zarzoso for his kind material help.

Notes

1 Linda Martz, *Poverty and Welfare in Habsburg Spain. The Example of Toledo* (Cambridge, Cambridge University Press, 1983), p. 1.

2 Brian S. Pullan, *Rich and Poor in Renaissance Venice: the Social Institutions of a Catholic State, to 1620* (Oxford, Basil Blackwell, 1971); Jean-Pierre Gutton, *La Société et les pauvres. L'exemple de la généralité de Lyon, 1534–1789* (Paris, Les Belles Lettres, 1971). For a recent overview on poverty in Early Modern Europe including a select bibliography, see Robert Jütte, *Poverty and Deviance in Early Modern Europe* (Cambridge, Cambridge University Press, 1994).

3 See Ramón Menéndez Pidal and José María Jover Zamora (eds), *Historia de España* (Madrid, Espasa-Calpe), particularly vols. XXIII (1989), XXIV (1979), XXV (1982), XXVI/1, 2 (1988, 1986), and XXVIII (1993), all of them concerning seventeenth-century Spain; John H.

Elliot, *The Count-Duke of Olivares: The Statesman in an Age of Decline* (New Haven, CT/London, Yale University Press, 1986); R.A. Stradling, *Philip IV and the Government of Spain, 1621–1665* (Cambridge, Cambridge University Press, 1988). A synthetic view for the whole period is provided by Henry Kamen, *Spain 1469–1714, A Society of Conflict* (London/New York, Longman, 1983).

4 Fermín Hernández Iglesias, *La beneficencia en España*, 2 vols (Madrid, M. Minuesa, 1876); Antonio Rumeu de Armas, *Historia de la Previsión Social en España. Cofradías – Gremios – Hermandades – Montepíos* (Madrid, Pegaso, 1944); María Jiménez Salas, *Historia de la Asistencia Social en España en la Edad Moderna* (Madrid, CSIC, 1958). The former also includes a broad preliminary section on Antiquity and the Middle Ages (pp. 9–159).

5 *De la Beneficencia al Bienestar Social: Cuatro Siglos de Acción Social (Ponencias Presentadas al Primer Seminario de Historia de la Acción Social)* (2nd edn, Madrid, Consejo General de Colegios Oficiales de Diplomados en Trabajo Social y Asistentes Sociales, 1988); Elena Maza Zorrilla, *Pobreza y Asistencia Social en España, Siglos XVI al XX. Aproximación Histórica* (Valladolid, Universidad de Valladolid, 1987).

6 Most of these histories consist of or include monographical studies on single hospitals, although they are very unequal in perspective and thoroughness of treatment. Among the most outstanding are those by Alberto Marcos Martín, 'El sistema hospitalario de Medina del Campo en el siglo XVI', *Cuadernos de Investigación Histórica*, 2 (1978), 341–62; Juan I. Carmona García, *El Sistema de Hospitalidad Pública en la Sevilla del Antiguo Régimen* (Seville, Diputación Provincial, 1979); Concepción Félez Lubelza, *El Hospital Real de Granada. Los Comienzos de la Arquitectura Pública* (Granada, Universidad de Granada, 1979); William J. Callahan, *La Santa y Real Hermandad del Refugio y Piedad de Madrid, 1618–1832* (Madrid, Instituto de Estudios Madrileños-CSIC, 1980); Carlos Ferrándiz Araujo, *Historia del Hospital de la Caridad de Cartagena (1693–1900)* (Murcia, Imprenta Provincial, 1981); Delfín García Guerra, *El Hospital Real de Santiago (1499–1804)* (n.p., Fundación Pedro Barrie de la Maza, 1983); Dieter Jetter, *Geschichte des Hospitals. Vol. 6. Santiago, Toledo, Granada: drei spanische Kreuzhallenspitäler und ihr Nachhall in aller Welt* (Stuttgart, Steiner, 1987); María Teresa López Díaz, *Estudio Histórico-Farmacéutico del Hospital del Amor de Dios de Sevilla (1655–1755)* (Seville, Diputación Provincial, 1987); Carmen López Alonso, *Locura y Sociedad en Sevilla: Historia del Hospital de los Inocentes (1436?–1840)* (Seville, Diputación Provincial, 1988); Teresa Santander, *El Hospital del Estudio. (Asistencia y Hospitalidad de la Universidad de Salamanca), 1413–1810* (Salamanca, Centro de Estudios Salmantinos-CSIC, 1993). For a useful (but by no means exhaustive) collection of documents concerning Early Modern hospitals in Spain, see Carmen Muñiz Fernández, 'Hospitales españoles (Información para su historia)', in Rafael Muñoz Garrido and Carmen Muñiz Fernández, *Fuentes Legales de la Medicina Española (siglos XIII-XIX)* (Salamanca, Universidad de Salamanca, 1969), pp.107–74.

7 Michel Cavillac, 'Introducción', in Cristóbal Pérez de Herrera, *Amparo*

de Pobres (Madrid, Espasa-Calpe, 1975), pp. vii–cciv; M. Cavillac, 'La reforma de la beneficiencia en la España del siglo XVI: la obra de Miguel Giginta', *Estudios de Historia Social*, 10–11 (1979), 7–59; Juan Antonio Maravall, 'De la misericordia a la justicia social en la economía del trabajo: la obra de fray Juan de Robles', *Utopía y Reformismo en la España de los Austrias* (Madrid, Siglo XXI, 1982), pp. 207–46.

8 Domingo de Soto, *Deliberación en la causa de los pobres. (Y réplica de Fray Juan de Robles, O.S.B.)* (Madrid, Instituto de Estudios Políticos, 1965); Jacques Soubeyroux, 'Sur un projet original d'organisation de la bienfaisance en Espagne au XVIe. siècle', *Bulletin Hispanique*, *74* (1972), 118–24; Cristóbal Pérez de Herrera, *Amparo de Pobres*, ed. by Michel Cavillac (Madrid, Espasa-Calpe, 1975), pp. 1–304.

9 On poverty and the poor in the Spanish picaresque novel see among others José Antonio Maravall, *La Literatura Picaresca desde la Historia Social* (Madrid, Taurus, 1986); Bronislaw Geremek, *La Estirpe de Caín. La Imagen de los Vagabundos y de los Pobres en las Literaturas Europeas de los Siglos XV al XVII* (Madrid, Mondadori, 1991), particularly pp. 235–93, 402–12; as well as the bibliography referred to in both of these works.

10 Juan Antonio Maravall, *Estado Moderno y Mentalidad Social, Siglos XV–XVII*, 2 vols (Madrid, Revista de Occidente, 1972): vol. II, pp. 238–49, 261–8, 276–7, 279–80; Henry Kamen, *Spain in the later Seventeenth Century, 1665–1700* (London/New York, Longman, 1980), pp. 276–90; David Goodman, *Power and Penury: Government, Technology and Science in Philip II's Spain* (Cambridge, Cambridge University Press, 1988), pp. 209–15, 250–1.

11 Martz, *Poverty and Welfare*; Alberto Marcos Martín, *Economía, Sociedad, Pobreza en Castilla: Palencia, 1500–1814*, 2 vols. (Palencia, Diputación de Palencia, 1985); Maureen Flynn, *Sacred Charity: Confraternities and Social Welfare in Spain, 1400–1700* (London, Macmillan, 1989).

12 See among others Guenter B. Risse, 'Medicine in New Spain', in Ronald L. Numbers (ed.), *Medicine in the New World. New Spain, New France, and New England* (Knoxville, University of Tennessee Press, 1987), pp. 12–63, particularly 37–42; Gonzalo Aguirre Beltrán and Roberto Moreno de Arcos (eds), *Historia General de la Medicina en México. Tomo II: Medicina Novohispana. Siglo XVI* (Mexico City, Academia Nacional de Medicina – UNAM, 1990), particularly Chapters 19 ('Las comunidades mesoamericanas ante la institución de los hospitales para indios' by Miguel León-Portilla, pp. 217–27), 20 ('Los hospitales de la Nueva España en el siglo XVI' by Josefina Muriel, pp. 228–54); and 23 ('El concepto de caridad como fundamento de la atención médica en la Nueva España' by Carlos Aguado Vázquez and Xóchitl Martínez Barbosa, pp. 272–8). For an exhaustive list and a summary history of the hospitals established all over the Spanish Empire see Francisco Guerra, *El Hospital en Hispanoamérica y Filipinas 1492–1898* (Madrid, Ministerio de Sanidad y Consumo, 1994).

13 Jütte, *Poverty and Deviance*, particularly, pp. 8–61.

14 Jütte, *Poverty and Deviance*, p. 45.

15 See Maza Zorrilla, *Pobreza y Asistencia Social*, pp. 13–17.

16 Martz, *Poverty and Welfare*, p. 5. For additional information on this issue, see Maza Zorrilla, *Pobreza y Asistencia Social*, pp. 18–35.
17 Henry Kamen, *Golden Age Spain* (Basingstoke/London, Macmillan, 1988), p. 55.
18 Marcos Martín, *Economía, Sociedad, Pobreza*, vol. II, pp. 369–83.
19 *Novísima Recopilación de las Leyes de España Mandada Formar por el Señor Don Carlos IV*, 6 vols., Madrid, 1805–1807 [facsimile reprint Madrid, Boletín Oficial del Estado, 1975], vol. V, pp. 429–30: book XII, title XXXI, laws I and II.
20 Cavillac, 'Introducción', pp. lxxviii–lxxix.
21 Bronislaw Geremek, *Poverty: a History* (Oxford/Cambridge, MA, Blackwell, 1994), pp. 120–41, 253.
22 Cavillac, 'Introducción', pp. lxxix–lxxxviii.
23 Jiménez Salas, *Historia de la Asistencia Social*, pp. 127–8.
24 Juan de Robles, *De la orden que en algunos pueblos de España se ha puesto en la limosna, para remedio de los verdaderos pobres* (Salamanca, Juan de Junta, 20 March 1545), pp. 147–8; Martz, *Poverty and Welfare*, pp. 21–3, 119–20.
25 Cavillac, 'Introducción', pp. lxxxviii–lxxxix.
26 *Novísima Recopilación*, book vii, title xxxix, laws i–xiii (vol., III, pp. 703–6). On this poor law see Martz, *Poverty and Welfare*, pp. 18–21.
27 Martz, *Poverty and Welfare*, p. 21.
28 Domingo de Soto, *Deliberación en la causa de los pobres* (Salamanca, Juan de Junta, 30 January 1545); Juan de Robles. On Soto and Robles see Quintín Aldea Vaquero, Tomás Marín Martínez and José Vives Gatell (eds), *Diccionario de Historia eclesiástica de España*, 5 vols. (Madrid, CSIC, 1972–1987), vol. III, pp. 2096–7; vol. IV, pp. 2507–8. On the major issues of confrontation between these theologians, see Cavillac, 'Introducción', pp. xcvii-cvi; Maravall, 'De la misericordia'; Martz, *Poverty and Welfare*, pp. 22–30; Flynn, *Sacred Charity*, pp. 93–9; Maza Zorrilla, *Pobreza y Asistencia Social*, pp. 83–7; Jiménez Salas, *Historia de la Asistencia Social*, pp. 89–97.
29 Domingo de Soto, *Deliberación*, pp. 9–142, *passim*.
30 Juan de Robles, *De la orden*. In: Domingo de Soto, *Deliberación*, pp. 145–316, *passim*.
31 Rumeu de Armas, *Historia de la Previsión Social*, pp. 171–2. For the social context of the period between 1540 and 1565, see Cavillac, 'Introducción', pp. cvi–cx; Martz, *Poverty and Welfare*, pp. 30–2.
32 Gilles Wijts, *De continendis et alendis domi pauperibus,et in ordinem redigendis validis mendicantibus . . . consilium* (Antwerp, 1562); Lorenzo de Villavicencio, *De oeconomia sacra circa pauperum curam a Christo instituta* (Antwerp, 1564). On Villavicencio, see Aldea Vaquero *et al.*, *Diccionario*, vol. IV, pp. 2765–6; Cavillac, 'Introducción', pp. cvi–cvii. On Wijts, see Geremek, *Poverty*, p. 199.
33 *Novísima Recopilación*, book vii, title xxxix, law xiv (vol. III, pp. 706–7). On the 1565 poor law see Martz, *Poverty and Welfare*, pp. 32–4.
34 Menéndez Pidal and Jover Zamora (eds), *Historia de España. Vol. XXIII. La Crisis del Siglo XVII* (Madrid, Espasa-Calpe, 1989). For a synthesis see Kamen, *Spain, 1469–1714*, pp. 196–256, 291–3.
35 *Que los hospitales generales es buen medio para el remedio de los pobres,*

si la República en común se encarga del sustento dellos (Madrid, 1560) (Library of the Real Monasterio de El Escorial, ms. L–I–12). For an edition of this manuscript see Soubeyroux, 'Sur un projet original', pp. 121–4. On this document see also Martz, *Poverty and Welfare*, pp. 65–6.

36 On Giginta's biography see Cavillac, 'La reforma de la Beneficiencia', particularly pp. 7–25. On his reform, see ibid., particularly pp. 33–59; Martz, *Poverty and Welfare*, pp. 66–76; Flynn, *Sacred Charity*, pp. 99–102; Maza Zorrilla, *Pobreza y Asistencia Social*, pp. 88–90; Jiménez Salas, *Historia de la Asistencia Social*, pp. 99–102.

37 Flynn, *Sacred Charity*, pp. 99–100; Martz, *Poverty and Welfare*, p. 73. For the Portuguese model see Chapter by Isabel M.R. Mendes Drumond Braga in this volume.

38 Miquel Giginta, *Exhortación a la compasión de los pobres* (Barcelona, 1583); *Cadena de oro* (Perpignan, 1584); *Atalaya de caridad* (Zaragoza, 1587).

39 Martz, *Poverty and Welfare*, p. 70.

40 For my summary description of Giginta's proposals I have mostly followed Cavillac, 'La reforma de la beneficencia', pp. 33–46.

41 On this topic see the chapter by María Luz López Terrada in this volume.

42 On the *Montes de Piedad* in the Spanish kingdoms see Aldea Vaquero *et al.*, *Diccionario*, vol. III, pp. 1726–36.

43 On Pérez de Herrera's life and works see Luis Sánchez Granjel, 'Vida y obra del Doctor Cristóbal Pérez de Herrera' [1959], *Médicos españoles* (Salamanca, Universidad de Salamanca, 1967), pp. 41–64; Cavillac, 'Introducción', particularly pp. xi-lxxiii; Cavillac, 'Noblesse et ambiguités au temps de Cervantes: le cas du docteur Cristóbal Pérez de Herrera (1556?–1620), *Mélanges de la Casa de Velázquez, 11* (1975), 177–212; Cavillac and Jean-Paul Le Flem, 'La "Probanza de limpieza de sangre" du Dr. Cristóbal Pérez de Herrera', *Mélanges de la Casa de Velázquez, 11* (1975), 565–75; José María López Piñero *et al.*, eds, *Diccionario de la Ciencia Moderna en España*, 2 vols. (Barcelona, Península, 1983), vol. II, pp. 159–60; Teresa Santander, *Escolares Médicos en Salamanca (siglo XVI)* (Salamanca, Europa Artes Gráficas, 1984), p. 294 (no. 2421).

44 For a list of his writings, see Cavillac, 'Introducción', pp. cxcvii–ccii. On the *arbitristas* see Juan Ignacio Gutiérrez Nieto, 'El pensamiento económico y social de los arbitristas', in Menéndez Pidal and Jover Zamora (eds), *Historia de España. Vol. XXVI-1. El Siglo del Quijote (1580–1680). I. Religión, Filosofía, Ciencia* (Madrid, Espasa-Calpe, 1988), pp. 233–351.

45 For a recent critical edition of these *Discursos* by Michel Cavillac, see Pérez de Herrera, *Amparo de Pobres*, pp. 1–301.

46 For my brief report on Pérez de Herrera's proposals I have mostly followed Cavillac's thorough introductory study to his edition of Pérez de Herrera's 'discourses'. See Cavillac, 'Introducción', particularly pp. xxxii–lxxiii, cxxix–clxxix. See also Martz, *Poverty and Welfare*, pp. 86–90; Flynn, *Sacred Charity*, pp. 105–7; Maza Zorrilla, *Pobreza y Asistencia Social*, pp. 90–6; Jiménez Salas, *Historia de la Asistencia Social*, pp. 103–11.

47 María Luz López Terrada, *El Hospital General de Valencia en el Siglo*

XVI (Valencia, Universitat de València, 1987), pp. 892–905.
48 Ibid., p. 893.
49 Carmona García, *El sistema de Hospitalidad pública*, p. 183.
50 See Juan de Robles, *De la orden* (foreword). In Domingo de Soto, *Deliberación*, pp.161–2. The 1540 poor law seems by no means to have gone as far at this point as claimed by Robles. Yet, whether Robles referred to any order by Charles V other than that of 1540 is not clear to the best of my knowledge.
51 Cavillac, 'Introducción', pp. cvii-cix; Cavillac, 'La reforma de la beneficencia', pp. 34–5; Martz, *Poverty and Welfare*, pp. 38–44.
52 Aldea Vaquero *et al.*, *Diccionario*, vol. II, 1248–9, 1103–4.
53 Guerra, *El Hospital en Hispanoamérica*, pp. 98–100, 498–501, 395, 379–80, 92, 489.
54 *Viaje de Turquía (La Odisea de Pedro de Urdemalas)*, edited by F. García-Salinero (Madrid, Cátedra, 1980), pp. 113–18.
55 Jiménez Salas, *Historia de la Asistencia Social*, pp. 173– 82.
56 Martz, *Poverty and Welfare*, pp. 77–86; Marcos Martín, 'El sistema hospitalario', pp. 360–1.
57 Martz, *Poverty and Welfare*, pp. 64, 85.
58 See Cavillac, 'La reforma de la Beneficencia', p. 39; Martz, *Poverty and Welfare*, pp. 61–2. The brief of 1567 was later confirmed by Pope Gregory XIII in 1584. See Marcos Martín, 'El sistema hospitalario', p. 360.
59 Martz, *Poverty and Welfare*, pp. 79, 243; López Terrada, *El Hospital General de Valencia*, pp. 895–905; Jiménez Salas, *Historia de la Asistencia Social*, pp. 307, 334.
60 Flynn, *Sacred Charity*, p. 104; Santander, *El Hospital del Estudio*, pp. 19–20.
61 Martz, *Poverty and Welfare*, pp. 81–4; Pedro García Barreno, 'El Hospital General de Madrid. Su primer Reglamento (1589). Parte 1', *Arbor*, 153/603 (1996), pp. 55–112; particularly pp. 59–64.
62 Carmona, *El Sistema de la Hospitalidad Pública*, pp. 177–95; Martz, *Poverty and Welfare*, pp. 79–81.
63 Carmona, *El Sistema de Hospitalidad Pública*, pp. 249–53.
64 Marcos Martín, 'El sistema hospitalario', particularly pp. 341–3, 359–62.
65 Flynn, *Sacred Charity*, pp. 102–4.
66 Flynn, *Sacred Charity*, p. 105.
67 Cavillac, 'La reforma de la beneficencia', pp. 16–20; Martz, *Poverty and Welfare*, pp. 71–6.
68 Cavillac, 'Introducción', pp. xxxvii-l, clxxviii-clxxix.
69 Martz, *Poverty and Welfare*, pp. 86–90.
70 Aldea Vaquero *et al. Diccionario*, vol. I, pp. 224–5; Cavillac, 'Introducción', pp. clvi–clvii; Jiménez Salas, *Historia de la Asistencia Social*, pp. 212–13; Pérez de Herrera, *Amparo de Pobres*, pp. 120–5.
71 See Chapter 8 by María Luz López Terrada in this volume.
72 Jütte, *Poverty and Deviance*, pp. 115–16.
73 Aldea Vaquero *et al.*, *Diccionario*, vol. I, p. 219.

9

HEALTH CARE AND POOR RELIEF IN THE CROWN OF ARAGON

María Luz López Terrada

Introduction

Social attitudes to poverty changed radically throughout the sixteenth century, culminating in a negative appraisal of poverty which, unlike the medieval concept, deemed those in need to be a menace and danger to society. This change has been upheld from very different viewpoints by all the authors dealing with this subject, who consider it to be the outcome of multiple and converging reasons found in both the Catholic and Protestant worlds.[1] As mentioned by Michel Cavillac, in the 1580s the differences between the repression system established in the Protestant area and the organised 'protection' found in certain Catholic countries were subtle, since although they were based on different theoretical premises, the resulting practice was very similar.[2] In any case poverty was no longer deemed to be an ethical ideal from either standpoint, a fact which had far-reaching consequences in the measures taken to fight poverty, and also when creating and founding new hospitals in the area which concerns us here: the Crown of Aragon. I believe it necessary to point out that two separate questions are involved: healthcare for the sick, and the measures to curb and attempt to control the increasing problem of poverty. It must be remembered that in the sixteenth century, the medieval hospital began to diverge into two separate institutions: (a) hospitals in the strict sense of the word providing medical care for the sick and generally associated with taking in orphans, and (b) hostels or shelters for the poor.[3] To a certain extent however, both questions were none the less closely linked by the fact that both were community matters dealt with, not in theory but in practice, by the city authorities at a time when the Modern State was being built and had not yet assumed all its future functions. It must be borne in mind that as occurred in Reformation Europe, in the Crown of Aragon, at least in the cities of Barcelona and Valencia, the notion that poor relief, including medical care, was a community and not a church responsibility was definitely established during this period. Those who wished to bring some order into the areas of welfare and health, were guided by the same principles and were oriented to the same goals: elimination of all beggary, and unification of all facilities and resources (hospitals, domiciliary relief and the like) in the hands of municipal or national authorities.[4] Measures of this nature were taken almost exclusively by the city authorities in the Crown of Aragon due to its institutional structure and the survival of a political system under which cities enjoyed considerable autonomy from monarchical power and also had a well-developed capacity for self-government.

The repression of beggary on the other hand was a common feature of the policy implemented by all European cities which was virtually the same everywhere and based on the same principles. The arrival of pauperism and the problems it entailed during the transition between the fifteenth and sixteenth centuries is a detail mentioned in all the historical studies dealing directly or indirectly with this subject which include general papers,[5] more specialised research into poverty in the Modern Age,[6] and even studies on the history of medicine which deal with the history of hospitals.[7] The model of hospital health care for the sick however was different in each case since, as stated by Rosen over thirty years ago, the form, functions and structure of hospitals 'have always been intimately linked with the varying economic, political, social and cultural conditions that govern the life of man. . . . To be understood, the hospital has to be seen as an organ of society, sharing its characteristics, changing as the society of which it is a part is transformed, and carrying into the future evidence of its past'.[8] In this chapter I will attempt to reconstruct the hospital system in the Crown of Aragon, which dealt mainly – as was usually the case until the nineteenth century – with the poorest strata of society. The basic factor taken into account under the most usual approaches to medical healthcare, is the socioeconomic diversification found in all periods and cultures. The model applied to modern European society specifically, dating back to Ancient Greece and developed in the Medieval Christian West, has three-tier, diversified medical health care, one for each social stratum. It is possible to distinguish, in a very simple fashion, between the health care received by the ruling classes who had their private doctors, that of intermediate groups who received basically domiciliary medical care and that of the most vulnerable classes who went to hospitals.[9]

Nevertheless, when taking stock of the resources available in a society to combat disease, it is important to bear in mind, in addition to said diversification, the existence of other forms of medicine i.e. the pluralism of medicine.[10] Following this line of thought, one anthropological viewpoint has been that in any complex society it is possible to identify, apart from the official medicine at any given time, the self-treatment among the population at a popular and domestic level, and the use of non-official medical approaches providing curative alternatives based on a variety of more of less systematised premises.[11] Hence we are aware that while the study of hospital health care is not exhaustive as regards the medical resources available to the population and specifically to the lower socioeconomic groups, it will be exhaustive in terms of the official structure around which said health care is organised.[12]

The Crown of Aragon hospital system

The marriage of the Catholic monarchs in the second half of the fifteenth century brought about the unification of the Crown of Aragon and the Crown of Castile. The Crown of Aragon had come into being in the twelfth century when Catalonia and Aragon were unified, and expanded in a federalist development which in fact consisted of the personal and dynastic union of the different kingdoms which were gradually incorporated (Majorca in 1229, Valencia in 1238, Sicily in 1282, Sardinia in 1323 and Naples in the fifteenth century). Hence it consisted of a plurality of autonomous power structures, characterised by the different social and political codes under the ruling principle of monarchical sovereignty. The union of the Crown of Aragon with Castile took place in accordance with these juridical principles, consequently, although the Spanish monarchy of the sixteenth and seventeenth century was seen from an outside standpoint to have a single voice and a single will, it was in fact a personal, dynastic union of two separate kingdoms which each retained its own constitutional structure and organisation, but had common foreign polices led by the sovereign. Indeed it was only when Charles I, heir to both thrones, came to the throne in 1519, that the two territories were brought together under a single sovereign, although this was far from meaning national unity.

Under this double monarchy, the two crowns were not exactly evenly weighted. The balance tipped clearly in favour of Castile with an inclination to all things Castilian which grew throughout the seventeenth century. Indeed the kingdom of Castile was larger, had a bigger population and a more prosperous economy. The Crown of Aragon in the sixteenth and seventeenth centuries on the other hand conserved its political liberties and jurisdictions (*fueros*) to a greater extent, preserving itself from the trend towards royal absolutism and centralisation, and mantaining its federalistic tradition in sharp contrast with the events of the same period in Castile. Hence, what really existed were several concrete entities: the Kingdom of Aragon, the Kingdom of Valencia, the Principality of Catalonia, the Balearic Islands, etc. Each of these political and social communities had individual characteristics and their own institutions, economic activities and culture.[13]

Our aim, insofar as the sources and studies carried out to date permit, is to reconstruct the Crown of Aragon hospital system. First I will consider the unification of hospitals, particularly those in the three major cities in this area: Saragossa, Valencia and Barcelona.[14] Reference will however be made whenever possible to other places although the hospitals in smaller towns and cities were a reflection on a smaller scale of how the largest three were run, to which people were sent in certain circumstances in order to receive adequate attention, for example foundlings or the insane. Second I will consider the case of Valencia in detail.

Despite the dynastic unification at the end of the fifteenth century and the widespread embrace of the Catholic faith, I believe it possible to talk of the existence of two hospital models in the Hispanic monarchy: the Castile model and that of the Crown of Aragon. The latter is characterised by the fact that since the early sixteenth century the three major cities – capital cities of three of the peninsular kingdoms comprising the Crown – and certain smaller cities had had large hospital centres with great health care capacity and considerable revenue. This situation arose as a result of the hospital unification which had been taking place in the Crown of Aragon since the fifteenth century, which involved a fusion of the services, rents and revenues of the numerous small hospitals into one large hospital, usually known as a 'general hospital'.[15] This process, which apparently commenced in Italy,[16] also began at a very early date in the Aragonese Confederation. Whilst this was doubtless an extremely complex situation, attributed by certain authors to the demographic crisis caused by plague epidemics,[17] it can only be fully explained by taking into account the earlier municipalisation and secularisation processes of hospital medical care taking place in this geographical area since the fourteenth century,[18] together with the impulse these processes received from the political and economic power of the urban oligarchy, the political autonomy and socioeconomic dynamics of the cities where it occurred, and the changes in social attitudes to poverty. The earliest and most significant unification was that which produced the Santa Creu Hospital in Barcelona in 1401 during the reign of Martin the Human.[19] This was followed by the foundation of the Nuestra Señora de Gracia Royal General Hospital in Saragossa by Alfonso V in 1425, and almost 100 years later in 1512 by the fusion of the city of Valencia hospitals. The smaller cities of Tarragona and Jaca managed to carry out this process in 1465 and 1540 respectively. Both instances saw a fusion into just two centres: the one dependent on the municipality and the other on the church.[20]

The first outcome of these unifications was greater financial standing and increased institutional power, incorporating the hospital into the local economy and politics to a greater extent than was the case with the small private hospitals. The management structure of the three large Crown of Aragon general hospitals was very similar. The three hospitals were run by a mixed commission consisting of members of the Church and the urban oligarchy, the former being represented by the cathedral chapter of each city. In Barcelona the commission comprised two citizens and two members of the cathedral chapter. The Saragossa commission was identical but appointed by the king. In Valencia the proportion was different: one cathedral canon and three citizens. The hospitals in Tarragona and Jaca were also run by mixed management boards.[21] Thus unlike the Castilian hospitals which were controlled directly by the Church, none of these hospitals were controlled by fraternities or bishops, but were managed and run by persons belonging to the institutions involved in founding them: the City (through the urban oligarchy) and the Church (through the canons). And while the Crown had played a key role in unifying the Castilian hospitals, its participation in founding those of the Crown of Aragon was limited to granting privileges and arbitration. Until the eighteenth century, except in Saragossa,[22] the Crown did not intervene at all in their management, in keeping with the charter model, although conflicts often arose due to the continuous attempts of the Crown to interfere in hospital management and control. It was not until 1707 with the *Nueva Planta* Decrees and the development of decidedly centralist politics that a legal framework came into being which made royal interventionism possible. This was clearly demonstrated by the wording of the new constitutions and the successive attempts to end the use of Catalan in administrative documents in the Valencia and Catalonia institutions, and also in particular by the fact that in the mid-eighteenth century almost all the hospitals in the Crown began to admit military sick and were consequently renamed General and Royal Hospitals. The Church's participation in the administration of these hospital remained unchanged from their foundation until the end of the eighteenth century when the Church became increasingly involved in hospitals such as that of Valencia with canons from the cathedral or archbishops themselves entering the upper echelons of the management of the institution.[23]

Furthermore, the larger hospitals also offered advantages to patients. Since the new hospitals maintained a full-time staff, many of whom lived in the hospital, a patient could receive benefit from spiritual or physical consolation at any hour of the day or night. Generally speaking, as we will see in more detail in the case of Valencia, the new unified hospitals were responsible for taking in and curing the sick, occasionally dealing with out-patients' illnesses and housing problems, coping with endemic and epidemic public health crises and caring for foundlings and the insane. The three large Crown of Aragon hospitals resulting from unification all provided health care for the sick poor, wherever they came from. House priests in eighteenth century Saragossa for example included confessors in Basque, French and Italian and of course Castilian Spanish. These three hospitals on the other hand all had a considerable number of sick which, at least in Valencia where there are admission records, constantly increased over the years. At the end of the sixteenth century a healthcare crisis of the period was described in a very similar fashion in both the *Santa Creu* and the Valencia General hospitals by the administrators of both.[24] An idea of the size of these hospitals is provided by the fact that the Nuestra Señora de Gracia Hospital wards had 500 sick beds, plus those for foundlings and the insane, and the incredible figure of 17,186 patients treated in the year 1786. Likewise the constitutions of the Saragossa and Valencia hospitals made very similar provisions for admissions: upon arrival the sick were seen by a doctor, their details were put on record and a member of the nursing staff took care of their belongings, which in the event of death would become the property of the Hospital. The three institutions took in a considerable number – which varied according to the circumstances – of manual workers from other regions, for whom the healthcare provided by hospitals was one of the few chances of survival in the event of illness, since they had no access to mutual support from relations.[25] This situation deteriorated during epidemics when those arriving from other regions were trapped in the city by the measures taken by the authorities to combat contagion.[26]

The hospitals in smaller places on the other hand, treated virtually only the sick and poor from the locality, such as the hospital in Tarragona founded to care exclusively for the poor and sick inhabitants of that city. Indeed, at the hospital in Jaca on the Road to Santiago, which treated an average of 38 patients a year, the locals were cared for indefinitely whereas pilgrims only received three days' care.[27]

As mentioned earlier, one of the main goals of unification was to increase revenue and improve finances. The three large hospitals in the Crown had basically the same financial means. The main source of profit of all three came from the alms obtained in a wide variety of ways. The administrators of Valencia and Saragossa for example both greatly increased the amount of alms received (both money and in kind) by setting up a preaching and collection system throughout the kingdom. Another important source of income common to the three centres was the ownership of patrimonial property (houses and land) and annuities. They enjoyed royal and ecclesiastic exemptions and privileges which also increased their income, particularly the concession granted to the three hospitals by the King to operate the theatre houses and bull rings of the three cities. Finally legacies provided a considerable source of revenue throughout this period both in terms of money bequeathed and to an even greater extent by increasing the patrimony of goods and property. The smaller centres relied on the same types of revenue although in smaller quantities. The considerable volume of revenue handled by these institutions was not however without certain economic difficulties. The inflationary period of the second half of the sixteenth century saw the start of financial shortfalls which worsened considerably during the seventeenth century and motivated the search for new sources of income and attempts to curb expenditure. In any case the dawn of the eighteenth century found the three institutions engulfed in economic problems requiring an overhaul of these centres and their financing.[28]

The final noteworthy feature in common was the staff. Research on the three hospitals shows that each institution had virtually the same employees with slightly different titles. The ward seniors were called *pares* in Valencia and Barcelona. The *clavari* (director) in Valencia for example, was the majordomo in Saragossa and the prior in Barcelona. Likewise and more importantly from our viewpoint, in order to be able to provide medical care for the sick who were admitted, the healthcare staff of both the three large hospitals and the smaller ones included not only professionals (doctors, surgeons and apothecaries) but also a variety of menial healthcare workers. One must remember that doctors, surgeons and apothecaries, as in the Crown of Aragon at that time, were quite different professions with well established and completely separate training and qualifications.[29] Because of the similarity of this point in each case and its importance in characterising these hospitals as full medical institutions, I will consider it in greater detail in the case of Valencia. Hence these were modern hospitals to which two characterisations could be equally well applied: that of Santa María Nuova of Florence – 'an institution organized along therapeutic lines and dedicated exclusively to the care of the sick',[30] and that also from Luis Vives in the early sixteenth century, one of the great theoreticians and renovators of the new Renaissance concepts of health care and poor relief – 'In my opinion, a hospital is an institution where the sick are housed and healed, where a certain number of needy are provided for; where boys and girls are educated, foundlings raised, the insane locked up and where the blind spend their life. Let it be known to the city aldermen that a hospital is responsible for all these types of care'.[31] Although Vives' definition is often thought to reflect the healthcare situation of his birthplace, the city of Valencia, I believe the specific context in which the works of Vives should be situated in order to be read and assessed in their true historical perspective is that of the city of Bruges in the early sixteenth century. It is nevertheless feasible to apply this perspective to the healthcare model of the city of Valencia.[32]

The Valencia General Hospital

Valencia General Hospital came into being in 1512 as the result of an Arbitration Decision pronounced by Ferdinand the Catholic that all the hospitals of Valencia should be amalgamated into one. The fusion process, which began in the last quarter of the fifteenth century and finished in 1512, was basically carried out by the city Council and the governors of the Hospital de los Inocentes.[33] It must be remembered that both institutions were run by the same people: the city oligarchy or *ciutadans* who controlled the city economy and political scene,[34] hence the new institution was governed by this group acting via the hospital treasurer, deputies and administrators. However, despite the hospital consolidation taking place, as demonstrated by M. Gallent,[35] to fulfil a municipal agreement to unify all the hospitals within the city boundary, both the management and finances of the new institution were kept independent from the *Consell* (Council). Furthermore, until the end of the eighteenth century this institution was virtually autonomous from the Church and the King, as were the Barcelona and Saragossa general hospitals.[36]

The hospitals unified in 1512 were Los Inocentes (founded in 1409 to care for the insane), Santa Lucia or de la Reina (founded in the thirteenth century and dependent on the municipality), En Clapers hospital (built in 1311 as provided for in a citizen's will) and San Lázaro (a leper house built in the early twelth century). The other four centres in the city: the Poor Priests, San Antonio, En Conill and En Bou hospitals were not included in the unification.[37] These were smaller and provided limited healthcare, for example the En Bou hospital was only for fishermen. This process transformed the city of Valencia medieval healthcare system into an entirely new one by 1512 in which virtually all the healthcare was provided in the new General Hospital founded, as stated in the Arbitration Decision, to admit all types of sick.[38] Besides this general nature, it was also to be the only institution in the city of Valencia providing health care, and in accordance with the Early Modern hospital model, the central place in the city – until the foundation at the end of the seventeenth century of the Casa de Misericordia – to provide poor relief.[39] This centre was designed, as were all the healthcare institutions of the period, to admit the poor i.e. to provide medical care for the lowest social strata. Also, by incorporating Hospital de Inocentes, it also had the mission of relieving families of the responsibility and danger inherent in caring for an insane relation, alleviating society and clearing the streets of mad tramps, and attempting to care for and if possible cure these indigents and destitute.[40] Transforming all these small centres, most of which were unworkable, into a general hospital, required a thorough reorganisation of the healthcare system which remained basically the same until well into the nineteenth century when the Hospital underwent a radical transformation involving its healthcare structure and management methods and even the medical precepts on which it ran. There were none the less other beneficent institutions in the city at that time, but these provided limited medical care very different to that of the Hospital. The most important were the Cofradía de Orfenes a Maridar, the Fraternity of Santa María de los Inocentes y Desamparados and the Colegio Imperial de Huérfanos de San Vicente Ferrer, founded in the fourteenth, fifteenth and the first half of the sixteenth century respectively. The Casa de Misericordia founded in 1640 for the sole purpose of providing shelter and food for the needy,[41] marked a definite separation between healthcare institutions and those providing poor relief.

Early Modern period hospitals were divided into a series of sections or wards where the sick were cared for according to their affliction. In the sixteenth century there were fevers (*febres*), French disease (*mal de siment*) and wounded (*nafrats*) wards. Three wards from the unified hospitals were also retained: the insane ward (*dements*), which as mentioned earlier was that of the former Hospital de los Inocentes; the foundling ward (*borts*), which was the largest section in Hospital de la Reina; and the lepers ward, formerly the leper house. The latter was the only building not vacated: leprosy being considered to be a contagious disease it was thought advisable to keep the sick in the former leper house situated outside the city, although San Lazaro Hospital as such ceased to exist and became a section of the General. The fevers, French disease and insane wards were in turn divided into male and female areas. A convalescence section was added in 1589 which had already been operating for a few years, as an annex to the fevers ward. Likewise in 1665 the wounded ward was closed in order to extend the home for foundlings and to separate children with eye diseases and tinea (*mal de ull, foch o tinya*) from the healthy and thereby avoid contagion.[42] This structure remained unchanged during the eighteenth century although several new sections were created such as the so-called secret chambers where 'single women go in great secrecy to give birth following a moment of weakness'. Similarly there was a room to treat married women who could not be cared for at home during childbirth and another 'well hidden, ornate room where the ailments of noble ladies in need were treated'.[43]

The General Hospital was located on the site of the former Hospital de los Inocentes situated in the west of the city beside the city wall. In 1492, in order to increase Hospital de los Inocentes' healthcare capacity, the construction of a cruciform building was begun – which as its name suggests was a building on a cross-shape plan in keeping with the principles of hospital architecture at that time[44] – which was to be alongside the former lunatic asylum. Construction was halted before completion due to the institution's financial problems and the hospital unification process itself undertaken in those years. Having agreed upon unification, the works necessary to finish the cruciform building and fit it out as a General Hospital were completed in a three-year period. These works were finished quickly thanks to an extraordinary subsidy from the city authorities and by 1517 all the sick had already been transferred from the old hospitals to the new centre. From this date and during the following three centuries, many works and repairs of varying significance were carried out on the Hospital premises. The largest works included the construction of a new cruciform building between 1587 and 1600 and a new church built in 1687. Hence, in the period under study, Valencia General Hospital consisted of two cruciform buildings (one unfinished with just two arms) touching at the tips in a double-X shape. The fevers, French disease and wounded wards were located in the cruciform buildings, with the men upstairs and the women downstairs. The other sections, which underwent more changes, were located around the two cruciform buildings. The insane ward remained in the medieval building between the church and the city wall. All these buildings were separated by orchards and courtyards with such diverse uses as vegetable patches and a cemetery.[45]

By the late sixteenth century the hospital had 279 beds, some with more than one occupant. Straw mattresses were often laid on the floor in the different wards when many patients were admitted and there was a shortage of beds.[46] This situation changed over time and by the mid-eighteenth century the hospital had 580 beds with 'an iron headboard and footboard, four boards all varnished and painted green to avoid any filth; a mattress base, a mattress, two sheets and a blanket, bedspread and pillow'. All the beds were similar except those where viaticum was given, which 'had better bedclothes, always very clean, and two mattresses', and those for the dying which were the same but lower. Next to each bed the sick had 'a stool, bedpan, one glass for water and another for wine, all of which were cleaned twice a day'. According to sources, certain measures of hygiene were applied in the eighteenth century such as changing bed linen every week, dressing the sick in white shirts and 'keeping completely separate beds and clothes for those with contagious diseases',[47] while in previous centuries the sheets, mattress supports and mattresses were apparently washed just once a year and the sick often went naked. The insane were in separate wards, men being totally isolated from women. Likewise the aggressive and non-aggressive insane lived apart. The former were confined to several small rooms or cells known as gabies situated side by side along a corridor separated by adobe partitions. Each cell was independent and access was via a door with iron bars and a padlock. Each cell had a wooden plank bed and chains nailed to the walls with an iron ring on the end to hold the lunatic down during a fit.[48] The peaceful lunatics who lived on the insane ward were free to move around the hospital and could even help finance the centre by going into the city to beg on certain feast days.[49]

The Hospital management structure remained unchanged from its foundation until 1785 when the royal inspector Pedro José Mayoral drafted new constitutions. In principle, the management was in the hands of four administrators elected each year: a canon from Valencia Cathedral, two *jurats en cap* – city aldermen chosen to represent gentlemen and citizens – and one of the ten Inocentes Guild deputies. The latter exercised considerable control over everything happening in the General Hospital since although they had no specific functions, one of them was the administrator and another the *clavari*, an annual post consisting of management tasks with direct control of financial administration and staff supervision. As mentioned earlier, it can be seen that this institution was independent of the city authorities, the Church and the monarchy.[50] According to research by M. Vilar, the earliest royal interferences in hospital management date from 1668 when the king appointed a royal inspector to control the hospital more directly and avoid any abuse or lack of control.

This inspector kept the monarch constantly informed in writing of everything going on in the institution, down to the pettiest detail.[51] However, the monarchy's increasingly centralising trend, which did not accept the totally autonomous fashion in which the institution was run, came to light during the eighteenth century. Unlike what happened in other institutions, Philip V's *Nueva Planta* decree abolishing Valencian privileges, did not bring about any noteworthy changes in hospital management. It was not until 1757 that any attempt was made to dismantle the existing structure. In his royal letters patent of 15 December of that year Ferdinand VI attempted to radically change the management style, substituting the four administrators by a board of thirteen administrators headed by a royally-appointed minister. This reform was given such a cold reception in the city that none of those appointed by Ferdinand VI to manage the hospital would accept the post, hence the reform was not implemented. The definitive administration reform took place during Charles III's reign when new constitutions, drafted by Canon Pedro José Mayoral as a result of a visit made in 1775, were pronounced in order to remedy the institution's pitiful conditions. The outcome of this visit was the 1785 constitutions drafted by Mayoral himself which were approved with slight amendments by the king. These new ordinances marked the end of the Hospital's renaissance organisation which was now controlled by a Board appointed almost entirely by the king, under the leadership of a clergyman, also royally assigned. Consequently, in addition to losing the political autonomy enjoyed to date, this centre, which had always been a wholly secular institution also came to have some ecclesiastic governors.[52]

As mentioned earlier, most of the sick admitted to this institution belonged to the lowest social classes. The 'average patient' was a sick person who worked for a living and was prevented from doing so by sickness and therefore had no income or, to a lesser extent, someone living on charity. In the late sixteenth and early seventeenth century for example, this centre provided medical care for many French emigrants – poorly qualified workers[53] with no family to care for them in the event of illness and who in addition became penniless once obliged to stop working. Hence their only chance of survival or bring cured was being admitted to hospital. It must be remembered that local craftsmen had not only families but also guild support.[54] Consequently the geographic origins of the sick were very heterogeneous and varied according to demographic and economic circumstances. In the case of the insane, the situation was different since 77.81 per cent of those admitted in the seventeenth century – the only period for which admission records survived – came from the Crown of Aragon and most of these were from the Kingdom of Valencia. Only 9.67 per cent were from Castile and 5 per cent from other recorded places, with the remainder being of unspecified origin.

The number of male and female patients varied over the period under study. Broadly speaking the figures tended to increase although the number of annual admissions varied greatly, being directly related to seasonal factors such as epidemics, the king's visits to the city or famine in neighbouring areas. As many as 4,000 admissions could be recorded in such years, as opposed to the normal figure of about 1,000 per annum.[55] We know that the number of sick increased considerably in the eighteenth century. Hence in the middle of the century every year the Hospital was receiving some 500 sick in the fevers, French disease and wounded wards, plus 150 insane, and was feeding approximately 400 foundlings, while the annual yearly figure for number of patients was about 4,000.[56] All the sick on the other hand, except the insane and brothel prostitutes,[57] went to the hospital of their own free will and received free medical care there. Once again the insane were an exception, since only manifest abject poverty of the insane and his relations could exempt them from paying for the hospital stay.[58]

A very revealing fact which demonstrates the medical nature of the hospital and the fact that it was not merely a centre to isolate the insane from society and lock them up, was their admission by the Inquisition. Between 1580 and 1680, 33 persons on trial were sent to the Hospital by the Inquisition Court. According to H. Tropé, who studied each of these cases, the inquisitors mainly considered the Hospital to be a therapy centre to which the accused insane were admitted for treatment before receiving due punishment when discharged. When the Holy Office physicians diagnosed insanity and were unable to punish an offence for the time being, the accused was admitted to hospital, to be held in custody, treated and, if possible, cured. While awaiting their cure, the trial was suspended and the Hospital became a faithful Inquisition collaborator: the *pares de orats* (heads of the insane ward) to whom the insane were delivered, undertook to keep the inquisitors regularly informed of the patient's progress. They were even occasionally required to appear in court, as were the Hospital physician and administrators, to give information about the accused's state of health. Once cured, the accused reappeared in court and the trial continued until the final sentence was passed and punishment imposed. Only two things could prevent the trial from being completed: death in Hospital or escape.[59]

The Hospital had many employees to care for the sick, almost half of whom had medical-care posts. Service employees (cooks, bakers, poultry farmers, etc.) accounted for a third. There were few ecclesiastic staff until 1585 – just a vicar and a chaplain – but after this date when four chaplaincies were founded by the bequests of two city noblewomen, the hospital came to have nine priests, a vicar, four confessors and another four non-confessor chaplains. Bureaucracy was entrusted to employees responsible for administration and management. Although generally speaking the posts were virtually the same from 1512 to 1785, certain minor changes due to new needs took place, such as the increase in physicians or surgeons and likewise a series of new employees on the different wards. It may be said that the healthcare staff throughout this period included both crystallised professions defined socially by regular teaching and qualifications (physicians, surgeons and the apothecary) and menial tasks carried out by persons with no training whatsoever (nurses, service staff, etc.). A strict hierarchy applied to this group, at the top was the physician who visited the sick twice a day and gave the necessary orders to the surgeon who applied the treatments, to the apothecary who prepared the medicines and to the *pares* and *mares* or ward seniors in charge of the different infirmaries. There was also an intern (*bachiller*), assisted by a medical student (*vellant*), who acted to a certain extent as a doctor on duty, being responsible for examining patients upon arrival, remitting them to the corresponding ward, reporting to the physicians every day and supervising the prescriptions sent to the dispensary. All the healthcare staff except physicians were obliged to live on the premises with their families. As may be expected, wages varied considerably and fluctuated from one period to another. The highest wages were paid to physicians, surgeons and the apothecary, and the lowest to the ward domestic staff. In addition to the wages paid in money, all staff also received rations, i.e. amounts paid in kind in different products particularly food. The type and amount of the ration varied according to the category and responsibility of the post.

A key issue which can be roughly reconstructed from available sources, is the medical treatment given to those admitted to the institution. According to the medical precepts of the period, food was of crucial importance in caring for both the healthy to prevent illness, and for the sick to be cured. Hence documentation shows that not all the sick had the same menu, since each patient received the food deemed most suitable for his illness and condition, which was always supervised by the *bachiller* or hospital intern. Generally however the diet was mainly based on the Valencian food system: wheat bread, mutton, chicken, eggs and wine, and also fish during religious fasting periods and vegetables grown in the *huerto* (vegetable patch). Most food was boiled or roasted, and a great deal of soup – which the dietary practice of the period deemed to be vitally important for the sick – and boiled fruit were also served. Very little milk was served due to the physicians' notions concerning its use, and it was only given as medicine.[60]

On the other hand, the sick received the medical or surgical treatment prescribed according to their affliction. The Hospital had a dispensary which complied with the regulations of the City Apothecaries Guild and the medical treatises of that time. All the medicines in the dispensary had specific therapeutic indications and were effective to a great extent. The two great novelties in sixteenth century therapeutics – American products and chemical medicines – did not make their appearance in the dispensary until the mid-seventeenth century. The insane, also deemed to be sick, benefited by these therapeutics too. A variety of operations were also performed both on persons admitted and those who came specifically to be operated on by the surgeons in the institution. Finally, mercurial inunction cures for the French disease were applied in spring and autumn.[61] I believe that the account given so far demonstrates that

Valencia General Hospital was an institution of a decidedly medical nature, like Nuestra Señora de Gracia Hospital in Saragossa and Santa Creu Hospital in Barcelona, providing healthcare and treatment for the poor sick.[62] This fact is clearly shown by the following considerations:

1 Those admitted to hospital were ill, apart from the foundlings, and the majority were farmworkers and craftsmen who came of their own free will to be cured of some illness, including the insane. The Hospital was not a 'refuge for all'.
2 The medical and surgical treatment administered showed that the sick poor were not simply taken in to be sheltered but that the fundamental reason was to cure them. In other words the intention of the hospital governors was above all to provide healthcare to those admitted although in certain cases this meant isolating them from society when deemed necessary for society as in the case of the insane or sufferers from the French disease.
3 The healthcare model established in the sixteenth century was preserved until the mid-nineteenth century when the hospital system was radically transformed, as shown by the fact that the separation of ailments into different wards organised at the start of the sixteenth century remained intact and unchanged until the second half of the nineteenth century.
4 The hospital had a considerable number of health care staff including professionals and ancillary posts. Furthermore, the latter were highly specialised.
5 The hospital had a close relationship from the start with the city municipal university, the Studi General. On the one hand, most of the physicians were also university professors and on the other, there is clear evidence of the use of the Hospital to teach medicine. We can confirm this point by the presence of the *bachiller*, who cared for the sick in exchange for the medical practice he obtained, and the existence on the hospital premises of a *caseta de notomies* (autopsy quarters) since at least 1586.[63]
6 Finally the medical nature of the Hospital is clearly highlighted when dealing with hospital hygiene and planning problems, with the phrase *pulisia del hospital* ('hospital police') being coined at the end of the sixteenth century with regard to the hospital hygiene problems arising when building or restructuring new wards.[64]

In addition to all these considerations, the Hospital served an important purpose in urban community health measures as a whole. There were two specific instances which underlined the Hospital's role in municipal public health problems. The first, somewhat removed from the aims of this chapter, was the collaboration between the city and this centre during plague epidemics,[65] and the other was the participation of its administrators in expelling vagrants from the city, which I will now discuss in detail. The expulsion of vagrants from cities was a measure adopted frequently by urban authorities throughout Europe to curb the growing numbers of poor and beggars. Apparently, according to Braudel, this procedure was particularly common in Mediterranean cities:

> Cities were obliged to maintain public order and to rid themselves, for public health reasons, of the swarming masses of poor: beggars, insane, true and fake cripples, persons without work or gain who crowded squares, taverns and convent soup kitchens. They were expelled but replaced by others. These angry expulsions, indicate the extent of the impotence felt by respectable cities faced with a constant invasion.[66]

The expulsion of vagrants was closely linked to public healthcare problems caused throughout Europe by the growing numbers of poor.[67]

Within the sphere of the Crown of Aragon, I have precise information on the situation in the city of Valencia,[68] where the poor were controlled and received relief from a series of municipal magistrates, such as the *afermamossos* in charge of supervising the unemployed, the *pare de orfens* or official responsible for orphans and the *procurador de miserables* who safeguarded the living conditions of poor prisoners and gave them help and legal aid. Parishes had a 'poor father' responsible for aiding parishioners in times of hardship with food, alms and clothing, and also providing the sick with a doctor, surgeon and medicine.[69] Different local regulations to control beggary were also established such as granting permits to the poor of a particular city. All other poor were deemed to be indigents and as such were repressed by law, particularly by periodic expulsion edicts issued mainly by the Viceroy and occasionally by the city authorities.[70] One such edict issued jointly by the municipal governors and the city hospital administrators in March 1554[71] is of particular interest to our field of study. First it banned foreign beggars from begging for more than three days due to the neediness found in the Kingdom of Valencia and also in Aragon and Catalonia. Secondly it mentions the great number of persons trying to live on charity, differentiating between *pobres mendicants* (poor beggars) and *vagamundos* (vagrants). The latter were accused not only of having no intention of working but also of attempting to invoke Christian mercy by inflicting fake wounds on their arms and legs, placing a considerable economic burden on the Hospital. For all these reasons it was established that foreign beggars should be fed for three days in the hospital and then be obliged to leave the city. Those who did not do so would be taken to the said institution and punished. Beggars from the kingdom on the other hand were also to go to the Hospital where they would be given everything they needed. Finally it was established that anyone sheltering any poor person – differentiating once again between vagrants and beggars – would be fined, since the hospital was the only place authorised to take them in. I believe that this edict clearly demonstrates the fundamentals of late sixteenth century municipal authority policies throughout Europe on the problems arising from growing numbers of needy. These fundamentals, i.e. the provision of relief for poor from the vicinity by more or less specialised institutions and the repression of beggary and expulsion of the poor from other areas particularly those called vagrants, clearly demonstrate poor relief to be a public responsibility, a community matter.[72] A very different question was, as we have seen earlier, healthcare for the sick, regardless of their origins. I believe this fact to be crucially important in order to conclude, as does Linda Martz with regards to Toledo, that there was no material difference between the measures taken in Catholic and Reformation Europe. In the same way, Pullan has demonstrated clearly that cities and countries both Catholic and Protestant, reacted in a very similar way with regard to the poverty and vagrantcy crises, or that Geremek's conclusions concerning European marginalisation as a whole, apply perfectly to the case of Valencia:

> the same chronological journey, the same human drama, the same attempts to deal with the situation and the same impotence when faced with successive crises, were to be found everywhere. Urban reforms, regardless of their effectiveness and duration, had the same resources and the same means: list the poor, expel as many vagrants as possible, select and identify the beggars entitled to aid, centralize charitable and hospital institutions under the control of the municipal authorities, ensure financing for health care . . .[73]

Notes

1 Although the most traditional historiography shows considerable differences in the community welfare found in Protestant Europe and in Catholic Europe, recent studies have a different viewpoint and consider that a veritable revolution in poor relief occurred throughout the continent. See for example J.P. Gutton, *La Société et les pauvres en Europe (XVIe-XVIIIe siècles)*, Paris, PUF (1974); C. Lis and H. Soly, *Pobreza y Capitalismo en la Europa Pre-industrial*, Madrid, Akal (1984); B. Pullan, *Rich and Poor in Renaissance Venice. The Social Institutions of a Catholic State to 1620*, Oxford, Blackwell (1971); L. Martz, *Poverty and Welfare in Habsburg Spain. The Example of Toledo*, Cambridge, Cambridge University Press (1983); J.P. Gutton, *La Société et les pauvres. L'Exemple de la généralité de Lyon*, Paris, Les Belles Lettres. (1971) and N.Z. Davis 'Poor relief, humanism and heresy: the case of Lyon,' *Studies in Medieval and Renaissance History*, 5, (1968) pp. 217–75.

2 M. Cavillac, 'La reforma de la beneficencia en la España del siglo XVI: la obra de Miguel de Gigintia', *Estudios de Historia Social*, 10–11, (1979) pp. 7–60.

3 J.M. López Piñero, *Historia de la Medicina*, Madrid, Historia 16 (1990), p. 37.

4 G. Rosen, 'The hospital. Historical sociology of a community institution', in E. Freidson (ed.) *The Hospital in Modern Society*, London, Macmillan, (1963), pp. 1–63 especially p. 15.

5 H. Kamen, *El Siglo de Hierro*, Madrid, Alianza Universidad (1977), pp. 456–75; F. Braudel, *El Mediterráneo y el Mundo Mediterráneo en la Época de Felipe II*, Madrid, FCE (1976), vol. II, pp. 118–22.

6 In particular J.P. Gutton, *La Société et les pauvres en Europe (XVIe-XVIIIe siècles)*, pp 51–92; B. Geremek, 'Criminalité, vagabondage, paupérisme: la marginalité à l'aube des temps modernes', *Revue d'histoire moderne et contemporaine*, 21, (1974), 337–75; J. Soubeyroux, 'Sur un projet original d'organisation de la bienfaisance en Espagne au XVIe siècle', *Bulletin Hispanique 74*, (1972), pp. 118–24; M. Cavillac, 'La reforma de la beneficencia', pp. 37–9; C. Lis and H. Soly, *Pobreza y Capitalismo en la Europa Pre-industrial*, Madrid, Akal (1984); J.L. Bertran Moya 'Pobreza y marginación en la Barcelona de los siglos XVI y XVII', *Historia Social*, 8, (1990), pp. 101–21.

7 G. Rosen, 'The hospital', p. 15.

8 G. Rosen, 'The hospital', p. 1–2.

9 P. Lain Entralgo, *La Relación Médico-enfermo. Historia y Teoría*, Madrid, Revista de Occidente (1964); López Piñero, *Historia de la Medicina*, pp. 170–1.

10 In the words of López Piñero 'the arrival of modern medicine did not mark the end of the use of magical and religious beliefs to fight disease' which have survived and are still found today in folk medicine and a more complex series of medical systems based on a mixture of religion and the occult, López Piñero, *Historia de la Medicina*. p. 24.

11 E. Perdiguero, 'A propósito de "el Baldaet". Curanderismo y asistencia ante la enfermedad', *Dynamis*, 12, (1992) pp. 309–10.

12 For alternative medicine in the sphere and period of our study, see M.L.

López Terrada, 'El pluralismo médico en la Valencia foral. Un ejemplo de curanderismo', *Estudis*, 20, (1994), pp. 167–81.

13 F.C. Casulla 'L'ordinamento della Corona d'Aragona nei secc. XIV e XV'. *La Corona d'Aragó. El Regne de València en l'Expansió Mediterrània (1238–1492)*,Valencia, Corts Valencianes (1991), pp. 75–80; S. Garcia Martinez, *Valencia bajo Carlos II. Bandolerismo, Reivindicaciones Sociales y Servicios a la Monarquía*, Villena, Ayuntamiento de Villena (1991); P. Iradiel, 'Valencia y la expansión mediterránea de la corona de Aragón'. *La Corona d'Aragó. El Regne de València en l'expansió mediterrània (1238–1492)*, Valencia, Corts Valencianes (1991) pp. 81–8; J. Perez, 'España Moderna (1474–1700). Aspectos políticos y sociales'. In J. Le Flem *et al.* (eds), *La Fustración de un Imperio (1476–1714)*, Barcelona, Labor (1982), pp. 136–259; J. Regla, *De les Germanies a la Nova Planta*, Barcelona, Edicions 62 (1989).

14 For information on the Santa Creu Hospital, Barcelona, see J. Danon Bretos, *Visió Histórica de l'Hospital General de Santa Creu de Barcelona*, Barcelona, Fundació Salvador Vives Casajuana (1978). For the Nuestra Señora de Gracia General Hospital, see J. Gimero Riera, *La Casa de Locos de Zaragoza y el Hospital de Nuestra Señora de Gracia. Apuntes Históricos, 1425–1808–1908*, Zaragoza, G. Gasca (1908); A. Baquero, *Bosquejo Histórico del Hospital Real y General de Nuestra Señora de Gracia de Zaragoza*, Zaragoza, Institución Fernando el Católico (1952); F. Zubiri Vival, 'Ordinaciones del Hospital Real y General de Nuestra Señora de Gracia de Zaragoza', *Zaragoza*, 24, (1966), pp. 95–124; and A. Fernandez Doctor and A. Martinez Vidal 'El médico en el Hospital de Nuestra Señora de Gracia de Zaragoza en el siglo XVIII', *Dynamis*, 5–6, (1985–86), pp. 143–58. For the Valencia General, see M. L. López Terrada, 'El Hospital General de Valencia en el siglo XVI (1512–1600)', doctoral thesis, Valencia (1986); M. Vilar Devis 'El Hospital General de Valencia en el siglo XVII (1600–1700)'. doctoral thesis, Valencia (1990); C. Ciscar Vilalta, 'El Hospital General de Valencia en el siglo XVIII (1700–1800): El edificio, el gobierno, el personal y la asistencia', doctoral thesis, Valencia, (1992).

15 Martz, *Poverty and Welfare*, p. 34.

16 See J. Henderson 'The hospitals of late-medieval and Renaissance Florence: a preliminary survey', in L. Granshaw and R. Porter (eds) *The Hospital in History*, London, Routledge. (1989), pp. 64–92.

17 See J.M. Comelles *et al.*, *L'Hospital de Valls*, Valls, Institut d' Estudis Vallencs, (1991), p. 111.

18 For example in Valencia, see A. Rubio Vela, *Pobreza, enfermedad y asistencia hospitalaria en la Valencia del siglo XIV*, Valencia, Instituto 'Alfons el Magnànim' (1984).

19 Danon Bretos, *Visió Histórica*, p. 18.

20 For Tarragona: J.M. Miquel Parellada and J. Sanchez Real, *Los hospitales de Tarragona*, Tarragona, Diputación de Tarragona (1959); for Jaca: J. Carrasco Almazor *et al.*, *La Vida hospitalaria en Jaca*, Jaca, no publisher, (1983).

21 Cf. notes 14 and 20.

22 In other aspects such as control of the medical profession, royal

intervention was also more pronounced in Aragon than in the other kingdoms of the Crown.

23 Cf. notes 14 and 20. For Valencia the policy implemented by the new dynasty in relation to the hospital, see M. Peset Reig and J.L. Peset Reig, 'Felipe V y el Hospital Real y General de Valencia', *Medicina Española*, 61, (1969), pp. 405–14.

24 Danon Bretos, *Visió Histórica*, p. 39.

25 As M. Jimenez Salas notes in *Historia de la Asistencia Social en España en la Edad Moderna*, (Madrid, CSIC, 1958): 'un mundo pobre y enfermo se albergaba en tales casas, propias de las ciudades importantes'.

26 For the Barcelona case, see Bertran Moya, 'Pobreza y marginación', pp. 110–11.

27 Cf. notes 14 and 20.

28 Cf. note 14.

29 L.M. López Piñero, *Ciencia y Técnica en la Sociedad Española de los Siglos XVI y XVII*, Barcelona, Labor (1979), pp. 49–57.

30 K. Park and J. Henderson 'The first hospital among Christians': The Ospedale di Santa Maria Nueova in early sixteenth-century Florence', *Medical History*, 35, (1991), 169.

31 J.L. Vives, *Obras completas*, translate by Lorenzo Riber, Madrid, Aguilar (1947), vol. I, 1392. For an analysis of the works of Vives from a health-care standpoint, see J.M. López Piñero, *Ciencia y Técnica*, pp. 34–9.

32 For other features of municipal welfare and health care in the city of Valencia cf. V.L. Salavert Fabiani and V. Graullera Sanz, *Professió, Ciencia i Societat a la València del segle XVI*, Barcelona, Curial (1990); V.L. Salavert Fabiani and J. Navarro, *La Sanitat Municipal a València (segles XII-XX)*, Valencia, IVEI (1992); López Piñero, *Historia de la Medicina*, p. 37.

33 M. Gallent Marco, 'El proceso de unificación de los hospitales valencianos (1482–1512)', *Estudios dedicados a Juan Peset Aleixandre* (1982, pp. 69–84), analyses the entire process, mentioning the various attempts and agreements which occurred in this period.

34 See J. Mouyen, 'Identificació i riquesa de l'oligarquía urbana', *Afers*, 23/24, pp. 201–42 (1996).

35 M. Gallent Marco, 'El proceso de unificación', p. 32.

36 It must be borne in mind that the local power itself was engulfed in the dialectics of local interest in defending to the hilt the extent of autonomy enjoyed versus the monarchical desire to control the municipality. In certain respects this is what occurred to those governing the hospital.

37 For medieval Valencian hospitals, see R.I. Burns, 'Los hospitales del Reino de Valencia en el siglo XIII', *Anales de Estudios Medievales*, 2, (1965), pp. 135–54; M. Gallent Marco, 'La asistencia sanitaria en Valencia (1400–1512)', doctoral thesis, Universidad de Valencia. (1980); F.P. Garcia Sabater, 'Memoria de un antiguo y olvidado hospital valenciano, el de en Bou', *Valencia Atracción*, 480, (1975), pp. 16–25; J. Guiral 'L'assistance aux pauvres à Valance – Espagne (1238–XVIe siècle)', *Actas de las I Jornadas de Metodología aplicada a las ciencias históricas*, (1975), pp. 323–6; J. Rodrigo Pertegàs, 'Hospitales de Valencia del siglo XV', *Boletín de la Real Academia de Historia*, 90 (2), (1927), pp. 561–602; A. Rubio Vela, *Pobreza I, enfermedad y asistencia hospitalana*

en la Valencia del siglo XIV, Valencia, Inst. 'Alfons el Magnànim' (1984). F. Vilanova 'El hospital de en Bou', *Revista Valenciana de Ciencias Medicas*, 16, (1914), pp. 175–86; R. Zaragoza Rubira 'Breve historia de los hospitales valencianos', *Medicina Española*, 47, (1962), pp. 152–60, 237–47, 275–6.

38 Archivo de la Diputación Provincial de Valencia (ADPV). Box IV–4/4.2. 1512 *Constitutions*, Chapter 44: 'que huy avant no hi haura ninguna hospitalitat particular, sino que sera hospital general'.

39 Ibid., chapter 1: 'en lo dit Spital General e no en altra part de la dita ciutat e raballs de aquella se tinga hospitalitat por als malats pobres'.

40 H. Trope, *Locura y Sociedad en la Valencia de los siglos XV al XVII*, Valencia, Diputació de València (1994), p. 182. This author maintains that the madhouse was not a hermetic place where people were imprisoned, but an isolation area with the dual mission of control and curing.

41 Salavert Fabiani and Navarro, *La sanitat municipal* p. 65.

42 López Terrada, 'El Hospital General de Valencia en el siglo XVI'; Vilar Devis, 'El Hospital General de Valencia'; Ciscar Vilalta, 'El Hospital General de Valencia en el siglo XVIII'.

43 I. Esplugues, *Relación y noticia de la fundación del Hospital real y general de la ciudad de Valencia.* (probably Valencia), 1739.

44 The cruciform pattern emerging from Florence then pervaded the rest of Europe. See John D. Thompson and Grace Goldin, *The Hospital. A Social and Architectural History*, Yale University Press, (1975); J. Henderson, 'The hospitals of late-medieval and Renaissance Florence: a preliminary survey', in: L. Granshaw and R. Porter (eds), *The Hospital in History*, London, Routledge (1989).

45 For a detailed study of the other works on the hospital premises see López Terrada, 'El Hospital General de Valencia en el siglo XVI'; Vilar Devis, 'El Hospital General de Valencia en el siglo XVII'; Ciscar Vilalta, 'El Hospital General de Valencia en el siglo XVIII'.

46 Apparently this often happened on the syphilis ward in spring and autumn, these being the times of year when mercury inunctions were applied. See López Terrada 'El tratamiento de la sífilis en un hospital renacentista: la sala del mal de siment del Hospital General de Valencia', *Asclepio*, 41 (2), (1989), pp. 19–50.

47 Esplugues, *Relación y noticia.*

48 Vilar Devis, 'El Hospital General de Valencia en el siglo XVII', pp. 1025–6.

49 Trope, *Locura y Sociedad*; Vilar Devis, 'El Hospital General de Valencia en el siglo XVII'; López Terrada, 'El Hospital General de Valencia en el siglo XVI'.

50 López Terrada, 'El Hospital General de Valencia en el siglo XVI'.

51 Vilar Devis, 'El Hospital General de Valencia en el siglo XVII'.

52 For the process of drafting the new constitutions and the preceding visit see Ciscar Vilalta, 'El Hospital General de Valencia en el siglo XVIII'.

53 Exact figures in López Terrada, 'El Hospital General de Valencia en el siglo XVI'; Vilar Devis, 'El Hospital General de Valencia en el siglo XVII' pp. 925–927. For French emigration to Valencia see Potrineau, 'La inmigración francesa en el Reino de Valencia (siglos XVI–XIX)', *Moneda y Crédito*, 137, (1976) pp. 103–33. Statements of the period

bear witness to the public contempt for these immigrants, one of the most explicit being that of Gaspar Escolano, author of a history of Valencia in the early 17th century: '. . . (there were) so many French, flocking like sheep to escape from the harshness of their kingdoms to the utmost tranquillity and Christianity they know Spain offers', (G. Escolano, *Decada primera de la Historia de la Insigne y Coronada Ciudad y Reyno de Valencia*, Valencia, Pedro Patricio Mey, (1610–11), vol. I, p. 100).

54 Salavert Fabiani and Navarro, *La sanitat municipal*, pp. 84–7.

55 López Terrada, 'El Hospital General de Valencia en el siglo XVI' and Vilar Devis, 'El Hospital General de Valencia en el siglo XVII' for detailed studies of annual admissions over the 16th and 17th century; and H. Trope, *Locura y Sociedad*, for studies of admissions and stays of the insane between the foundation of the Hospital de los Inocentes and the late 17th century.

56 Esplugues, *Relación y noticia*.

57 The insane were taken to the Hospital either by their families or by the municipal authorities and in some cases mentioned later were remitted by the Inquisition. Prostitutes on the other hand were required to see the surgeon appointed by the city for this purpose each week, and in the event of illness were obliged to stop work immediately and be admitted to the Hospital for treatment, to the syphilis ward as may be expected. See V. Graullera Sanz, 'Un grupo social marginado: las mujeres públicas (el burdel de Valencia en los siglos XVI y XVII)', *Actas du II colloque sur le Pays Valencien a l'Epoque Moderne*, (1980) and López Terrada, 'El tratamiento'.

58 Information on the insane is from H. Trope, *Locura y sociedad*, pp. 175–82.

59 Ibid., pp. 183–206. The paper which we have briefly summarised is based on both hospital and inquisition sources including certain trials.

60 López Terrada, 'El Hospital General de Valencia en el siglo XVI'; Vilar Devis, 'El Hospital General de Valencia en el siglo XVII'; Ciscar Vilalta 'El Hospital General de Valencia en el siglo XVIII'.

61 López Terrada, 'El Hospital General de Valencia en el siglo XVI'; López Terrada, 'El tratamiento', pp. 19–50. For the specific treatment administered to the insane, see Trope, *Locura y sociedad*, pp. 258–70.

62 J. Henderson 'The hospitals of late-medieval and Renaissance Florence', finds in Renaissance Florentine hospitals active medical care too, and S. Cavallo, in 'Charity, power, and patronage in eighteenth-century Italian hospitals: the case of Turin' in L. Granshaw and R. Porter (eds), *The Hospital in History*, London, Routledge. (1989) pp. 93–122, 97; explains that some charitable institutions in Turin seem to have been designated for the sick from the time of their foundation. As we said earlier, the Crown of Aragon hospitals in this period are very similar to the Italians.

63 This was the area where autopsies were carried out, according to López Piñero, *Ciencia y Técnica* p. 102; and was used by *Estudi* university professors. Luis Collado for example when referring to an item of vascular anatomy, mentioned in a 1588 manuscript that '*visus novis fuit in hospicum pauperum Valenciae 3 die mensibus, in loco ad anatomes exercendum*', quoted by L. Garcia Ballester, 'Las obras médicas de Luis

Collado (died 1569)', Nota a propósito de un manuscrito del British Museum (MS Sloane, 2489). *Asclepio*, 23, 263–70 (1971), 267–8. This date, thought to be the earliest reference to the autopsy quarters, can be brought backward to 1586 because a lawsuit concerning the construction of a new ward in that year made frequent reference to it, situating it next to the hen run and the plaster works.

64 López Terrada, 'El Hospital General de Valencia en el siglo XVI', pp. 605–7.

65 López Terrada, 'La colaboraciòn de la ciudad de Valencia y el Hospital General ante las epidemias de peste del siglo XVI', in M. López Piñero, H. Capel and J. Pardo (eds), *Ciencia e ideología en la ciudad*, pp. 37–45 Valencia, Consellería d'obres pùbliques, Urbanisme i transports (1992); Vilar Devis, 'El Hospital General de Valencia en el siglo XVII'.

66 Braudel, El Mediterráneo, p. 118. Such expulsions were not limited to the Mediterranean area but were also frequent in the Crown of Castile. For concrete measures taken by a city to combat begging, see B. Bennassar, Valladolid en el Siglo de Oro, Valladolid, Fundación Municipal de Cultura (1983) on Valladolid, and L. Martz, *Poverty and Welfare*, on Toledo.

67 B. Geremek 'Criminalité, vagabondage, paupérisme', p. 359.

68 For Barcelona, see J.L. Bertran Moya 'Pobreza y Marginación' p. 118, correlating the expulsions carried out by the *Consell de Cent* and the plague epidemics.

69 Salavert Fabiani and Navarro, *La sanitat municipal*, p. 63.

70 Braudel, *El Mediterráneo*, pp. 119–120; M.D. Minguillon Ortega, 'El justicia criminal de Valencia durante el reinado de Felipe II: delitos y sentencias', licentiate thesis, Universidad de Valencia (1981), 72. These authors gathered specific information on the expulsions of unemployed persons carried out in 1576 and 1583 respectively. See also Salavert Fabiani and Navarro, *La sanitat municipal* p. 64.

71 A.D.P.V. IV–2/2, folios 76v–77v: 'Los dits administradors . . . provehixen que faça la crida ordinaria per a bandejar los pobres vagamundos'. The crida is reproduced in full in López Terrada, 'El Hospital General de Valencia en el siglo XVI' p. 120.

72 M. Cavillac, 'Introducción', to C. Perez de Herrera, *Amparo de pobres*, Madrid, Espasa-Calpe. (1975), pp. 1–195, especially p. 81.

73 Geremek, 'Criminalité, vagabondage, paupérisme', pp. 364–5.

10

POOR RELIEF IN COUNTER-REFORMATION PORTUGAL: THE CASE OF THE *MISERICÓRDIAS*

Isabel M. R. Mendes Drumond Braga

Translated by Christine Salazar

During the Counter-Reformation era, Portugal was an integrated part of the network of kingdoms which formed Catholic Europe. Therefore the worries, problems and – in the case with which we are dealing here – the forms taken by assistance to the poor, did not differ fundamentally from those in the other Southern-European countries. Nevertheless, there was scope for some variety on various levels, the most notable being, in the field of poor relief, the creation of the Misericórdias.

The Lisbon Misericórdia, founded in 1498, served as a model, in organisational terms, for all the others. It was established in the reign of King Manuel, and the foundation took place under the auspices of Queen Leonor, widow of the previous monarch, João II. The role played by the queen is not quite clear however, i.e. one does not know whether Queen Leonor took the initiative or whether she limited herself to being the voice of those involved with the problems of poor relief.

It must not be forgotten that the foundation of the Misericórdia dovetails with a tradition of lay philanthropy shared with the rest of Christendom. It was a period of peace, centralisation and wealth as a result of overseas expansion, but it was also a period characterised by various reforms in the field of administration. One need therefore not be surprised if the reform of poor relief – which had already begun earlier – took on larger proportions during Manuel's reign.

On the other hand, the extension of the network of Misericórdias (throughout the entire kingdom as well as the Portuguese territories scattered around the globe) during the sixteenth and seventeenth centuries coincides with a strong Church presence in society. Obviously this is not a new factor, but respect for the sacraments became more widespread – something which has to be seen in relation to the greater pressure exerted on priests as far as the fulfilment of their functions was concerned. Also, the creation of new dioceses in Portugal as well as overseas allowed a better religious coverage of the population and more efficient action on the part of the clergy.[1] The latter was becoming more and more disciplined and determined in the fulfilment of its functions after the Council of Trent, despite initial opposition to the reforms on the part of some sections.[2] On the other hand, the Inquisition, pastoral visits, the celebration of synods and the creation of institutions such as the Mesa da Consciência e Ordens, all attempted to confront attitudes among lay people and among members of the Church that could be considered outside orthodoxy. One should also remember the growth of the clergy, and especially of the religious orders, which would give the Crown scope for intervention.

At the end of the fourteenth century and the beginning of the fifteenth, Portugal witnessed a decline of the establishments for poor relief. This was due to poor management by the administrators (*provedores*) as well as the economical and monetary crisis, combined with a decline in population and an increase in armed conflicts. This situation permitted (especially in the fifteenth century) an increase in royal intervention in the administration of hospitals, which resulted in the nomination of persons trusted by the monarch for ensuring the management of the establishments (causing protests by the court councils), and in an increased number of *compromissos*, or regulations, that facilitated royal control and minimised abuse by the *provedor*.[3]

It was, however, only from 1498 that important modifications took place in Portugal as far as relief was concerned. In fact, it was at that date that a confraternity was created in Lisbon, under the invocation of Nossa Senhora, Mãe de Deus, Virgem Maria da Misericórdia (Our Lady, Mother of God, Virgin Mary of Mercy). It was therefore generally referred to as the Misericórdia. It gave impulse to the reform of relief, already begun in relation to the concentration of hospitals, when Misericórdias were formed in quick succession in the kingdom of Portugal as well as in the Portuguese territories in Africa, Asia and America. These were lay confraternities under the afore-mentioned invocation, with direct protection by the king. It is true that in medieval Portugal there had been many confraternities for devotion, charity and mutual help as well as socio-professional ones,[4] but it is also true that the Misericórdia presented characteristics different from these earlier ones, such as privileges granted by the king, and the social, economical and spiritual assistance being given to the entire community and not only to the limited core of the brethren.[5]

Although the Misericórdias were modelled on the one in Lisbon, each of them functioned autonomously, with its own statutes – the *compromissos* – subject to royal confirmation. Even where the *compromisso* of Lisbon[6] was adopted, the Misericórdias were local, independent institutions, based however on common principles, thus guaranteeing uniformity among them.[7] Indeed, these principles were the fourteen works of mercy, divided into spiritual (instructing the ignorant, counselling those requiring it, admonishing those who err, comforting the afflicted, forgiving offences, suffering wrongs patiently, and praying for the living and the dead) and corporal works of mercy (nursing the sick, clothing the naked, giving drink to the thirsty, harbouring strangers, assisting prisoners and captives, and burying the dead).

Because of that, it fell to the Misericórdias to, for example, conduct the funerals of confraternity members and their relatives, as well as of the poor and those condemned to death; also, the assistance to poor prisoners, the treatment of those who were sick and poor, home-help for the poor, and the giving of dowries to orphan girls. These activities were performed by the confraternity members as voluntary work, mainly in specialised institutions administered by the Misericórdia, such as general hospitals, orphanages and hostels for women.[8] The carrying-out of these activities by the Misericórdia members gave them a community-oriented aspect, guaranteeing something like a nationwide social service not subject to the central bureaucracy.[9]

The Misericórdias also accumulated considerable possessions, both through direct donations of goods and real estate, and through acquisitions made by the administrative bodies using funds from earlier legacies in the form of chapels and masses. Many donors attempted to preserve in some way the donated goods by establishing an entail, thus making them inalienable and only to be administered by the Misericórdia. It needs to be kept in mind that the Misericórdias, being in charge of funerals and burials, were guaranteed the accumulation of considerable pious legacies and inheritances, as well as having royal authorisation to claim alms for which purpose they had authorised lawyers, called *mamposteiros*.[10]

Belonging to the local Misericórdia meant enjoying the benefits of an Order. Although the proportion of nobles to commoners varied, the brethren were not allowed to be manual workers. In this case, however, the term 'noble' did not necessarily imply noble blood: churchmen, the well-to-do and some professional groups were also included under this heading.[11] The brotherhood was governed by an assembly of thirteen; ten of these made up the *Mesa* and the rest were the provost, the scribe and the treasurer.

Several conditions were required for admission to the Misericórdia, such as being neither Moorish nor Jewish, nor being married to persons of such blood, leading an honest and God-fearing life, serving the institution without hope of gain, and being able to read and write. It was also advisable to have a stable personal financial position.[12] The restrictions regarding Moorish and Jewish blood were introduced at the Lisbon Misericórdia at the end of the sixteenth century, and were current practice in the entire system during the first quarter of the seventeenth century. This complied with a principle in effect in Spanish and Portuguese society, namely *limpenza de sangue* (purity of blood), which tended to discriminate against converted Jews, Moors, blacks, mulattos and gypsies, preventing them from entering municipal councils or chambers, universities, military orders and cathedral chapters. It is known, though, that in many cases – including the Misericórdias – blood barriers were transgressed.[13]

That the exclusion was resented by the minorities is clear from the fact that some elements of those minorities did not abstain from criticising the Misericórdias in a derogatory way. One example is the case of some converted Jews (who had obviously not assimilated their catechism). They were accused of uttering disrespectful opinions about the institution, saying things such as: 'Look what rags they are adoring' – referring to the flag of the Misericórdia carried in procession by Old-Christians. Another apparently did not shrink from saying that he 'didn't give a shit for the Misericórdia'.[14]

It seems beyond doubt that, in addition to providing an important aid network, the Misericórdias also represented a strong local power factor, in competition with other authorities such as the civic councils, or even the bishop or the chapter.[15] Although the Misericórdias were created at a time of royal centralism, they must not be confused with it since they began to contribute to the strengthening of local government. The figure of the king did, however, have its importance, be it on a symbolical level – the royal crest on portals, and the king's picture on the flags – or on the level of protection. The monarch not only gave support to these institutions, but he also gave direct incentive to their propagation by writing to the chambers suggesting the creation of local Misericórdias. It was clearly his intention to endow the kingdom with a body of uniform institutions, in order that eventually it would become easier for the royal authority to penetrate the sphere of local government.

There was yet another characteristic aspect to these brotherhoods, i.e. the laicisation of aid. Poor relief was effectively, and progressively, withdrawn from the control of the Church authorities. Nevertheless, the aims of the brotherhood were closely related to the Christian faith. Despite the participation of clergymen in the Misericórdias (and in powerful positions at that), these duties were performed in the context of an institution that functioned under royal patronage.[16]

It is impossible to quantify which spiritual works of mercy had the greatest relevance in the mentality of the time (what was considered the worst poverty was the kind that led to the perdition of the soul), but it is easier to make some conjectures regarding the corporal works of mercy. The creation of Misericórdias went hand in hand with the annexation of the local hospitals to the respective Misericórdias, a process which became more pronounced in the second half of the sixteenth century. This made it possible to extend aid to a larger number of people by having it centralised in a hospital of greater resources and proportions, which replaced small individual hospitals. The forms of social solidarity developed by the medieval confraternities were continued, but now they were adapted to the needs of a larger population.[17]

It fell to the State to take measures in exceptional cases, such as during and after epidemics. Indeed, from an early date the treatment of the sick had become a preoccupation of private persons as well as the Crown. In 1526 Pedro Vaz was nominated Inspector-General of Health; he had travelled to various Italian cities with the purpose of studying solutions adopted by them in the case of epidemics. It should not be forgotten that from at least the fifteenth century the Portuguese Crown took some measures against the plague. Given that the true causes of the plague were then unknown, it is not surprising that in most cases these measures proved powerless. Among them was the escape of people from affected areas to safe zones, which at times led to a spread of the plague. It seems, however, that the evacuation of infected areas was actually established by the authorities, under royal orders and upon medical advice.[18] Other measures required the isolation of those infected and of the infected areas. Ports were particularly subject to control, given that the authorities had to check where a ship had come from, and prevent its entry, if it came from an area hit by the plague. Those travelling by land, too, had to declare to the authorities where they came from, having to pay fines (which were used for the benefit of captives) if they lied about this point.[19]

The Crown also had the task of creating emergency hospitals (although most of the patients stayed in their own homes), which were destroyed after the end of the epidemic. At least that was what happened in the second half of the fifteenth century.[20] Other measures aimed at restricting the spread of the plague were the closing-down of schools, the prohibition of public festivals and the burning or disinfecting of the clothes that had belonged to the dead. As a contagious disease, the plague, just like leprosy, belonged to the realm of public health and was therefore the domain of royal and municipal authorities.

Throughout Early Modern times, the number of medical graduates increased as well. Some studied in Portugal, others abroad, especially at French and Spanish universities, or even at the hospital of the monastery of Guadalupe. On the other hand, after the final removal of the Portuguese university of Lisbon to Coimbra in 1537, the presence of various Spanish doctors became common. Other than these, there were also the barber-surgeons, midwives and apothecaries, who were distributed unevenly throughout the kingdom, showing greater concentration in the cities.[21] The practice of medicine by unqualified practitioners was very widespread, while the Crown permitted individuals without university training to treat certain diseases, if they had been examined and approved by the Surgeon-General.[22]

Thus exceptional measures in times of crises were the reserve of the Crown and the local authorities, while the Misericórdias – through the hospitals they administered – were in charge of the day-to-day assistance to the sick, in particular to those who were needy.

Since the beginning of the sixteenth century, it had been the local authorities in Portugal who were in charge of the upbringing of abandoned children, but in the major cities and towns of the kingdom the chambers transferred this task to the local Misericórdias, although the former continued to fund this activity. During the seventeenth and eighteenth centuries contracts between the two institutions were common.[23]

In the seventeenth century, Portugal was already using the 'wheel' for receiving abandoned children – a mechanism which would be used in Spain, Italy and Southern France (later in all of France), but not in England, where there was no anonymity in abandoning children.[24] The wheel was a hollow wooden cylinder, revolving upon an axle, and situated in a window. It had a single opening, thus making it impossible for the person leaving the child and for the one receiving it to see each other. The arrival of a child was signalled by a bell, and the child was immediately taken in and cared for by the nurses.[25] Assistance included baptism, if the sacrament had not been administered, and the entire care was entrusted to a nurse who would bring up the child at her home.

The council's obligation regarding the support of abandoned children finished when the children reached the age of 7. From then on, the children were under the tutelage of the judges of orphans, whose responsibility was limited to introducing the children into the labour market. Unlike Italy, where the hospitals tended to keep abandoned children up to adult age – especially girls, of whose marriage the institution was in charge – in Portugal the judges had to find somebody to take the children in, i.e. a family who would employ them and care for them. The judges' duties terminated when the children attained majority at the age of 20, five years earlier than other young people.[26]

For orphans the situation was different. In the case of children who were to inherit, legal mechanisms had to be created to safeguard the administration of these inheritances, to avoid the orphans being cheated out of their patrimony. Orphans were under the protection of the judges of orphans, who were in charge not only of abandoned children over the age of 7 and of the disabled, but also had control over guardianships and trusteeships, the registering of all the orphans in the locality, the confirmation or nomination of guardians and trustees, and the inventorying of goods. They had to guarantee that the education, upbringing and marriage of the orphan corresponded to the quality and condition of the person, and to judge civil-law cases in which under-age orphans were involved. In the case of poor orphans, the aim was to teach the boys a trade and the girls housework.[27]

In the case of female orphans, dowries and hostels were used; in fact, the Misericórdias instituted dowries and imposed rules of conduct. It was understood that those provided with dowries had to remain virgins, could not leave the place where they lived without authorisation from the Misericórdia, and had to inform it of the day on which they intended to marry.[28] In some cases there were also local safe houses, i.e. houses in which the women were enclosed in order to protect them from society, although reintegration into society by marriage was desired.[29] In the safe houses the women received elementary instruction: reading, writing, religious doctrine, sewing and embroidery. Most of these houses were founded after the Council of Trent,[30] and they contributed to maintaining chastity, a virtue that was highly prized during the Counter-Reformation. It has to be added that widows or unmarried women who were exposed to poverty because of the lack of a husband or a father were also the object of the Misericórdia's aid, as long as they preserved irreproachable behaviour.[31]

Independently of the Misericórdias, the first institution intended for orphans which functioned in Portugal entirely under the responsibility of the State was founded in 1780 and called Casa Pia de Lisboa. It was an agglomerate of different establishments committed to various categories of the needy, namely beggars, the elderly and children without protection. At the time, the idea of charity and social aid being obligations of the State towards the citizens was beginning to present itself.[32]

According to their statutes, the Misericórdias were also bound to assist prisoners. In their case, the aid given had to take into account the degree of poverty and the worthiness of the cause. It was the task of the Misericórdias to guarantee expenses incurred for lawsuits for release, and for food, which was provided twice weekly, on Sundays and Wednesdays.[33] During some periods, e.g. at the end of Holy Week, the prisoners were given a festive meal. Some Misericórdias were also in charge of the cleanliness of prisons and of the sustenance of imprisoned slaves, although their masters later had to reimburse the institution.[34]

As for those condemned to death, they had to be accompanied by brethren of the Misericórdia, who provided them with food and spiritual assistance. The brethren then saw to it that, after death, the bodies were collected and buried in consecrated ground. The Misericórdia then had mass said, and annually on All Saints' Day, a procession was held in memory of those who had been executed.

Because of Portugal's geographical situation and because of its expansion to other continents, many were taken prisoner by Moslems. Factors contributing to facilitate the capture of Christians by Moors were the raids, especially on the Algarve coast, fishing and travel on the Atlantic, and the Moors' continued presence in fortified places in North Africa. This situation had first begun to produce a reaction in the twelfth century, when the religious orders for the release of captives were founded, and was still present in Early Modern times.[35] The Crown had always preferred general ransom to individual liberation, making the former its responsibility from 1461 to 1561. From then on the task finally became the monopoly of the Trinitarian order, although the sources of funds varied – such as collections of alms, donations and legacies by bequest, the goods of those who died intestate, goods found without owners, as well as fines.[36]

Nevertheless, some Misericórdias also attended to the ransoming of captives. Following its *compromissos*, the Porto Misericórdia stipulated that priority be given to women and children, and that help for ransoming be given by preference to those from the city, and only then to those from outside.[37] As for the Setubal Misericórdia, such transactions only took place when there was a bequest especially destined for this purpose.[38] In effect, although the ransoming of prisoners was a work of charity, it was mainly in the hands of the State[39] and not of the Misericórdias.

In conclusion, the most notable aspect of aid in Portugal was the incorporation of a number of institutions under the administration of the Misericórdias. In little more than a century the Misericórdias took root on the Atlantic islands, in Africa, India and China, hand in hand with the settling of Portuguese in the new territories. One hundred and twelve were founded between 1498 and 1599. During the second half of the sixteenth century and all of the seventeenth, the tendency towards restricting admission to the brotherhood grew. As the number of brethren increased, at the same time their social origin became narrower, and thus the Misericórdia became more and more strongly controlled by a restricted elite. This situation contributed to their decline in the eighteenth century, when some houses were reduced to lending money at interest in order to support their income.

The Misericórdias, created well before the beginning of the Counter-Reformation, within a mental framework close to that of Catholic Reform, nevertheless emphasised modes of behaviour that were not alien to those the Counter-Reformation defended. It is not quite possible, though, to draw conclusions about the influence of either process on the other. It should be noted that in 1562 – on the occasion of a Portuguese delegation participating in the Council of Trent – the Pope created the system of 'confraternities under royal protection'. This meant that the foundation of these institutions depended on the king, and that the bishops had the right to intervene only in questions of church maintenance and cult ornaments. In practice, royal protection meant that life inside the Misericórdias was not subject to scrutiny by the Church authorities; thus charity became laicised, although the principles of its exercise were of a religious nature.[40]

If we consider the particular position of the Iberian Peninsula, and specifically of Portugal, as far as the religious problems of sixteenth-century Europe are concerned, it needs to be pointed out that the problem of Protestantism which fired the Counter-Reformation elsewhere, had little impact. It is clear that Protestantism was limited to some foreigners and (even more rarely) to Portuguese living abroad or in close contact with foreigners.[41]

In Portugal the problems were different. Throughout the kingdom there was a certain malaise within the Church, leading to ascetic movements as well as monastic and pastoral renewal. Nevertheless, the questions that preoccupied the Church and the Crown, as far as religious debate was concerned, were the conversion to Islam of those taken captive by Moslems, and the presence within Portugal, of Jews and Moors converted to Christianity.[42] Eventually the latter question served as a pretext for the establishment of the Holy Office, which was a mixed tribunal. In Early Modern Portugal the relevance of these questions relegated any other religious problems or debates to a lower order of priority.

The Counter-Reformation can be understood as the amalgam of the procedures carried out in order to contend against the Protestants, while insisting, on the level of doctrine, that salvation can be obtained through grace accorded by God through men, in particular through works of mercy and the practice of the sacraments. The Catholic Reform movement too, can be seen as a renewal of the Church of Rome, insisting that every believer know the catechism and his own religion; for this purpose missions were organised, attempting to teach by prayer and promoting performance of the sacraments with decency, but also with splendour.[43] It is clear that the two movements were interconnected.

The Counter-Reformation accompanied aid with a preoccupation with suppressing deviant behaviour, combining charity to the poor with a desire to save their souls. This aspect is visible in the works performed by the Misericórdias, for example for the condemned, prisoners, poor orphans and abandoned children. On the other hand, the preoccupation with confidentiality and spiritual intimacy expressed in the creation of the confessional – was mirrored in the discretion with which abandoned children were received (through the 'wheel', as explained above).

In the same way, the safeguarding of female honour through the use of the safe houses, attempted to ensure chastity, a virtue much valued during the Counter-Reformation. Through the clergy, the Counter-Reformation aimed at creating a population that was better behaved than during the Middle Ages, i.e. less violent, less prone to vengeance, more chaste and better educated. The education given to orphans, the assistance to prisoners and those condemned to death, and the practice of the spiritual works of mercy were in perfect accordance with these aims.

In fact, although they were created before it, and especially before its repercussions, the Misericórdias harmonised perfectly with the spirit and the principles of the Counter-Reformation, which established salvation by good works, given that the brethren gave their aid as voluntary work. It seems to us that the Counter-Reformation did not so much condition or determine poor relief in Early Modern Portugal as progress side by side with it. Finally, the enormous success of these institutions in Early Modern times resulted from the agreement between the royal concept of aid and the common culture of aid which reinforced the existing hierarchies and kept the difference between rich and poor distinct.

Notes

1 Elvira Cunha de Azevedo Mea, 'A Igreja em Reforma', in *Portugal do Renascimento à Crise Dinàstica*, edited by João José Alves Dias (= *Nova História de Portugal*, under the direction of Joel Serrão and A.H. de Oliveira Marques, vol. 5), Lisbon, Presença, 1998, pp. 413–46.

2 Marcello Caetano, 'Recepção e Execução dos Decretos do Concílio de Trento em Portugal', *Revista da Faculdade de Direito da Universidade de Lisboa*, vol. 19, Lisbon, 1965, pp. 7–88; Amélia Maria Polónia da Silva, 'Recepção do Concílio de Trento em Portugal: As Normas Enviadas pelo Cardeal D. Henrique aos Bispos do Reino em 1553', *Revista da Faculdade de Letras História*, 2nd series, vol. 7, Porto, 1990, pp. 133–43; Maria Fernanda Enes, *Reforma Tridentina e Religião Vivida (Os Açores na Época Moderna)*, Ponta Delgada, Signo, 1991, pp. 14–25; Isabel M.R. Mendes Drumond Braga, 'A Visita da Inquisição a Braga, Viana do Castelo e Vila do Conde em 1565', *Revista de la Inquisición*, vol. 3, Madrid, 1994, pp. 29–67.

3 Maria José Pimenta Ferro Tavares, *Pobreza e Morte em Portugal na Idade Média*, Lisbon, Presença, 1989, pp. 142–5; Paulo Drumond Braga, 'A Crise dos Estabelecimentos de Assistência aos Pobres nos Finais da Idade Média', *Revista Portuguesa de História*, vol. 26, Coimbra, 1991, pp. 175–90.

4 On medieval confraternities see Maria Ângela Godinho Vieira da Rocha Beirante, *Confrarias Medievais Portuguesas*, Lisbon, [no publisher's name], 1990; Maria Helena da Cruz Coelho, 'As Confrarias Medievais Portuguesas: Espaços de solidariedade na vida e na morte', *Confradias, Gremios, Solidariedades en la Europa Medieval,* Estella, [no name], 1992.

On confraternities in the Early Modern period, see Guilhermina Mota, 'A Irmandade de Nossa Senhora do Carmo da Marmeleira Mortágua (Primeira Metade do Século XVIII)', *Revista de História das Ideias,* vol. 9, no. 2, Coimbra, 1987, pp. 267–308; Pedro Penteado, 'Confrarias Portuguesas na Época Moderna: Problemas, Resultados e Tendências de Investigação', *Lusitania Sacra,* 2nd series, no. 7, Lisbon, 1995, pp. 15–52.

5 Laurinda Faria dos Santos Abreu, *A Santa Casa da Misericórdia de Setúbal de 1500 a 1755. Aspectos de Sociabilidade e Poder*, Setúbal, Santa Casa da Misericórdia, 1990, p. 23.

6 *Um lnstrumento Português de Solidariedade Social no Século XVl. O Compromisso da Misericórdia de Lisboa*, Lisbon, Chaves Ferreira Publicações, 1992.

7 Isabel dos Guimarães Sá, *A Circulação de Crianças na Europa du Sul. O Caso dos Expostos do Porto no Século XVIII*, Lisbon, Fundação Calouste Gulbenkian, JNICT, 1995, p. 101.

8 Ibid.

9 Laurinda Abreu, *op. cit.*, p. 23.

10 Costa Godolphim, *As Misericórdias*, Lisbon, Imprensa Nacional, 1897, p. 41; Laurinda Abreu, *op. cit.*, pp. 47–53; Isabel dos Guimarães Sá, *A Circulação de Crianças*, p. 101.

11 A.J.R. Russel-Wood, *Fidalgos and Philanthropists. The Santa Casa da Misericórdia of Bahia. 1550–1755,* London/Melbourne/Toronto, 1968, p. 23; Laurinda Abreu, *op. cit.*, p. 133.

12 Laurinda Abreu, *op. cit.*, p. 24; Isabel dos Guimarães Sá, *A Circulação de Crianças*, p. 102.

13 Claude Chauchadis, 'Les Modalités de la Fermeture dans les Confréries Religieuses Espagnoles (XVIe–XVIIIe siècles)', *Les Sociétés Fermées dans le Monde Ibérique (XVIe–XVIIIe siècles),* Paris, CNRS, 1986, pp. 91–3.

14 Paulo Drumond Braga, *A Inquisição nos Açores*, Ponta Delgada, Instituto Cultural de Ponta Delgada, p. 327.

15 José Damião Rodrigues, 'Poder e Solidariedade: as Misericórdias na Época Moderna (Séculos XV–XVIII)', *Terceira Idade. Poder, Conflito e Solidariedade,* Povoação, [no name], 1993, p. 13; Isabel dos Guimarães Sá, *A Circulação de Crianças*, p. 102.

16 Laurinda Abreu, *op. cit.*, p. 23.

17 Laurinda Abreu, *op. cit.*, p. 133; José Damião Rodrigues, *op. cit.*, p. 21.

18 Maria José P. Ferro Tavares, 'A Politica Municipal de Saúde Pública (Séculos XIV *XV)', Revista de História Económica e Social*, vol. 19, Lisbon, 1987, p. 20.

19 Isabel M.R. Mendes Drumond Braga, 'Para a História do Medo no Portugal Quinhentista: Peste e Religiosidade', *Revista de Ciências Históricas,* vol. 8, Porto, 1993, p. 85.

20 Maria José p. Ferro Tavares, *op. cit.*, p. 25.

21 Isabel M. R. Mendes Drumond Braga, 'A Saúde Pública e os seus Agentes em Portugal: o Caso dos Boticários (1521–1557), *Asclepio*, vol. 46, fascicle 2, Madrid, 1994, pp. 57–75.

22 Idem., *Ibidem*, pp. 60–1.

23 Isabel dos Guimarães Sá, *A Circulação de Crianças*, pp. 33, 90.

24 Idem., *Ibidem*, p. 38.

25 Idem., *Ibidem*, pp. 37, 106; Idem., 'Abandono de Crianças, Infanticídio e Aborto na Sociedade Portuguesa Tradicional através das Fontes Jurídicas', *Penélope,* vol. 8, Lisbon, 1992, pp. 75–89; Maria de Fátima Marques Dias Antunes dos Reis, 'As Crianças Expostas em Santárem em Meados do Antigo Regime (1691–1710). Elementos Sociais e Demograficos', master's dissertation in Modern History, presented at the Faculty of Letters, University of Lisbon, 1988, p. 107.

26 Isabel dos Guimarães Sá, *A Circulação de Crianças*, pp. 61, 91, 108.

27 Ana Maria Marques Guedes, A Assistência e a Eiducação dos Orfãos durante o Antigo Regime. O Colégio dos Orfãos do Porto, master's dissertation in Modern History, presented at the Faculty of Letters, University of Porto, 1993, pp. 42, 98.

28 Laurinda Abreu, *op. cit.*, p. 75.

29 Isabel M.R. Mendes Drumond Braga, 'A Misericórdia de Ceuta e a Protecção às Donzelas 1580–1640', *Congresso Internacional de História Missionação Portuguesa e Encontro de Culturas. Actas, vol.* 3, Braga, 1993, pp. 455–63; Ana Maria Marques Guedes, *op. cit.*, p. 70.

30 Ana Maria Marques Guedes, *op. cit.*, pp. 77–9.

31 Isabel dos Guimarães Sá, 'Entre Maria e Madalena: A Mulher como Sujeito e Objecto de Caridade em Portugal e nas Colónias (Séculos XVI–XVIII)', O *Rosto Feminino da Expansão Portuguesa. Actas, vol. 1,* Lisbon, Comissão para a Igualdade e para os Direitos das Mulheres, 1995, p. 330.

32 Ana Maria Marques Guedes, *op. cit.*, p. 85.

33 Costa Godolphim, *op. cit.*, p. 46; Laurinda Abreu, *op. cit.*, p. 102; Isabel dos Guimarães Sá, *A Circulação de Crianças*, p. 123; Maria Ângela V. da Rocha Beirante, *Santarém Quinhentista,* Lisbon, [no name], 1981, pp. 244–6.

34 Fernando Cecílio Calapez Correia, *A Cidade e o Termo de Lagos no Periódo dos Reis Filipes,* Lagos, Centro de Estudos Gil Eanes, 1994, p. 288.

35 Isabel M.R. Mendes Drumond Braga, 'Mulheres Cativas e Mulheres de Cativos em Marrocos no Século XVII', *O Rosto Feminino da Expansão Portuguesa. Actas,* vol. 1, Lisbon, Comissão para a Igualdade e para os Direitos das Mulheres, 1995, pp. 439–48.

36 Isabel M. R. Mendes Drumond Braga, 'Contribuição Monetária das Comarcas Portuguesas para a Obra de Redenção de Cativos (1523–1539)', *Brigantia,* vol. 14, no. 1–2, Bragança, 1994, pp. 23–34.

37 Isabel dos Guimarães Sá, *A Circulação de Crianças*, p. 123.

38 Laurinda Abreu, *op. cit.*, p. 12.

39 Maria Ângela Beirante, 'O Resgate dos Cativos nos Reinos de Portugal e Algarve (Séculos XII-XV)', *Actas das III Jornadas de História Medieval do Algarve e Andaluzia,* [Loulé], Câmara Municipal, 1989, pp. 273–81; Isabel M. R. Mendes Drumond Braga, 'O Primeiro Resgate Geral de Cativos após a Restauração (Tetuão 1655)', *Itinerarium,* vol. 40, Braga, 1994, pp. 117–30; Paulo Drumond Braga, 'Os Trinitários e o Resgate de Cativos: O Caso de 1728–1729', *Congresso Internacional de História Misionação Portuguesa* e *Encontro de Culturas. Actas,* vol. 3, Braga, 1993, pp. 484–9; Isabel M. R. Mendes Drumond Braga, *Entre a Cristandade e o Islão (Séculos XV–XVII). Cativos e Renegados nas*

Franjas de duas Sociedades em Confronto, Ceuta, Istituto de Estudios Ceutíes, 1998.

40 Isabel dos Guimarães Sá, 'As Misericórdias e a Protecção Régia. Etapas de uma Relação Privilegiada', paper presented at the 'Encontro sobre as Transformações na Sociedade Portuguesa 1480–1570', Lisbon, Fundação das Casas de Fronteira e Alorna, 18–21 November 1996 (photocopied text).

41 Paulo Drumond Braga, 'Carta de D. Manuel I a Carlos V sobre a Rebelião de Lutero (1521)', *Itinerarium*, vol. 145, Braga, 1993, pp. 33–43.

42 Jorge Borges de Macedo, 'Damião de Góis et l'Historiographie Portugaise', *Damião de Góis Humaniste européen*, [Paris], École Pratique des Hautes Études, 1982, pp. 74–7.

43 Eugénio dos Santos, 'Missões Populares e Festa Barroca: Um Aspecto da Sensibilidade Colectiva', *I Congresso Internacional do Barroco. Actas*, vol. 2, Porto, Reitoria da Universidade do Porto, Governo Civil do Porto, 1991, pp. 641–8.

11

PERSPECTIVES ON POOR RELIEF, HEALTH CARE AND THE COUNTER-REFORMATION IN FRANCE

Colin Jones

The complexity of the influence of the Counter-Reformation in poor relief and health care is particularly evident in the case of France. The Catholic revival did not imprint itself on virgin soil here – any more than in any other major state – but was itself deeply inflected not only by the presence of a strong Protestant minority within the country, but also by the distinctive prior histories of poor relief and health care within the French church and state. In this chapter, my aim is to provide a broad overview of the varying contexts in which the Counter-Reformation operated. As we shall see, it is tempting to narrate the history of poor relief and health care in the sixteenth and seventeenth centuries in terms of a dynamic and symbiotic triangular relationship involving church, state and local government.[1]

There was a strong tradition of intervention of the French monarchy in religious and therefore charitable affairs dating back to the Middle Ages. The kings of France claimed to rule by divine right – and indeed had long been held to cure cases of scrofula – 'the King's Evil' – by the royal touch.[2] This thaumaturgic power was divinely bestowed on a new ruler at his coronation, traditionally held at Reims, in a ceremony whose liturgy evoked an episcopal consecration. Indeed, by virtue of his crowning, the king became 'outside bishop' (*évêque du dehors*), a kind of honorary super-primate of the French church. In a long-enduring struggle, which had included the Papacy's 'Babylonian Captivity' in French-controlled Avignon in the fourteenth century, the king had wrested significant concessions from the Pope. The Pragmatic Sanction of 1438 and then in 1516 the Concordat of Bologna granted French rulers extensive powers including rights of appointment to major benefices. It was customary to view the 'Gallican Church' – as the Catholic church in France, was generally named – as quasi-independent from Rome. The four 'Gallican Articles' which in 1682 were made state law in France actualised and gave further expression to a long-existing tradition of autonomy, evident in the persistent refusal of the king to make the decrees of the Council of Trent state law.[3] The resolutions made at Trent in regard to poor relief as everything else only filtered slowly onto the French ecclesiastical agenda, through being accepted by diocesan synods in the last years of the sixteenth century and the early decades of the seventeenth. An important step was taken in 1614 when the Assembly of the Clergy – the Gallican Church's national representative institution – gave the resolutions its approval. But this fell short of formal state commitment and endorsement of the Tridentine package of measures. It meant that in Counter-Reformation issues such as poor relief, the monarch was always a major player.

The temptation for French rulers to convert to Protestantism was arguably lessened by the considerable powers which the Concordat of Bologna accorded them. When a Protestant actually acceded to the throne – the Bourbon, Henry of Navarre, who succeeded the last of the Valois dynasty, the childless Henry III in 1589 – he did not spend long before passing into the Catholic camp. It was a case of *politique oblige*: the new Henry IV (1589–1610) abjured his Protestantism and was received into the Roman church. The Bourbon dynasty's attachment to Catholicism did not, however, prevent the formation within France of a very substantial Protestant grouping.[4] By 1560, there were some 2,150 Huguenot (i.e. Protestant) communities scattered throughout France. Though arithmetically this was meagre when set against the total number of France's 36,000-odd communities, in fact the strategic importance of the Protestant implantation was far more extensive as a result of their geographical expansiveness, their concentration in bustling cities rather than in rural fastnesses, and the inroads which Protestants made within the social elite: in the mid-sixteenth century, maybe a half of the nobility and one-third of the bourgeoisie were Protestant. Taken together, Protestants formed a group too strong (save latterly) to be liquidated (as in Italy and Spain), yet not strong enough (as in Germany, England, etc) to take over the central apparatus of the state.

Alongside these important contextual factors regarding the trajectory of Counter-Reformation in France, a further point deserves emphasis, namely the deep felt bitterness and aggressiveness which characterised inter-confessional relations within France. The state was indeed almost torn apart in the Wars of Religion (1561–98) following the death of Henry II in a jousting accident in 1559, after which the crown passed into the hands of two successors – Francis II (1559–60) and Charles IX (1560–74) who were minors, and a third – Henry III (1574–89) – who was both ineffective and childless.[5] Weakness at the centre created a forum for dynastic wrangling between the nation's grandees, anxious to expand their power at the expense of central government. The Edict of Nantes of 1598 purportedly brought confessional peace: Protestants were accorded freedom of conscience, and the right to worship within designated localities, including over 150 fortified townships. But religious division was still intact and bitterness intense and enduring. The accession of Louis XIII (1610–43), a fervent Catholic, led to reductions in Protestant liberties, notably in the Peace of Alès of 1629. The Huguenots were by now clinging on to a perfervid royalism themselves, as surety against an increasingly militant Catholic church, and they were conspicuously absent from the numerous anti-governmental uprisings and riots in the middle decades of the century, centred on the civil wars of the Fronde (1648–53). Protestant liberties were still under attack by largely covert means, however, well in advance of the decision of Louis XIV (1643–1715) in 1685 to revoke the Edict of Nantes. The 1685 Edict of Fontainebleau formally ended Protestant worship within France.[6] Maybe a quarter of a million Protestants left the country rather than accept their enforced transformation into 'New Converts' to Catholicism. Resistance was greeted, on the individual level, with numerous imprisonments, while armed rebellion in the Cévennes mountains in the so-called 'Camisard War'of 1702–4 brought a repression which Protestant exiles abroad used to fashion a formidable propaganda campaign against the putative 'tyranny' and 'despotism' of Louis XIV.

In placing the acerbity of Protestant–Catholic relations in France in the era of the Counter-Reformation at the heart of my analysis, I am consciously going against the grain of the bulk of research since the 1960s and 1970s which has tended to stress parallelism rather than conflict between the two sides. The influential work of Jean Delumeau in particular, views the Counter-Reformation project as transcending the bounds of the confessional struggle, and being characterised by a more general move to 'Christianise' western society from above – an elite movement in which Protestants and Catholics partook.[7] There is a good deal of value in this, largely sociological analysis, on which indeed I will be drawing. Equally, however, it is crucial not to lose sight of – as the sociological view sometimes does – the enduring bitterness of the anti-Protestant struggle in conditioning all aspects of its Tridentine social policies, poor relief included. There were fewer stronger stimulants to Catholic charity, for example, than the presence within the same locality of a Protestant community. Neither Protestant nor Catholic elites wanted their poorer brethren being attracted into the opposing camp by the lure of more or better-attuned charitable provision, and so an emulative process of bidding and counterbidding occurred between the two sides – a process which continued well into the seventeenth century. At Nîmes, for example, as Wilma Pugh has shown, there was not only a very high volume of giving: in 1640 between 90 and 100 per cent of all wills contained charitable measures. In addition, there was a marked cross-fertilisation of ideas about how best to provide aid, which led to a particularly broad range of imaginative charitable initiatives being launched here.[8] (It would also be instructive to know the extent to which local paupers were aware of this process and adjusted their own demands for charity to the politico-confessional squabbles going on over their heads.)

Current historiography has highlighted the extent to which the locality – certainly the township, often the parish or the village as well – was the theatre in which Protestant and Catholic elites staged their competition for the hearts and minds of the poor. It also needs to be stressed that the locality already had a record as an arena for elite emulation in this sphere. Protestantism was only one influence in the great bout of innovation in poor relief schemes which characterised the period from the second to the fourth decades of the sixteenth century. A programme of reform prevailed in a great many towns and cities throughout Europe from Augsburg to Zurich by way of London, Paris, Nuremberg, Ypres, Madrid, Toledo, Venice and a great many places besides. The movement was led by municipal lay elites – the church, including even bishops, who traditionally were held to hold a brief for the interests of the poor, were largely sidelined. These municipal programmes of relief were exemplified by – and often copied verbatim from – the poor-law tract, *De Subventione pauperum* (1526), by Christian humanist Juan-Luis Vives. They emphasised system and rationalisation in poor-relief provision, and envisaged expropriating existing hospital foundations if necessary; setting the poor to work; and making a clear and rigid distinction between the 'deserving' poor (to be aided) and the 'undeserving' (to be punished if they resisted work). The schemes were often funded from a local poor-rate – though some churchmen opposed replacing voluntary almsgiving by such a tax obligation – and often supplemented by expropriated properties of run-down charitable institutions.[9]

Three further aspects of municipal dynamism in poor-relief matters in the early sixteenth century should also be stressed, namely, governmental support, plague measures and the municipalisation of hospitals. In the thirteenth century, the Crown had established the principle that all hospitals which could not demonstrate their origins were to regarded as royal foundations, and as such prone to visit, correction and jurisdiction of the agents of the Grand Aumônier, the king's personal chaplain.[10] The Crown also used its own judicial officials as stalking horses in this regard. The Edict of Orleans in 1561 established the principle that hospital administration was to be in lay hands, and this and other measures bolstered the claims of local magistrates to audit and inspect charitable institutions. The central government's national legislation was often, it is true, imperfectly implemented – the Ordinance of Moulins in 1566 which had stated that all parishes were to look after their own poor, for example, was widely disregarded. Yet municipal officials did benefit from having the central government behind them in their struggles to wrest charitable hegemony away from the church.

The early sixteenth century also witnessed, second, local lay officials taking a key role in organising against what was undoubtedly the biggest periodic threat to the poor – as to the community as a whole – namely bubonic plague.[11] The creation of municipal boards of health and/or of 'health captains' became the vogue: 1531 saw the first health board established in Paris, for example, to deal with all aspects of a plague epidemic (quarantines, isolation of infected households, street cleaning, organisation of plague hospitals, hiring of plague staff, burial and disinfection services, police surveillance, etc). Third, municipalities also became more involved in the take-over of run-down, unattended or poorly-managed hospitals and leper-houses.[12] The diminution in the incidence of leprosy had put a question-mark against the future of the latter – which had numbered well over 2,000 in France as a whole. The decline of the great medieval nursing communities had also caused the deterioration in the fortunes of many charitable establishments: the Order of the Holy Spirit, which had serviced 400 hospitals in France alone in the fourteenth century, was found in only a dozen by the seventeenth and the once dynamic Order of Saint-Lazare, which had specialised in leper foundations, was little more than a cipher. Nursing orders which had survived – such as the Augustinian sisters who ran the

Paris Hôtel-Dieu – were seriously demoralised.[13] Many charitable institutions thus vegetated unattended or poorly served, while others were put to extraneous uses – private residences, almshouses, schools, hostels, even brothels. Many municipalities were keen to bring within their reform initiatives the charitable potential these properties constituted. From the 1490s, town officials had begun to avail themselves of the unused hospitals as exclusion centres for syphilitics when the 'French' (or was it 'Neapolitan'?) Pox' arrived.[14] A similar process of enlistment had occurred in fifteenth-century Dijon as regards plague. The hospital administrators at Dijon realised that the admission of plague victims would lead to the death of most other inmates and the certain destruction of most of the furnishings, and tried to keep them out. The Dijon townspeople rioted, however, to force the hospital to accept the diseased.[15]

Historians have tended to emphasise the determining influence on this early sixteenth-century poor-relief reform movement of a growing social and economic crisis involving the effects of war, famine and epidemic disease and characterised by mass urban pauperisation. While it would be foolish to deny the importance of the pressure from below in stimulating this round of charitable reform, it is also worth noting the extent to which the struggle emerged from intra-municipal strife which predated the hard economic times. Since the Middle Ages, poor relief had been one way in which emerging elites had striven to mark their arrival on the local scene, and to boost their prestige. In the thirteenth century, for example, communes in the Midi had seen new urban oligarchies limiting the church's power over poor relief provision by placing themselves in a managerial role.[16] A similar ambition to circumscribe ecclesiastical hegemony in the administration of poor relief was evident in the wave of reform innovation in the early sixteenth century predating the Reformation.[17] Rivalry between Protestant and Catholic fractions of the elite over the organisation of poor relief was, we might argue, simply a latterday epiphenomenon of a long running saga of intra-elite rivalries and urban power-struggles.

The early stages of Reformation and Counter-Reformation thus took place in the context of pre-existent patterns of elite rivalry within a boisterous and dynamic urban culture heavily committed to poor-relief reform. Yet, it should be pointed out, it was confessional strife (along with continuing economic problems) which in its turn helped crack apart this strong municipal investment in poor relief. The Wars of Religion fractured any sense of consensus in many townships within which formerly fairly sedate forms of elite emulation had previously occurred. Secular elites had been able to prevail over churchmen so as to increase their own involvement in poor relief, but from the 1560s the municipalities began to fall apart at the seams under confessional pressure and economic and social ills. Popular riot and turbulence added to the problems of municipal governments. Whereas riot had earlier stimulated imaginative relief programmes – Lyons' great Aumône Générale of 1534 followed on from the riot of the Grande Rebeine of 1529, for example – in the later period it seemed rather to paralyse reforming intentions.[18] Lack of money also contributed to a growing drying up of initiative. A serious resurgence of plague epidemics in the late sixteenth and early seventeenth centuries not only disrupted municipal action, but also caused many townships to fall desperately in debt. Municipal finances were frequently ruined not only by the hiring of trained medical personnel to care for plague victims, but also by the buying up of grain stocks to allow the people to live during a period of cessation in normal trading relationships.[19] War too took a material toll. Municipalities had found it difficult to maintain or restore charitable properties and hospitals damaged by civil and foreign turbulence. When King Philip II of Spain besieged Saint-Quentin in 1557 towards the end of the Italian Wars (1494–1558), for example, he gave orders that adjacent churches and monasteries were to be spared but that hospitals could be destroyed. Similarly, the siege of Protestant Montpellier in 1562 led to the levelling of the numerous hospitals in the suburbs of the city.[20]

The financial weakness which afflicted municipalities from the middle of the sixteenth century onwards allowed the vanguard position in charitable reform to pass out of their hands into the control of supra-local agencies, the state and the Catholic church. These latter increasingly assumed the innovatory role left vacant by the now beleagured municipalities. The impact of war, religious strife and civil and foreign war provided an auspicious setting for monarchs still anxious, for example, to take over the property of disaffected hospitals and leperhouses. In 1612, Louis XIII established a special commission – the Chambre de la Générale Réformation des Hôspitaux et Maladeries de France – with wide-ranging powers to reform superannuated leperhouses and defunct hospitals. With Cardinal François de La Rochefoucauld, the Grand Aumônier, at the helm from 1618 to 1645, the commission made significant inroads on local institutions.[21]

The growth of the absolutist state brought a new and more cogent set of objectives and considerations into play within the field of poor relief.[22] The monarchy's wish to build up the economy if necessary through its own intervention – through state manufactories, trading companies, aggressive tariff policies and so on – had an impact on poor relief policies, in that it was held that effective social welfare measures would set the poor to work and increase the number and effectiveness of producers. A further motivation now in play was the wish of central government to devise a more developed welfare infrastructure for its standing army. The build-up in France's armed forces in the seventeenth century – from 20,000 in 1629, the army had grown to 150,000 in the late 1650s, and was over a quarter of a million by the end of the century – stimulated government into making provision for sick, ailing, disabled and retired soldiers. Efforts to establish a veterans' hospital in 1584 and then in the 1630s came to nothing. From the 1630s onwards, however, sick and ailing soldiers placed more pressure on hospital capacity and served as a convenient pretext for extending state intervention in local charitable provision, especially in war-zones. And in 1670 the great Hôtel des Invalides was established in Paris.[23]

If the weakness of the municipalities allowed central government to adopt a more advanced position on poor relief from the late sixteenth century and in particular in the seventeenth century, it also allowed greater scope to the church. The latter had often been the victim of municipal initiatives in poor relief throughout the sixteenth century. Now, increasingly regenerated in the wake of the Council of Trent, the church had a chance to make up lost ground. Significantly, the monarchy offered support to the ecclesiastical hierarchy. Primed after Trent to recover their moral responsibility for charitable provision as 'fathers of the poor', bishops resumed their traditional responsibilities over hospitals and charitable institutions, and played a key role in marshalling the diverse clerical energies unleashed by the Catholic revival. From the 1620s and 1630s onwards, bishops were more likely to be resident in their sees; more thorough-goingly committed to their ecclesiastical tasks; and making regular diocesan visitations (which invariably included visiting charitable institutions and the auditing of their accounts). The bishop rather than the town council was now the monarchy's favoured agent for poor relief reform.

Sixteenth-century national legislation favouring municipal control over poor-relief programmes was now conveniently forgotten. From the 1620s, the state, acting through its local administrative officials, the Intendants, began to impose on municipalities a more severe financial tutelage.[24] Symptomatic of the power-shift at local level was the fate of the element of municipal compulsion which had often accompanied earlier poor-relief rationalisation schemes, in both Catholic and Protestant communities. The Tridentine church prized voluntary charitable giving over compulsory poor rates and opposed any element of obligation. Yet so forceful was the religious revival of these years, that the move away from local poor-rate systems seems scarcely to have been noticed. What I have called elsewhere a 'charitable imperative' – a moral obligation to give, preferably generously, to the proven needy – emerged to attenuate the financial and institutional consequences of the disinvestment in the principle of compulsion. Indeed, the reimposition of ecclesiastical hegemony over local poor-relief measures was accompanied by one of the most rich and diverse outpourings of charity in the history of Catholicism.[25]

Hardly surprisingly, a grateful Catholic church played an important part in polishing and foregrounding the religious dimension of France's divine-right monarchy: the arch-panegyrist of Louis-Quatorzian absolutism was, fittingly, a prelate – Bishop Bossuet of Meaux. The alliance between central government and church hierarchy was not without its strains and tensions. The state continued, as we have noted, to withhold its formal support from to-the-letter endorsement of the Tridentine decrees. There was also disagreement over some policy issues: in particular a powerful lobby of religious activists within the lay and ecclesiastical elites – the *dévots* – found it hard to stomach the government's running an independent foreign policy involving alliance with Protestant princes, high tax policies and measures of internal centralisation. Despite these tensions, however, what is truly striking about the relationship between Catholic church and state for most of the seventeenth century was the very extensive community of interest which they shared, and which was the cornerstone for a remarkable efflorescence of charitable initiatives.

This is not the place to rehearse the manifold features of this religious and charitable revival in France – the role of the new orders, the regeneration of the bishops' bench, the reform of the secular clergy, the enlistment of elite energies, and so on. Nor is there space to cover all the variegated forms assumed by the charitable imperative, as Catholics gave freely both from their pocketbooks and of themselves. What, in the context of the present chapter, is particularly worthy of note was the extent to which the charitable imperative took the form of a Christocentric project which had a curative as well as a caritative dimension. The Catholic activist, lay or clerical, represented him- or herself as following the lead given by Christ – the *imitatio Christi* was arguably the master metaphor in the church's Christianisation project. As Pierre Fourier, when he was a priest in eastern France, claimed, his role as *curé* involved him being 'shepherd of his people, father, mother, captain, guard, guide, sentry, physician, barrister, attorney, intermediary, nurturer, example and mirror' to all and sundry.[26] Particular stress was put on the role of the Christian as surrogate physician, comprehending the idea of Christ the healer who had cured the sick, the lame, the blind, the possessed. Spiritual health thus overlapped with physical well-being as tasks of the Christianising project. Saint Vincent de Paul – one of the most influential reformers in this field – told his followers that a missionary must do 'what the Son of God did on earth – work for one's neighbour, visiting and curing the sick (and) instructing the ignorant for their salvation'.[27] Cure and care, both spiritual and material, were thus part of Catholic conversion strategy: as a seventeenth-century handbook for parish priests put it, 'it is certain that by the cure of the body one can as often cure souls as with sermons and good advice'.[28]

Regular orders, both old and new, showed an engagement within this Christianising (and Catholicising) strategy by developing a commitment to medical care. Though a conciliar ruling of 1215 had prohibited ecclesiastical involvement in the spilling of blood, there always remained a smattering of priests who formally trained as physicians and even a few who practised as surgeons. The hospital order of the Antonines were specialists in cases of gangrenous ergotism and their mother-house at Vienne proudly displayed from the rafters the mummified limbs of grateful amputees. The Brothers of Saint John of God – or Brothers of Charity – had been introduced into France from Italy in 1601 by Queen Marie de Medici. By the reign of Louis XIV they were to be found throughout France in 27 institutions, including the famous Hôpital de la Charité in Paris. Besides an early commitment to care for the insane, the Brothers were especially renowned for their lithotomy techniques.[29]

The seventeenth century further witnessed the emergence of members of the regular orders as medical practitioners working as apothecaries in charge of the dispensaries in the convents and monasteries under their care. Initially intended to serve the needs of the community, the monastic dispensary in the seventeenth century became a semi-public institution where the laity could seek medical advice and purchase home-made remedies. The Jesuits confined most of their medical activities to their extra-European missions; but the confirmation of 'Jesuit's Bark' as an effective febrifuge helped the prestige of this sector and their dispensaries were much visited. Two Dutch visitors to Paris in 1657 found a veritable chemical laboratory, sporting two skeletons and a pickled corpse, when they visited the Petits-Augustins' monastery; the Jacobins, for their part, offered 'Osiris Philosophical Waters'; and the Carmes Déchaussées a 'Sovereign Water against Apoplexy and Vapours'. Women's convents were also engaged in such trade – the Miramions had a well-stocked dispensary for example.[30]

Monks' medicine was spiritual as well as material. Regular orders were often the custodians (as well as the publicists) of saints' relics which were widely attributed curative powers. The Counter-Reformation was indeed a golden age of the saint's relic, a heyday for the miraculous in general – and most of the miracles involved bodily healing. It is important not to see this healing cult of the miraculous as merely, as many historians would have it,[31] a 'popular' (i.e. 'superstitious') phenomenon, sprung from the rock of ages. It was not, for example, in the mists of time but rather very precisely from 1625 that the healing shrine of Saint-Anne-d'Auray dates. In that year, a statue of the virgin was dug up accidentally there and miracles soon blossomed: from 1634 to 1647 there would be practically a miracle a week on the site.[32] The 'popular' element in such beliefs can also be exaggerated. To judge by those alleged to be cured at such healing shrines, the middling and upper classes were if anything often over-represented. The lines of the scrofula victims awaiting the thaumaturgic 'Royal Touch' also included individuals from all ranks of society. Much the same can be said of another putatively 'popular' set of beliefs, attaching to the cult of the ex-voto. At its outset around 1600, the ex-voto was a practice endorsed by the elite as much as the masses: court artist Philippe de Champaigne even painted one for his daughter, a Jansenist nun in the aristocratic milieu of the Port-Royal convent.[33] In this context one can comprehend the stress on divine healing in Catholic proselitising strategy: 'Show us your miracles', was the missionary's regular cry when confronted by sceptical Protestants. 'Folk religion' was not simply attacked by the forces of Counter-Reformation; it was also, to a considerable extent, generated by them in the heat of conflict.[34]

The world of print, often portrayed as a solvent of 'popular superstitions', played a considerable role in bolstering this miraculous view of healing. The piety-drenched, miracle-strewn literature of the Bibliothèque bleue – the cheap, roughly-bound handbooks and chapbooks which constituted the raw reading materials of rural

France – were of particular importance in this respect. Tales of saints' lives and miraculous cures jostled alongside practical guides to health like Madame Fouquet's *Recueil de receptes charitables* and the *Médecine des pauvres.* Recent scholarship on this source has stressed first that the Bibliothèque bleue does not contain timeless forms of piety and lore, but, rather, contains the distinctly and historically located ethos of post-Tridentine piety; and second that this was not – as was once held – merely the province of the illiterate and semi-literate classes. This outcrop of so-called 'popular culture' was frequently to be found on the bookshelves of the great – with Madame de Sévigné, for example, at the head. Indeed, the strictly medical works within the collection had close links to the core of the medical community: Madame Fouquet's anthology had been composed under supervision of a Montpellier medical graduate, Delescure, while many of the other titles were also the work of medical graduates. It would be instructive to view the phenomenon of the Bibliothèque bleue as a successful arm of the marketing of both Counter-Reformation piety and elite medical views.[35]

If the regular orders and the world of print were in the vanguard of one version of ecclesiastical medicine, others, both secular clergy and the laity, followed in their wake. The national Assembly of the Clergy in 1670 was to pass a resolution, which subsequently received royal endorsement, urging bishops to establish dispensaries of popular remedies in each parish.[36] Before the bishops had got hold of this theme, however, there had been a call for improvement in medical care at parish level propagated by post-Tridentine religious activists. The *dévots* believed in religious work going on within every possible framework. The seigneurie was a favoured organ of relief endeavour: witness, for example, the Duc de Luynes' booklet, 'Instruction for Teaching Those Who Have Lands of Which They are Seigneurs What They May Do For the Glory of God and the Relief of Their Neighbours', which restated the charitable duties of the seigneur (and, especially, of his wife) in emollient, post-Tridentine language.[37] It was in both the seigneurie and the parish that new forms of charitable confraternities operated, often on the model of the confraternity of Ladies of Charity, established in 1617 in Châtillon-les-Dombes by the young parish priest that was Vincent de Paul. In the 1620s, the model was picked up by Parisian well-to-do ladies who sought to achieve their own sanctification by visiting the poor in their homes and providing them with both bodily and spiritual care.

The parish was moreover a favoured locale of religious activity for perhaps the most important and influential *dévot* lobby, the famous Company of the Holy Sacrament, or the *cabale des dévots.*[38]. This clandestine caucus, cloaked beneath a shield of anonymity, included eminent churchmen (Vincent de Paul, Olier, Bossuet), and powerful laymen from the old aristocracy (Conti, Nemours, Liancourt, etc) and the high Robe nobility (Séguier, Noailles, Lamoignon, d'Argenson, etc). Operating in Paris from the late 1620s down to its dissolution in the 1660s, the Company also had around 60 local branches, which worked hand in hand with other networks of *dévots* such as the Jesuit-inspired Confraternities of Messieurs and the Ladies of Charity. The Company's hand was found behind just about every imaginable and major item of social and religious reform throughout this period, including the assault on Protestantism. Members saw themselves as 'good angels' – the term was their own[39] – acting to re-Christianise artisanal confraternities, to check on public morals, to reform prostitutes and the sexually disorderly, to support educational initiatives, to engage in famine relief, to establish parish confraternities for home relief and medical care, to galvanise alms-giving, to drive Protestants out of public life (a task to which they devoted especial care) – to use every imaginable means, in fact, to combat paganism, ignorance and heresy.

The context in which this wide-ranging programme was devised and tested was French involvement after 1635 in the Thirty Years War (1618–48) and the Franco-Spanish War (1635–59) when the north-eastern part of France (and latterly, the Ile-de-France) was devastated by the passage and fighting of armies.[40] The stimulus to charity in this period was intense. The poor seemed the unwitting victims of the random violence of a rapacious soldiery which destroyed the material and spiritual frameworks of everyday life. Peasants and poor townspeople were driven to starvation and every imaginable form of aberrant behaviour including murder, infanticide and cannibalism. An impressive relief operation for the war-torn provinces was organised out of Paris by individuals linked to the Company of the Holy Sacrament. Prominent here was the *Magasin charitable*, a kind of clearing bank for charitable contributions plus a baroque Oxfam acting as a relay centre for second-hand clothes and effects which were shipped out regularly to the needy. The Ladies of Charity were supposed to have spent over half a million livres in relief work for Champagne and Picardy between 1648 and 1660 – total expenditure was even greater. The work was also impressive for being widely-publicised: the organiser of the *Magasin charitable*, Maignart de Bernières, published regular descriptions, or *Relations*, which served as fund-raising, tub-thumping publicity material, encouraging what we may call a culture of conspicuous donation in which the well-off were primed to give to the pathetic species of impoverished humanity, bereft of material and spiritual succour, luridly portrayed in the pages of the *Relations*.

Victims of violence, however, the poor were also its sometime perpetrators. These same were, after all, the years of widespread riot and revolt caused by aggressive taxation policies, and culminating in the civil wars of the Fronde. In this regard, the poor were figured as wild, dangerous and unconstrained – the carriers of a kind of disorderly yeast, which incorporated riot and disease (the equation between poverty and plague was a frequently made one).[41] The very success of their work on the theatres of warfare in eastern France and the Ile-de-France pushed the *dévots* in the Parisian elite into an ever greater enterprise – the confinement of the poor in the so-called *grand renfermement des pauvres*.[42] The Company of the Holy Sacrament had for long preached the virtues of confinement of the poor in 'general hospitals' ('*hôpitaux généraux*') as a panacea for poor relief. The signal virtue of the 'general hospital' was its multifunctionality. It could serve as refuge for the needy poor, victims of life's hardships. But it could also house the wilfully disorderly poor, who could be disciplined into good Christian living. The institutions allowed economies of scale in poor relief, allowing charitable provision to go further than if each pauper remained within the wider community. They could distinguish more clearly just who among the poor was deserving and who undeserving, and measure out their treatment in proportion to their divergent needs. They allowed the provision of work for inmates – seen as both a spiritual and a material therapy for the poor. And the poor and their numerous children could be supplied with an unremitting diet of spiritual care: the institutions were to run to a liturgical metronome. Significantly too, the institution dovetailed neatly with the exigencies of the state: general hospitals held out the promise of becoming conscript manufactories, assisting the state's balance of trade, training workers in useful occupations and boosting local businesses. Above all, they seemed an admirable (and relatively cheap) way of achieving social discipline and spiritual harmony in what still seemed a very unstable political and social landscape.

The Company of the Holy Sacrament had made the confinement of the poor its official policy in the early 1630s, and in the following decades its members throughout France acted to encourage local initiatives in this direction. The example of the Charité hospital which had been established at Lyon in 1614 was held out as the model to follow. By the early 1650s, a good head of steam had built up within Paris for the headquarters of the Company to throw its weight behind its imposition of the general hospital model in the capital. In 1656, a royal edict established an Hôpital Général in Paris – it was opened in 1657. In 1662, a further decree ordained the creation of similar institutions in every major township. Counter-Reformation militants had thus been crucial in making of the principle of confinement the state's official medicine for poverty. This symbiosis between Counter-Reformation church and absolutist state went on to bring about, in the second half of the seventeenth century, moreover, one of the most major transformations in the structures of poor relief in French history. It was in the 1670s and 1680s in particular that government really buckled down to the task, initiating reforms, coordinating local confinement policies, and providing publicity to explain the best means of establishing such institutions. At local level, it was bishops (rather than town councils) whom the government targeted as the leaders of the movement and who chaired the new hospital boards. The state also sponsored what we may call the technicians of confinement, notably the Jesuit fathers Chaurand, Guevarre and Dunod, who acted as roving state emissaries, organising the establishment of numerous hospitals throughout France.[43] They placed emphasis on the fiscal advantages of confinement to local elites: by stimulating local charity, establishment costs could be mimimized; by ensuring that inmates worked, the institutions could not only be self-sufficient but even help the locality's balance of trade; while the confinement of the poor would mean that the 'charitable tax' imposed on the rich by street beggars would cease. In addition the Hôpital Général would ensure that paupers emerged from it better Christians and more docile and less rumbustious subjects. Streets would be cleared of the moral contagion embodied by the down-and-out, who would also be less health-threatening for the social elite. As a proponent of a Hôpital Général at Metz put it, 'everything in these institutions, as in the best regulated monasteries, is clean, whereas formerly beggars lodged in stinking and infected holes and were the first to be attacked by contagious diseases, and communicated them to the wealthy by creeping amongst them in the streets, in the churches and at their doors'.[44]

By 1700, this multiform movement of confinement which combined spiritual, charitable, repressive and medical aims had sunk deep roots. Over a hundred institutions had been established throughout France. The Parisian prototype contained getting on for 10,000 inmates, and the total number of the confined came to exceed 100,000 individuals. The intellectual dominance of the confinement model was so extreme moreover, that it was extended to a range of other categories of perceived social problem: sexually disorderly women, gypsies, witches, lunatics – and of course Protestants.[45]

If the Counter-Reformation frequently represented itself in terms of a healing role, that work of therapy could be stretched to include some rather unpleasant spiritual surgery. It was precisely as a means of healing the wounds within a severed Christian body that Tridentine activists justified the work of outright repression aimed at the Huguenots. The phrase, 'one king, one law, one faith', justified the wholesale erasure of Protestant identity. Long before the Revocation of the Edict of Nantes in 1685, local Catholic activists had led virulently anti-Protestant campaigns. Thus while their parents were variously exiled, executed or imprisoned, Huguenot children were separated from their families and placed within Hôpitaux Généraux as a means of ensuring their conversion. Adult Protestants entering hospitals were subjected to bouts of proselytising: births and deaths registers proudly displayed Protestant abjurations of their faith. Those who resisted in Montpellier but who died, risked becoming the first port of call for cadaver-seeking surgical and medical students.[46] By the 1680s, moreover, virtually all property formerly owned by Huguenot communities – and this included Protestant churches and cemeteries as well as charitable resources and hospitals – had been sequestrated to the benefit of local hospitals, and particularly Hôpitaux Généraux. Besides making these expropriations, the state also renewed its efforts to divert the property of leperhouses and defunct local hospitals into the coffers of the larger hospitals,[47] yet it would still be true to say that the extensive redrawing of the hospital map at the turn of the century was achieved at the direct expense of a now-outlawed Protestant community. The most significant programme of poor-relief in the wake of the Counter-Reformation was partly at least ensured by the rankest of religious intolerances steered through jointly by church and state.

It would be wrong to imagine that these major and largely repressive institutional changes encapsulated the whole of the contribution of Counter-Reformation militants to the reorganisation of poor relief. There was a less violent mood at work, in character altogether more fraternal – though maybe 'sisterly' would be a better designation. We see something of this undercurrent in the circumstances surrounding the establishment of the Paris Hôpital Général, which almost miscarried due to a split within the ranks of the activists over the degree of compulsion involved in such a confinement. Vincent de Paul welcomed the idea of the hospital as a refuge for paupers – his Hôpital du Saint-Nom de Jésus established in 1653 was very much organised on these lines, with aged paupers as its clientele. The saint saw in the pauper a hapless victim, not a social aggressor, and he was less than enthusiastic about the forcible confinement of Parisian paupers and the expulsion of outsiders to their homes. He reacted against the idea of the hospital as a kind of compulsory lazaretto for the morally and spiritually diseased which was current among many members of the Company of the Holy Sacrament. 'To establish a General Hospital, shut up in it the poor of Paris and do nothing for those in the countryside is certainly not to my liking', he wrote. 'Paris is the sponge of the whole of France: it attracts most of the gold and silver of the country, If the poor cannot enter Paris, what are they to do, especially those poor people of Champagne, Picardy and other provinces ruined by war?'[48]

Perhaps the clearest manifestation of this less repressive, more overtly compassionate stream within Counter-Reformation piety was the renovation of religious communities devoted to charitable purposes. The Brothers of Charity were one case in point, but the vast bulk of such individuals were females.[49] The religious revival did stimulate out of their erstwhile torpor many older hospital nursing communities: the Augustine sisters at the Paris Hôtel-Dieu, for example, were regenerated in the 1630s. Critical here however was the creation of new communities devoted to poor relief and health care. The role of the Daughters of Charity (*Filles de la Charité*) established by Saints Vincent de Paul and Louise de Marillac in 1633 was particularly important in this respect. They owed their inception to the fact that the middle and upper-class ladies of religious confraternities devoted to charity were repelled by the dirty work of visiting, cleaning and caring for their pauper charges. Realising that the poor were suffering from the fact that these Ladies made their own servants do this work in their place, Vincent de Paul and Louise de Marillac formed the idea of a kind of trained spiritual servant class, drawn from the lower orders (and thus used to hard work), but subjected to the kind of intense spiritual training formerly only given to the (largely middle-class) women of the monastic orders. Crucial too was his, and Louise de Marillac's, conception that this care should be located not simply within hospitals and convents but out in the world, in the diseased and dirty homes of the poor.

This is not the place to describe the tortuous and frequently cunning way which Vincent de Paul managed to circumvent the Tridentine emphasis on enclosure for all female religious. Suffice it to say that by the 1650s, this obstacle had been overcome, and numerous other similar female nursing communities – as well as a great many devoted less to care for the poor than to education – had been founded and were expanding fast.[50] By 1700, the Daughters of Charity – the only truly national of such bodies – served in excess of 200 institutions: some of these were hospitals, some charity boards presided over by Ladies of Charity, and some were seigneuries. In all of the institutions to which they and their ilk were attached, they conceived of their task as including the service of every aspect of the needs of the sick poor. Even though the overarching motivation was spiritual and proselytising, this meant a new level of commitment to the material care of sickness. They took with them to each new establishment a copy of Madame Fouquet's medical anthology, which seems to have stood as a vade-mecum for them in most medical matters. Each new establishment of the Daughters of Charity also received a little box of syringes and ligatures for minor surgical procedures. The sisters also invariably assumed control of the hospital's apothecary services. Though they were strictly enjoined to be respectful to medical staff within their institutions, these individuals were frequently conspicuous only by their absence. In practice, most of the medical services in most of the institutions in which they served were largely under the control of the sisters.

Nursing sisters also had a major influence on the hygienic state (and thereby therapeutic effectiveness) of institutions to which they were attached. They made of their takeover of these institutions a campaign of resacralisation of hospital space. They equated contagious disease with moral contagion – and were against both; their contracts of service stipulated that they were to be barred from treating contagious and shameful cases and pregnant women. Cleanliness was accorded a high – and a highly spiritual – value. The regulations of the sisters at Luzignan hospital for example enjoined them to uphold 'cleanliness and neatness in their persons in all things, as serving towards edification'. The Augustine sisters of the Miséricorde de Jésus declared open war on stench: sisters were, their constitutions stated, 'to keep the hospital very clean, to burn perfumes, to have filth emptied as swiftly as possible, to open windows to take in air, and never to leave any linen or indecent thing lying about'. Sisters of charity, Louise de Marillac told her charges, should view themselves as 'sunshine which passes continually over filth without being soiled by it in the slightest'.[51] Cleanliness and purity were not next to godliness for such women – they *were* godliness.

This massive extension of the role in medical care of religious personnel – notably nursing communities, but also as we have seen, male members of the regular orders as well as the 'good curé'[52] – had clear implications for the orthodox medical community. The question of how the medical community reacted to the recharged commitment of the church to bodily (as well as spiritual) healing was complicated, moreover, by the fact that, especially in the sixteenth century, a great many physicians in particular, but also apothecaries and surgeons were Protestants. The potential for conflict was reduced, however, by the church's strenuous efforts throughout the seventeenth century to bring back medical faculties and colleges – as well as guilds of surgeons and apothecaries – within the aegis of the church. It was also important in this regard that the bulk of the individuals to whom the religious wished to cater were largely outside direct competition with the medical community, and especially with its most prestigious and influential arm, the physicians. The poor who were the prime target of post-Tridentine care were largely out of the reach of physicians, who tended to live in cities and to charge high fees for their services. It was conventional legal lore that the church could and indeed should provide for the medical needs of the poor, albeit out of charity rather than a wish for material gain. Conflict was thus not necessarily built into the relations between the two communities. It was not out of the question for medical men to accept 'popular' remedies if they seemed to work and if they partook of the largely Galenic medical world which both medical men and their clients accepted. The physicians at the Hôtel-Dieu in Romarantin in the Orléanais freely admitted, for example, that the remedy for gangrenous ergotism in use in their hospital had been borrowed wholesale from the remedy-book of the local lady of the manor.[53] This kind of symbiosis with remedies drawn from what we might call the 'medical penumbra'[54] was all the more apparent with physicians influenced by Paracelsianism.

This does not mean that it was always plain sailing between churchmen and spiritually-motivated women on the one hand and the medical community on the other. The Parlement of Paris was primed by the medical faculty to attack the growth of the conventual pharmaceutical sector – but with little success. At Metz, local surgeons accused the Brothers of Charity of stealing their clients, admitting the wealthy into their hospital where they should only take paupers. The Dijon apothecaries took the Brothers of Mercy to court to prevent them retailing their wound ointment derived from the fat of executed criminals. The Montpellier apothecaries in the 1670s tried to coordinate a national campaign against competitors from the regular orders and even considered appeals to the royal council and the pope.[55] Some of the sharpest barbs were reserved for women engaged in medical care, echoing the insults launched by fourteenth-century physician Guy de Chauliac against 'women and idiots' meddling in medicine.[56] Attacks on the Daughters of Charity and others of the nursing communities were exacerbated by medical annoyance at the high degree of protection which such communities enjoyed from well-placed patrons. The Daughters of Charity, for example, numbered among their sponsors Louis XIII, Louis XIV, the latter's mother (queen regent Anne of Austria) and high nobles of both Sword and Robe. The high *dévot* caucus thus provided the protective shield within which this extension of medical care took place if and when medical men chose to contest the place religious personnel had earned in the dispensation of medicine.

Although we are noting this element of conflict between the medical and religious nexuses over the administering of health care, it would not be appropriate for us to conclude on it. Although contemporary physicians might be loath to admit it, there is a case for arguing that the Counter-Reformation, among its multifarious domains of action, was a major force of medicalisation within French society.[57] If we take the term medicalisation to mean not the internalising of physicians' lore so much as the wide diffusion within society as a whole of a range of practices, institutions and beliefs about health current among the social elite, then the statement looks helpful. If medicalisation there was in this period it is unlikely to have come from within the medical community, if only because of shortage of numbers. The medical community scarcely hit the 20,000 mark in this period – and the number of physicians was a small proportion of that figure. The clergy, in contrast, numbered 200,000 in the early seventeenth century, perhaps a quarter of a million at mid-century.[58] We can moreover add to the arithmetic the firm commitment of the post-Tridentine clergy towards care and cure of the poor, the revival of miraculous healing, the proliferation of popular medical literature, the birth and the diffusion of specialist nursing communities, the beginnings of a takeover of hospital care by such communities, and the enlistment of the charitable (and fitfully repressive) enthusiasms of sundry lay activists. Even if the motivation in question was largely spiritual rather than material, and targeted the body as a means of attaining the soul, it may still be possible to conclude that the Counter-Reformation helped to reshape from top to bottom the provision of health care in France as it did the structures of poor relief.

Notes

1 In this chapter, I will be drawing on my previous work on Early Modern France in the domains of poor relief (notably *The Charitable Imperative. Hospitals and Nursing in Ancien Régime and Revolutionary France*, London, 1989, and medical care (notably *The Medical World of Early Modern France*, Oxford, 1997, co-authored with Laurence Brockliss).

2 See Marc Bloch's classic treatment of the religious aura of Bourbon monarchs in his *The Royal Touch. Sacred Monarchy and Scrofula in England and France* (London, 1973).

3 On the impact of Trent in France, see J. Imbert, 'Les Prescriptions hospitalières du Concile de Trente et leur diffusion en France', *Revue d'histoire de l'Église de France*, 42 (1956) pp. 5–28. More generally too, see J. Imbert, *Le Droit hospitalier de l'Ancien Régime* (Paris, 1993).

4 For the history of Protestantism in France, see D. Ligou, *Le Protestantisme en France de 1598 à 1715* (Paris, 1968).

5 M.P. Holt, *The French Wars of Religion, 1562–89* (Cambridge, 1995). This is particularly useful in viewing the Wars not simply in terms of grandee power politics but also in highlighting the religious stakes at issue.

6 J. Garrisson, *L'Édit de Nantes et sa révocation* (Paris, 1985); E. Labrousse, *La Révocation de l'Édit de Nantes* (Paris, 1985).

7 J. Delumeau, *Le Catholicisme entre Luther et Voltaire* (Paris, 1971) – English translation as *Catholicism from Luther to Voltaire* (London, 1977) – has been followed by a host of local studies wielding a similar 'Christianisation paradigm'.

8 W.J. Pugh, 'Protestant and Catholic testamentary charity in the seventeenth century', *French Historical Studies*, 11(1980) pp. 479–504; W.J. Pugh, 'Social welfare and the edict of Nantes: Lyons and Nîmes', *French Historical Studies*, 4 (1974) pp. 349–76.

9 M. Bataillon, 'J.L.Vives, réformateur de la bienfaisance', *Bibliothèque d'humanisme et renaissance*, 14 (1952) pp. 141–58; M. Fatica, 'Il "Subventione pauperum" di J.L.Vives', *Società e Storia* (1982) pp. 1–30; and, for the early sixteenth-century campaign in general, R. Jütte, 'Poor Relief and Social Discipline in 16th-Century Europe', *European Studies Review*, 11 (1981) pp. 25–52. For the poor-rate, see M. Fosseyeux, 'Les premiers budgets municipaux d'assistance. La taxe des pauvres au XVIe siècle', *Revue d'Histoire de l'Église de France*, 1934. For the European context, see R. Jütte, *Poverty and Deviance in Early Modern Europe* (Cambridge, 1994).

10 M. Portal, 'Le Grand Aumônier de France (jusqu'à la fin du XVIIe siècle)', *Revue de l'Assistance publique à Paris* (1954); L. Le Grand, 'Comment composer l'histoire d'un établissement hospitalier', *Revue d'Histoire de l'Église de France*, 16 (1930), pp. 161–239, esp. pp. 218ff.

11 For the full range of responses, see F. Hildesheimer, *La Terreur et la*

pitié: L'Ancien Régime à l'épreuve de la peste (Paris, 1990); M. Lucenet, *Les Grandes Pestes en France* (Paris, 1985); and C. Jones, 'Plague and its Metaphors in Early Modern France', *Representations*, 53 (1996) pp. 97–127.

12 F. Bériac, *Histoire des lépreux au Moyen Âge: Une société d'exclus* (Paris, 1988); L. Le Grand, 'La désolation des églises, monastères et hôpitaux en France vers le milieu du XVe siècle', *Revue des questions historiques* (1898) pp. 180–8; F. Dissard, *La Réforme des hôpitaux et maladeries au XVIIe siècle* (1938).

13 P. Brune, *Histoire de l'Ordre hospitalier de Saint-Esprit* (Lons-le-Saulnier, 1892); M.C. Guérin, 'Une tentative de réforme militaire et hospitalière, 1672–93: son application en Normandie', thesis, École des Chartes, 1975; M. Fosseyeux, *Une Administration parisienne sous l'Ancien Régime: L'Hôtel-Dieu de Paris aux XVIIe et XVIIIe siècles* (Paris, 1912); and N.Z. Davis, 'Scandale à l'Hôtel-Dieu de Lyon', in *La France d'Ancien Régime: Études réunies en l'honneur de Pierre Goubert* (Paris, 1985).

14 See the overviews in R. Jütte, 'Syphilis and Confinement: Hospitals in Early Modern Germany', in R. Jütte and and N. Finzsch (eds), *Institutions of Confinement: Hospitals, Asylums and Prisons in Western Europe and North America, 1500–1950* (Cambridge, 1996); and J. Arrizabalaga, J. Henderson and R. French, *The Great Pox: The French Disease in Renaissance Europe* (London, 1997).

15 C. Aubertin and C. Bigarre, *Esquisse historique sur les épidémies et les médecins à Beaune avant 1789* (Beaune, 1885), pp. 28–9, 65.

16 See, for example, *Assistance et charité. Cahiers de Fanjeaux*, 13 (Toulouse, 1978).

17 Cf. the well-known move in 1505 by Parisian lay notables to replace the cathedral canons as administrators of the Paris Hôtel-Dieu: J. Imbert, *Les Hôpitaux en droit canonique (du Décret de Gratien à la sécularisation de l'Hôtel-Dieu de Paris en 1505* (Paris, 1947).

18 J.P. Gutton, *La Société et les pauvres. L'exemple de la généralité de Lyon, 1534–1789* (Paris, 1971); N.Z. Davis, 'Poor Relief, Humanism and Heresy: The case of Lyon', *Studies in Medieval and Renaissance History*, 5 (1968) pp. 215–75.

19 A. Croix, *La Bretagne aux XVIe et XVIIe siècles: La Vie, la mort, la foi* (2 vols.; Paris, 1981), especially pp. 524ff., 715ff.

20 Damourette, 'Hôpitaux et béguignages à Saint-Quentin au Moyen Âge', *Annales agricoles de Saint-Quentin*, 2nd series, 9 (1981) pp. 163–85, 179ff.; L. Guiraud, 'La Réforme à Montpellier', *Mémoires de la Société archéologique de Montpellier*, 2nd series 6–7 (1918): 6: 251 and 7: 78.

21 Dissard, *La Réforme des hôpitaux*; Portal, 'Le Grand Aumônier'. Cf. J. Bergin, *Cardinal de La Rochefoucauld: Leadership and Reform in the French Church* (New Haven, CT, 1987).

22 For an up-to-date summary of the development of the French state, see J.B. Collins, *The State in Early Modern France* (Cambridge, 1995).

23 For military welfare reforms, see C. Jones, 'The Welfare of the French Foot-soldier from Richelieu to Napoleon', in Jones, *The Charitable Imperative*.

24 R.J. Bonney, *Political Change in France under Richelieu and Mazarin, 1624–61* (Oxford, 1978), Chapter 14.

25 Jones, *The Charitable Imperative*. See also the broader discussion in C. Jones, 'Charity before c. 1850', in W. F. Bynum and R. Porter (eds), *Companion Encyclopaedia of the History of Medicine* (2 vols.; London, 1993). The poor-rates were also not much missed because they had fallen into abeyance in the period of civil and religious strife in the late sixteenth and early seventeenth centuries.

26 Cited in R. Taveneaux, L*e Catholicisme dans la France classique, 1610–1715* (Paris, 1980), p. 163.

27 P. Coste (ed.), *Saint Vincent de Paul. Correspondance. Documents. Entretiens* (14 vols.; Paris, 1920–5), ix, 15.

28 J. d'Aubry, *Le Triomphe de l'Archée et la merveille du monde, ou, La Médecine universelle et véritable* (1659: 4th edn, Paris, 1660).

29 H. Brabant, *Médecins, malades et maladies de la Renaissance* (Brussels, 1966), pp. 94–5; A. Chagny, *L'Ordre hospitalier de Saint-Jean-de-Dieu* (Lyons, 1951); G. Russotto, *San Giovanni di Dio e il suo ordine ospedaliero* (2 vols; Rome, 1968).

30 For Jesuits' Bark, see P. Delaveau, *Histoire et renouveau des plantes médicinales* (Paris, 1982), 186ff. For the monastic apothecaries, M. Fosseyeux, 'Les Apothicaireries de couvents sous l'Ancien Régime', *Revue de la Société de l'histoire de Paris et de l'Île-de-France*, 46 (1919).

31 This is especially the case with historians following the Christianisation paradigm of Jean Delumeau, who overstress the immemorial longevity of 'pagan' 'superstition'.

32 'Les Miracles de Sainte-Anne d'Auray', in J. Delumeau (ed.), *La Mort des pays de cocagne. Comportements collectifs de la Renaissance à l'âge classique* (Paris, 1976).

33 B. Cousin, *Ex-Voto de Provence: Images de la religion populaire et de la vie d'autrefois* (Paris, 1981), pp. 15ff.

34 For a fuller discussion of medicine and religion, see esp. Brockliss and Jones, *The Medical World of Early Modern France*, especially chapters 1 and 4.

35 R. Mandrou, *De la Culture populaire aux XVIIe et XVIIIe siècles* (Paris, 1969); G. Bollème, *La Bibliothèque bleue: La littérature populaire en France aux XVIIe et XVIIIe siècles* (Paris, 1971); and especially G. Dotoli, 'La Religion dans la "Bibliothèque bleue" au XVIIe siècle', in M. Tietz and V. Kapp (eds), *La Pensée religieuse dans la littérature et la civilisation du XVIIe siècle en France* (Paris, 1984). See too the broader context sketched out by Roger Chartier, 'Culture as Appropriation: Popular Cultural Uses in Early Modern France', in S.L. Kaplan (ed.), *Understanding Popular Culture: Europe from the Middle Ages to the Nineteenth Century* (Geneva, 1984).

36 J. Verdier, *La Jurisprudence de la médecine en France* (2 vols.; Alençon, 1762–3), I, 547.

37 Louis-Charles, duc de Luynes, *Instruction pour apprendre à ceux qui ont des terres dont ils sont seigneurs ce qu'ils peuvent faire pour la gloire de Dieu et le soulagement du prochain* (Paris, 1658).

38 A. Tallon, *La Compagnie du Saint-Sacrement (1629–1667)* (Paris, 1990). See too E. Chill, 'Religion and Mendicity in Seventeenth-century France', *International Review of Social History*, 7 (1962) pp. 400–25; and R. Elmore, 'The Origins of the Hôpital Général of Paris', PhD

dissertation, University of Michigan, 1975. For related Jesuit-inspired groupings, see too L. Châtellier, *The Europe of the Devout* (Cambridge, 1989).

39 Tallon, *La Compagnie du Saint-Sacrement*, 114 (citing the Marseille branch).

40 There is excellent untapped material on the social impact of war in the unpublished London University PhD thesis of E. Archer, 'The Assistance of the Poor in Paris and in the North-eastern Provinces of France, 1641–1660' (1936). See too G. Cabourdin, *Terres et hommes en Lorraine (1550–1635). Toulois et le comté de Vaudrémont* (Nancy, 1979); J. Jacquart, 'La Fronde des Princes dans la région parisienne et ses conséquences matérielles', *Revue d'histoire moderne et contemporaine*, 7 (1960).

41 Cf. Brockliss and Jones, *The Medical World of Early Modern France*, especially pp. 65–6, 82–3.

42 The classic text on the so-called 'Great Confinement' is M. Foucault, *Histoire de la folie: folie et déraison à l'âge classique* (Paris 1961) – abbreviated English version available as *Madness and Civilisation. A History of Insanity in the Age of Reason* (New York, 1973). Cf. C. Jones, 'The Construction of the Hospital Patient in Early Modern France', in Jütte and Finzsch, *Institutions of Confinement*, especially pp. 55ff.

43 The Chaurand and Dunod campaign may be followed in C. Paultre, *De la Répression de la mendicité et du vagabondage en France sous l'Ancien Régime* (Paris, 1906).

44 Archives départmentales de la Moselle: H 4677: cited in Brockliss and Jones, *The Medical World of Early Modern France*, p. 681.

45 For the statistics, see M. Jeorger, 'La structure hospitalière de la France sous l'Ancien Régime', *Annales. Économies. Sociétés. Civilisations*, 32 (1977) pp. 1025–51. For the other groupings, cf. Jones, *The Charitable Imperative*, pp. 217–18.

46 Brockliss and Jones, *The Medical World of Early Modern France*, p. 713.

47 D. Hickey, *Local Hospitals in Ancien Régime France: Rationalisation, Resistance, Renewal* (Montreal, 1997).

48 Coste, Saint Vincent de Paul.

49 For the revival of hospital communities, see especially Jones, *The Charitable Imperative* (in particular Chapter 3: 'Vincent de Paul, Louise de Marillac and the revival of nursing in the seventeenth century'); J.P. Gutton, 'La Mise en place du personnel soignant dans les hôpitaux français (XVIe-XVIIIe siècles)', *Bulletin de la Société d'histoire des hôpitaux* (1987) pp. 11–19; and Imbert, *Le Droit hospitalier*, 217ff.

50 See especially C. Molette, *Guide des sources de l'histoire des congrégations féminines françaises de vie active* (Paris 1974) for a helpfully full roster of these communities.

51 Brockliss and Jones, *The Medical World of Early Modern France*, 687; M. Flinton, *Sainte Louise de Marillac: L'Aspect social de son oeuvre* (n.p., n.d.), 235.

52 P. Sage, *Le 'Bon Prêtre' dans la littérature française d' 'Amadis de Gaule' au 'Génie du christianisme'* (Geneva, 1955).

53 C. Poitou, 'Ergotisme, ergot de seigle, et épidémies en Sologne au XVIIIe siècle', *Revue d'histoire moderne et contemporaine*, 23 (1976) pp. 354–68.

54 For this term, and a lengthy discussion of the relationship between this kind of medical practice and more 'orthodox' practitioners, see Brockliss and Jones, *The Medical World*, especially Chapter 4.
55 Ibid., p. 258.
56 Ibid., p. 266.
57 For a discussion of this slippery term, ibid., pp. 32–3.
58 Ibid., pp. 520–9 (medical community); Tavenaux, *Le Catholicisme dans la France classique*, 123–4 and note (clergy).

12

HEALTH CARE AND POOR RELIEF IN REGIONAL SOUTHERN FRANCE IN THE COUNTER-REFORMATION

Martin Dinges

Introduction

The title of this chapter alludes to three interrelated topics: health care, poor relief and the Counter-Reformation. I define health care as 'all measures taken either by the sick person or by another to maintain health or to recover from illness'. This definition includes prevention and therapy, provided by individuals and/or social institutions. For the notion of health the contemporary understanding is decisive. An adequate notion of Early Modern health care therefore includes spiritual aspects, dietetics and eventually medical health care in the strict sense.

The role of health care in poor relief may be defined as the relative importance of health care in all the welfare measures of a given society. This relative importance can first be observed in the field of representations of health, for example as an answer to the question whether health was an important issue in poor relief schemes. Here one has to consider the interpenetration of health care and spiritual care. Taken a step further, it could be measured as the part of a given welfare budget dedicated to health care.

A second point of interest is to get a more precise idea of the impact of the Counter-Reformation on health care and poor relief. Conceptualising the problem this way, we must recognise the fact that the reform of poor relief was not – as the older historiography of around 1900 put it – the effect of the Reformation, but had older roots in Catholicism. We can see more clearly now that there are features common to poor relief in Early Modern times: the growing influence of the state, increasing rationalisation, bureaucratisation and proto-professionalisation, and the stress on education.[1] The dissensions were less about poverty and begging than about the means to deal with them.

As the reform activities in poor relief had already started before the Reformation, it is more appropriate to consider the Catholic influence on poor relief and health care from its earlier beginnings in the fifteenth century. The notion of 'counter-reform' tends to conceal these earlier reform activities. After the Reformation all three major denominations had 'modernising effects' on both topics during the epoch of 'denominationalisation'.[2] It is therefore evident that the Counter-Reformation as the major cultural movement in the Catholic countries had an important impact on a crucial issue such as poor relief. More precisely, our purpose is to understand how the Catholic church managed to stay a major player in the field.[3] In sixteenth-century France, the major challenge to church influence was the state. It is therefore crucial to observe when and how the church won back general and institutional influence which it had partially lost since the end of the fifteenth century. This way we get a more precise idea of the direct influence on people, practices and institutions.

Second, the Counter-Reformation church found itself in a situation of denominational competition, which had an impact on health care. Was it seen in a different manner because of the rivalry between denominations? Was health care used as a means to foster Counter-Reformation propaganda? Was it instrumentalised in order to invite conversions? In what way were Counter-Reformation intentions important for health care – not only in comparison between countries, but also in local society?

Third, we have to consider how the renewed influence was finally used to help the poor, and specially those who were ill and poor. Were new institutional or personal means mobilised? Did this change poor relief and health care? Did the image of the poor and of illness change, for example into a more spiritual representation, during the Counter-Reformation?

These questions can be answered most easily in a regional or local context, as Beckerman-Davis has claimed for the example of Toulouse.[4] As the contribution of Colin Jones gives the general overview of the situation in France, I shall describe and analyse what people did at grass roots level. Therefore, I shall discuss some of the aforementioned problems for Southern France,[5] basing myself mainly on my own research on Bordeaux,[6] and including studies on Aix-en-Provence, Grenoble, Lyons, Marseille, Avignon, Montpellier, Nîmes, Toulouse, Vic-en-Bigorre and Montmorillon.[7]

I shall first look rapidly at self-help of the poor when ill, continue with indoor relief, then pass on to outdoor poor relief, and finish with some remarks about the penetration of Counter-Reformation ideas on poor relief and health care into people's minds and practices as expressed in donors' wills.

Self-help as the first and dominant strategy for coping with illness

Our contemporaries, within the social security systems of the welfare state, are left to their own devices far more than Early Modern individuals, who were more strongly integrated into a social network of kinship, family, household, neighbourhood, professional sphere as well as of other, for example, voluntary religious associations and communities.[8] From these they could expect services, and especially assistance in the case of illness, and for these they, too, performed such services. Notarial acts and – in particular wills and inventories of estates – make it easier to grasp at least the outlines of these networks of self-help for France than for countries further north. Thus there is evidence for mutual nursing – for example, for sixteenth- and seventeenth-century Bordeaux, within the following social relationships:[9] between husband and wife, parents and children, siblings living at a great distance from each other, between employers and servants, landlords or landladies and lodgers, and colleagues at work. What is remarkable is that care for the sick is not only performed by persons part of whose role it is to look after the sick, such as by mothers for their children, wives for their husbands or servants for their employers. Evidently the role of members of the family or the household in health care is predominant. It was common to cope with illness in this framework, and for practical reasons it was easiest to mobilise the closest persons for help. Such bonds were sufficiently strong to make people, for example, travel from a distance of forty kilometres, or to motivate them to invest a substantial part of their limited fortune in order to save another person.

Although assistance from outside the person's household, such as from the neighbourhood or working environment, was less frequent, it was not unheard of. It was particularly important for apprentices or migrant workers, who had come from outside the community and did not yet know a sufficient number of people locally who could help them. In the case of illness, even very recently-formed relations of employment could result in protracted assistance that was necessary for the stranger's survival. In this respect long-term residence is helpful, but not essential, for the accumulation of 'social capital' that can be mobilised in the case of illness.

The expenses resulting from illness, combining loss of income and cost of treatment, could be very high, and it is known that even poorer patients attempted to consult good doctors.[10] The sick therefore often borrowed money, a fact that is also evident from wills. The same social relationships that proved useful for sick care were relied on here, too. However,the possibility of relieving the household budget by reducing expenses, especially rent payments, was also an important feature, and it was common to allow at least delayed payments. Along with those, there were also various forms of small loans, which were also used in the case of illness. In notarial acts one can find mentions of pawnbroking and even a 'hypothecary' loan for a bed. Thus those affected mobilised all their resources in order to be able to help themselves. Self-help in the case of illness was also expected by the authorities.[11] The statutes of municipal hospitals explicitly limited the circle of persons to be admitted to those who could not find help elsewhere.[12]

One supplementary resource during illness could be the income of a family member who had been sent to beg in the streets, or more precisely in the churches. There beggars were and continued to be a common feature throughout Early Modern times, even though the church and Catholic authorities tried from time to time to liberate the sacramental space from the 'plague of beggars'. As the repression of begging was a little less rigid in Catholic countries than it was in Protestant ones, it is possible that the Catholic background – not the Counter-Reformation in itself – had an indirect positive influence on the chances of the poor to gain a supplementary income by this means.

It is difficult to find out what was the concrete nature of the help given in the households in the case of illness. The notaries provide nothing more precise than the basic fact of 'caring'. Descriptions of popular medical practices could be found in the judicial records on malpractice and on superstition, which have not been systematically scrutinised for our topic in Southern France. Used in a careful manner, they would at least provide an outside view of 'popular medical culture'.

Books on the *médecine des pauvres*, even though written by learned authors with a university background, at least provide some points of reference; the genre had been popular since 1504, and the titles demonstrate the close connection between health care and poor relief, such as, Philippe Guibert's *Le médecin charitable enseignant la matière de faire et préparer en la maison avec facilité et peu de frais les remèdes propres à toutes sortes de maladie selon l'avis du médicinaire* (Paris, 1627). The fifteen editions printed between 1627 and 1678 in Paris, Lyons and Rouen also bear witness to the considerable demand for this kind of guide to self-medication.[13] A later, equally successful, work, in print from 1714 until 1839, shows a closer connection between the church as institution and health care: *La médecine et la chirurgie des pauvres, livret de santé du moine Dom Nicolas Alexandre* (even the title mentioning a Benedictine monk as author). He collected information about popular practices, and knew academic medicine, its concepts of illness, humoral pathology, French university medicine of the last 200 years, as well as the latest actual scientific research, but he was also well acquainted with the rural world. One may well make a case here that works of that kind only continued old Benedictine traditions, and that the Counter-Reformation is only to be seen as the successor of such traditions. It is also true that in these books and therapeutic precepts, prima facie, no contents specific to the Counter-Reformation can be isolated, and thus the link with the movement of Catholic reform is a rather loose one. On the other hand, from the viewpoint of the church as offerer, there was competition on the medical market between offers of magical and religious healing, while the sick availed themselves of these either alternatively or simultaneously. So far no research has been done on the tendencies of the Counter-Reformation to establish the monopoly of means of healing in this sector. The same is true for the – presumably increasing – role of healing saints and of therapeutic pilgrimages, encouraged by the church, after 1600.[14]

The advice for behaviour in times of plague, given in the plague rules by the physician Briet (who had been commissioned by the city council of Bordeaux), were also meant to increase the possibility for self-help in the household. Along with morning prayers, he recommended the warming and frequent changing of underwear. However, judging from the inventories, the poorer city dwellers did not have this option, given that they did not own a second set of clothes for changing.[15] He recommended a breakfast consisting of a well-buttered slice of bread and an egg, together with some water mixed with wine, a little 'bol' (bole) and grey amber. For lunch he advises against meat and the rotten cheese which people – according to Briet – ate at the time. For the physician Briet the recommendation of prayers was as self-evident as the formulation of certain dietetic precepts. However, his advice to refrain from meat seems strange, at least for poorer households, since meat was only very rarely on the menu there. The question whether he was equally wrong in assessing the readiness of the population to pray in case of illness cannot be answered, but the evaluation of representative collections of popular proverbs supports the hypothesis.[16] Altogether, however, Briet's text is an example of how cautious one needs to be in drawing conclusions on the actual medical behaviour of a population from prescriptive writings.

Inventories of estates could provide further access to medical practice in the household, but, unfortunately, for Bordeaux this approach is disappointing: in the households of the lower half of society there is only evidence of water basins, which could have been used for hand-washing, but there is no mention of a single brush for clothes, nor of any drug or medical object. Thus one must conclude that even for everyday hygiene practices – beyond the use of cloth and underwear – there is little to be learnt from our source.[17] Thus self-help in the case of illness was historically a relatively constant behaviour pattern, but little can be said with precision on domestic medical practices in the South of France.[18] It appears that the influence of the Counter-Reformation was overall rather limited. As for sectors in which it was felt at all, one needs to mention forms of religiously inspired healing by practices which evoked the help of the saints for certain diseases, as well as pilgrimages related to them. It is certain that the importance of both spheres for everyday lay medical practices grew within the period under review.[19] Along with these, an institutional setting that could develop Counter-Reformation influence in everyday life was community care (described on pp. 259–66) which had direct influence on the households.

It was only when the environment of the poor had been exhausted that outside help was considered. However, in Early Modern times self-help was put under pressure: the demographic situation (families torn apart by plagues or increased migration) and the state of the economy (increase of structural unemployment, e.g. during cyclical crises) deteriorated. These factors diminished – temporarily or permanently – the capacity for social help, and the need for welfare benefits and care in the case of illness increased. If one takes the availability of beds in institutions as an indicator, the picture for Bordeaux, showing parallels with other cities, is the following: the hospital and the work-house of this city provided beds for 0.15 per cent of the population in 1525, 0.5 per cent in 1600, and 1.9 per cent in 1675, but for a smaller percentage again in the extremely rapidly-growing city of the eighteenth century.[20] These numbers at least give a frame of reference for institutional sick-care. Thus both supply and demand increased for public welfare services, although most cases of illness were still dealt with by the poor affected by it themselves – usually in their own home.

Institutions for indoor relief for the sick poor

For the cases that could not be cared for at home, there were hospitals, as in Bordeaux; around 1520 they presented the confusing picture of a large number of small institutions, rarely dominated by a larger one. The legacy of the Middle Ages survived in pilgrims' hospices and institutions for foundlings (Saint Jacques), as well as in houses for the elderly and for the treatment of particular diseases, such as Saint Anthony's fire, leprosy or bubonic plague (the latter outside town).[21] The resources of the old Benedictine Hospital Sainte-Croix were channelled into this last institution; in the case of an actual outbreak, huts were constructed.[22] Nothing is known of a hospital for the treatment of syphilis, and those infected were presumably cared for in small private institutions, the evidence for which is only transmitted by some notaries in Toulouse. Around 1520 there was no indication as to which one of the many hospitals was likely to become a nucleus of centralisation, but finally the hospital administered by the city's most important chapter was chosen for that purpose. The structure of hospitals in Bordeaux was comparable to that of Toulouse, but, although the same centralising tendencies were at work in Bordeaux, they were finally not as effective as they were in the capital of Languedoc.[23]

The hospitals for lepers and those suffering from ergotism or bubonic plague represented specialised institutions, defined, at least in their function, by certain medical problems, even though presumably the 'treatment' given to the sick there did not differ much from general poor relief and welfare. Against this background the hospital reforms of the 1530s aimed at a concentration of resources from two points of view. On the one hand, they wanted to ensure that only the actually needy were cared for, on the other, they intended to concentrate all the scattered sources of revenue from the various institutions for social welfare and poor relief.

The impulse given locally was mainly based on political, not denominational, elite competition. In Bordeaux, the active elements in the reforms were the high judges at the royal court of justice, the parlement, who increasingly enforced their influence against the city council. In particular from the 1530s onwards – not least with the help of considerable pious endowments from within their wealthy environment – they acquired growing influence on the administrative council of the hospital of Saint-André, thus forcing the canon of Saint-André into a less and less influential minority position. Thus indirectly the great legacies based on the increasing piety of individuals led to a strengthening of the lay element and to a pushing back of the church as an institution from the administration of the hospital that, more and more, was becoming the nucleus of the city's health care. While in 1520 it offered a maximum of forty places (not beds), in 1560/70 there were between 130 and 150, and in 1600 between about 150 and 200.[24] Even in the seventeenth and first half of the eighteenth centuries the numbers do not increase much beyond the latter ones.

The reforms led to a stricter control of hospital administration,[25] expressed first of all in a stricter regulation of admissions. According to the 1542 city statutes, only local patients, who were unable to work and no longer had any other possibility of self-help, were to be admitted.[26] In Aix-en-Provence it was persons suffering from venereal diseases, with chronic or infectious diseases, and 'those who have a fever or are wounded'.[27] In fact, the inmates of the Bordeaux hospital in the seventeenth century were children, aged people and mainly young men, who were mostly not born in the city and had migrated, often from far away. In opposition to the statutes, an important section of the inmates was composed of the typical unskilled migrant workers working in the leather or wood manufacture or in the harbour. They were lacking social capital in the city, which would otherwise have provided for health care.[28]

The sources supply information on medical treatment and daily routine at the Hôpital Saint-André for a later period only. The internal conditions as we know them well for the seventeenth century mirror the concept of disease inspired by Catholic reform. In the following I shall attempt to locate the contemporary concept of health care more precisely by investigating its practice. When looking at the 'medical' personnel, one notices the prominent position of the two (!) priests, who, from the beginning, are situated in the uppermost pay group among the qualified expert staff. In 1620 their wages corresponded to about two-thirds, from the middle of the century about half, of the general manager's income, and were permanently 10 per cent below the physician's.[29] This shows the continued great importance of spiritual care.

As for doctors, during the sixteenth and up to the second decade of the seventeenth centuries there were only the two city physicians, who were also in charge of the hospital and were meant to visit it at least twice a week.[30] It would appear that, while the doctor was only employed at the hospital part-time, he only paid passing attention to the inmates of that institution, preferring his fully-solvent private clientele.[31] The (unrecorded) amount of the basic wage paid by the city would have been an important variable in this. The fact that at the beginning of the seventeenth century a physician was employed exclusively for duty at the hospital, shows the increase of duties in this institution, and offered the opportunity for more intensive medical care.

The remaining medical personnel were surgeons and nursing staff. Along with the fixed employment of a hospital physician, the increase of specialised medical personnel, as well as the growing number of messenger boys and surgeon's journeymen and apprentices (especially from the 1640s), points to the growing importance of health care in a narrower, 'modern', sense, given that during the seventeenth century the number of inmates did not increase accordingly. Certainly the percentage of medical staff within the total hospital personnel increased. It would also seem that the training of medical recruits played an ever greater part at the Saint-André Hospital, showing tendencies towards 'proto-professionalisation'.

A matter of interest in this context is the nursing staff classed as 'lower personnel' in the hospital accounts. In 1602 fifteen persons are listed without precise description of their duties. In 1644 more information is provided regarding various sectors of manual duties in the hospital, but the 'female nurse for the scrofulous' is the only one among the nursing staff whose duties are clearly designated, like the mattress-maker's, the washer-woman's, the scullion's or the grave-digger's. Only in 1672 do we find additional mention of four further 'female nurses', as well as of a herb collector, who was supposed to purchase herbs for medicinal use on the market. It would appear that the authors of the pay lists themselves only slowly, in the course of the seventeenth century, developed a clearer understanding of specific duties requiring special qualifications within the nursing professions, which then found its linguistic expression. In relation to other academically or manually skilled professions, this kind of personnel is very low-paid; during the entire century the amounts did not surpass 6 per cent of the hospital director's salary, including payment in kind.[32] Although the security of a regular meal per day made work at the hospital attractive, there appears to have been a great turnover when the job market was favourable. Nothing can be deduced from the sources regarding the qualification of the nursing personnel, but it appears to have been, as elsewhere, very low.

In Bordeaux, the named doctors, surgeons, nurses, apothecaries, as well as their assistants, apprentices and messenger boys – altogether at least thirty-four persons – cared for from 150 to a maximum of 200 hospital inmates. In 1720 the ratio was thirty-four staff to an annual average of 197 patients.[33] As in the 1760s, this corresponded to one hospital employee (including administration, priests, etc.) per six patients. A comparison of this personnel ratio with other towns in Southern France is not possible, as, for example, for Aix only the total number of patients per year is known, but not the length of stay. There, for 758 patients per year (1780/83), there were 'four doctors, two surgeons, one apothecary and thirty-six nurses'. According to Fairchilds, this corresponds to a ratio of nurses to patients that was higher by one third than that of the Paris Hôtel-Dieu.[34]

The multi-layered Early Modern concept of health care also becomes apparent from an observation of the daily routine in the wards. Every morning mass was said there for the patients at the altars, of which there was one in every ward. The altar paintings showed representations of Christ's Passion, of the Virgin Mary and other saints who triumphed over suffering, be it as doctors (Cosmas and Damian) or as organisers of welfare (Vincent de Paul). The virtue of chastity (Susannah) was also propagandised, a fact that was not surprising, given that the beds were often occupied by two patients – albeit never of different sex. Given that paintings with these subjects were not put up in the hospital wards as the fortuitous result of donations, they must be considered a deliberate choice, for a great number of other paintings, not particularly valued for altars, were stored in chests in side rooms. The hospital's self-image as a healing institution with Christian – i.e. Catholic – motivation, having a medical and a welfare function, and at the same time aiming for the moral improvement of its inmates, becomes evident in the iconographical 'programme' that can be tracked for the year 1739.[35] The subjects of the paintings would not have been without effect, for, apart from the altar decorations, these representations were the only visual stimuli to inspire the sick poor to meditations reaching beyond the hospital's daily routine.

The latter was conspicuous by its problematic hygiene conditions. The wards, seven in 1739, with twenty to thirty-four beds each, were, at least occasionally, 'overcrowded, poorly ventilated, and generally there was little understanding of the infectious nature of disease'.[36] The custom of occupying each bed with two patients, one a convalescent and the other severely, and often contagiously, ill (albeit never a man with a woman), has already been mentioned. At Aix-en-Provence, too, only the specialised hospitals offered the standard of one bed per patient.[37] For Bordeaux there are no records for anything resembling the horrible conditions of hygiene for new-borns that Fairchilds reports for Aix.

At least the beds had curtains that were changed according to season, ensuring thermal insulation and a minimum of privacy, and the wards were heated. However, the innovation, of 1739, of emptying the privies three times daily gives a poor testimony for earlier times. It is obvious that there must have been an unpleasant smell and a risk of infection. The patients' clothes were kept at the entrance to the wards or in lofts and sometimes in storage rooms, not usually in chests, so parasites would have spread unchecked. Patients' old clothes were used for wound dressings.[38]

Medical care cannot be reconstructed in detail, but, from the beginning of the seventeenth century onwards, the hospital accounts provide a list of drugs bought by the hospital pharmacy: among others, large quantities of theriac. There are other, quite general, insights into medical practice: sugar was bought exclusively for medical purposes, for the manufacture of medicinal syrups. Dressings were made with milk; after 1739 they were to be changed twice daily. Knives and scissors were bought for the surgeons, and pharmacopoeias and glass bottles for the apothecaries. It can be concluded from the 1739 inventory, quoted several times, that hygienic conditions had been very bad and the standard of nursing very basic.

Thus another important effect of the Counter-Reformation had not yet made itself felt at the Bordeaux main hospital at this point, i.e. the Catholic nursing orders, confraternities and lay associations had not yet gained a foothold at the Bordeaux city hospital.[39] It was only at this rather late point that it was recognised there, too, that good nursing could not be organised without these persons working from religious motivation – and thus presumably with greater motivation than the ordinary wage-earners. The sisters brought to the hospital ideas of spiritually motivated cleanliness, which they put into practice by the daily cleaning of the wards and of the privies.[40] By doing so they appear to have made an important contribution towards a reduction of the mortality rate in this institution, from around 30 per cent in the sixteenth down to 10 to 20 per cent in the eighteenth century.[41]

Despite the problematic hygiene conditions, specialised surgery is reported even for small rural hospitals.[42] The records of the hospital at Montmorillon (Poitou) mention fifteen amputations, thirteen of them successful, between 1660 and 1790. Apparently, deliberate preference was given to patients from the lower or middle classes, who were young and considered robust (one fifth of them women), in whom decay ('gangrène, putréfaction tissulaire, corruption') of the affected limb had already begun. They had to agree to the operation,[43] which was usually performed four days after their admission to hospital. With an average of thirty-seven days, the convalescing period of amputees was longer than that of other patients. What is relevant for our topic – other than the successful performance of the operation even in that period – is the fact that the operating surgeon was an Augustinian friar specialising in this difficult medical field, like many of his fellow members of the order. This highlights a further link between spiritual and medical/surgical healing, which, in this form, can be considered a characteristic of the Counter-Reformation.[44]

Along with the spiritual and medical healing activities performed by Counter-Reformation poor-hospitals described so far, the great importance of dietetics should not be forgotten. Considering the sizeable proportion of food expenses within the hospital budget, one could even speak of 'nutrition therapy' as the main path towards recovery for the sick poor.

Percentages of the expenses at the Saint-André hospital

Budgetary year	*1602*	*1622*	*1647*	*1672*
Personnel	13.4	6.9	9.6	7.5
Wood	5.9	6.6	7.8	10.4

Source: M. Dinges *Stadtarmut in Bordeaux 1525–1675*. Alltag, Politik, Mentalitäten, Bonn, 1988, p. 408.

The table shows the continuous reduction in expenses for personnel in contrast to the increasing expenses for covering the need for fuel. In each year, however, expenses for food were the largest item, with percentages between 50 and almost 70 per cent.[45] By comparison, the expenses for pharmaceutic products were always well beneath 1 per cent. The same is true for the expenses for spiritual healing, where only the personnel costs, for the priests, were of any importance. The great importance attributed to food is also reflected, other than in the percentage of expenses, in the frequency of written regulations dealing with it, be it a question of eliminating abuses such as misappropriation, regulating the portion of payments in kind within the wages, or determining the rations for the patients (which, however, rarely related to actual practice).[46]

In contrast to this, the sources for Bordeaux provide no information on doctors' dietary prescriptions. However, the account books regularly show differentiation in food acquired for the healthy or for the sick inmates, recognisable in particular from different types of meat. Thus the sick were given beef, the healthy pork. In the case of illness among the leading hospital personnel, a cock would be bought exceptionally, specifically for fortifying the convalescents.

Even in the seventeenth century, the continuing influence of impulses of pre-Tridentine Catholicism can be detected to great extent in the everyday nursing care at the Bordeaux main hospital. Indirectly, it was Catholicism itself that fostered the large building extensions of the sixteenth century and the decrease of the institutional influence of the official church. Some impulses inspired by the Counter-Reformation only made themselves felt in the eighteenth century: the development of iconography is part of these, as well as the late introduction of a nursing order in 1739.

Thus the representatives of the church in the seventeenth century did not succeed in institutional innovation at the centre of the welfare efforts, but only in spheres of action newly discovered and purposely developed by the church. The background to this was that the influence of the Council of Trent remained very limited in France for a long time, both in hospital matters and elsewhere.[47] The Council's decrees never became effective in France from a legal point of view for the state church, particularly because (among other reasons) the regulations on the patrimony of hospitals and the jurisdiction on the control of accounts touched on prerogatives of the French kings. Therefore, after unsuccessful negotiations with the crown, the Catholic church only introduced the regulations in modified form, beginning in the 1580s, in provincial councils at Bordeaux, Borges, Toulouse and Narbonne, and more or less limited itself to improving the administration of the hospitals in their charge. It seems to me, therefore, that the reformatory impulse, spreading from these regional synods – in part directly inspired by Charles Borromaeus – to the clergy and finally to lay people, was more important than the administrative tightening of existing church patrimony.[48]

In Bordeaux, the reformatory impetus inspired by the Counter-Reformation was set in motion by Archbishop François de Sourdis (archbishop 1599–1628), who had spent some time in Milan and, while there, had come to know the reform activities of Charles Borromaeus.[49] Supported by the now regular regional synods, this self-confident, power-conscious holder of the bishopric began his offensive in the sphere of poor relief. Simultaneously with mobilising lay people for the development of a communal poor relief system (see pp. 259–66) from 1600, he demonstrated successful city politics to the city council. Using his private means, he had the malaria-infested swamp directly behind the city wall, drained, a project that had been discussed for decades by the jurade and the parlement without being realised. In order to save the network of canals from decay, he founded a charterhouse there, the monks in which were to be in charge of the maintenance. While the attempt at repelling malaria was an impressive feature of health politics, the foundation of a small specialised hospital for fifteen cripples, near the charterhouse, clearly showed the claim of this prince of the church to play a part in the decisions in matters of poor relief, too. The name, Hôpital Saint-Charles, expresses not only homage for the example of the Milanese Charles Borromaeus, but at the same time a programme, also recognisable in the, now weekly, distribution of alms to fifteen men and ten women: charity inspired by Christian faith was again to become a factor of politics. It deliberately continued the ill-famed distributions of alms as an opportunity for poor relief – destined for specific groups, and carefully controlled. However, this was only the prelude to a much more far-reaching institutional innovation that the bishop wanted to enforce under his leadership. The concept of an 'Hôpital des Métiers', i.e. of a workhouse for the poor, had been around for some time. When, in 1624, the pious legacy of the widow Anne de Tauzia (see Figure 12.1) fell due, de Sourdis pressed for the construction of such an institution, which promised to be a considerable contribution towards the solution of welfare problems. Using a starting capital of five-and-a-half times the yearly budget of the city's largest hospital (Saint-André), de Sourdis even wanted to begin the construction by himself, but the city council blocked the buying of the land. The parlement showed little readiness to accept a new political actor in the poor relief sphere. De Sourdis was forbidden unauthorised construction in 1639, and in 1645 the parlement secured the majority in the board of trustees – only to delay everything again. It was only after the Fronde and the ensuing local Ormée revolt, which lasted until 1653, that the city's other political powers, too, realised that the projected institution (now to be called Hôpital de la Manufacture) might have a socially calming effect, or even contribute to a re-education of those unwilling to work.[50] While the bishop's claims for the leadership of public opinion and plenipotentiary decision in welfare matters were pushed

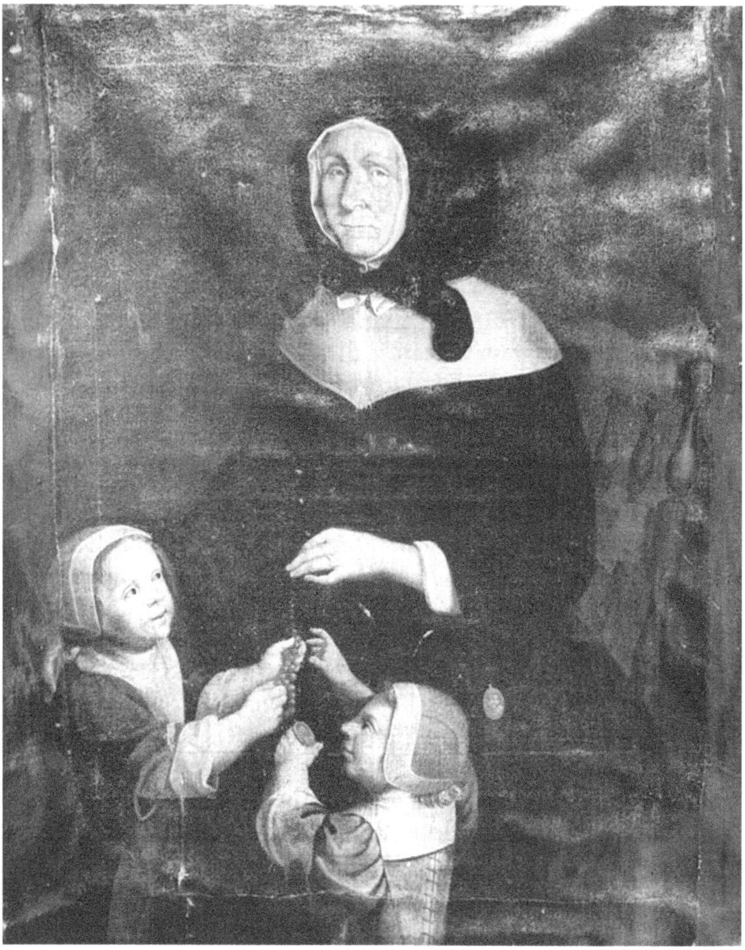

Figure 12.1 Anne de Tauzia (as widow Madame de Brezetz), *c*. 1560–1624, was a very rich noblewoman married to a councillor of the parliament. She is a good example of that important part of the city's elites which after 1600 joined in the Counter-Reformation spirituality. Her important will of about 30,000 livres allowed the foundation in Bordeaux of the General Hospital called 'La Manufacture' from 1619. She also continued the tradition of dressing and feeding the poor: she ordered the giving of clothes and a piece of bread to 100 women and 100 men, insisting that this distribution had to be carried out in good order. Painter unknown, dated second quarter of the seventeenth century. Courtesy of Inventaire générale Aquitoine cliché Dubau/Chabot.

Source: Reproduced by permission of Ministère de la Culture

back, he was, nevertheless re-admitted as the innovative initiator and as a junior partner on the board of trustees. Also, the Bordeaux Manufacture was under the direction of a clergyman, and, right from the foundation, a religious order played an important role in the care for the inmates.[51]

Similarly to the situation in Bordeaux, it can be observed in many Southern French towns that Catholic reform elites – clergy as well as lay people, among the latter not infrequently high judges or their wives – were of great importance in the spread and realisation of *hôpitaux généraux*. One well-known case is the part played by the clergyman Saint Vincent de Paul in the 1656 legislation on the topic.[52] The considerable influence of local Catholic activists, working in the vanguard of the generalisation of a new hospital model that would finally be supported by the monarchy, has been overlooked so far. Thus, for example, in Marseille the canon Emmanuel Pachier managed to win the support of people from all parts of the city and collect enough money, in about 1640, to put into practice a decree made in 1621 by the city council for the construction of an Hôpital général de la Charité.[53] Elsewhere it was the local Compagnies de Saint Sacrement, founded in 1672, who got under way measures for the Catholic disciplining of the poor by other means. Furthermore, three Jesuits who conducted a propaganda campaign for general hospitals – Fathers Guevarre, Chaurand and Dunod – were instrumental in the implementation of this legislation. They had taken over the model from the Capuchins, a fact that suggests, among other things, that the Catholic reformers were rather successful in applying innovative methods in the use of media and in propaganda. Sometimes the Jesuits would have advertising brochures for the new institution printed in advance, then preach for periods between three days and three weeks, and finally give the decisive impulse for the construction of a general hospital by conducting a successful collection.[54] It is due mainly to them that the development of general hospitals finally proceeded from the 1680s onwards. The long-term effects continued up to 1712 in the 'late- developing' city of Grenoble, when they finally achieved what local forces had not been able to do.[55] The co-operation of local, regional and supra-regional forces of a varied nature, often of wealthy lay people, canons, members of religious orders and the congregation, is characteristic of the functioning of Counter-Reformation influences.

In the workhouses it was possible to accommodate more paupers than in previous other institutions, and usually to care for them regularly there. It is more difficult to judge whether the new foundations had any influence on health care. It was the conscious aim of these institutions to provide moral improvement, through work and prayer, for the poor unwilling to work or for those who had failed, in particular, prostitutes who were new in their profession or already willing to leave it; thus there were no medical aims as such. It is possible, however, that they had indirect effects, in the sense that the newly established workhouses would take over from the hospitals of the older type part of the clientele not in need of medical treatment, so that perhaps the hospitals were in a better position for focusing on their medical duties. At least according to the statutes, this appears to have been the idea in Lyons: the sick, *malades*, were to be cared for at the Hôtel-Dieu, the incurably ill and the innocents (foundlings) at the Charité.[56] It is difficult to determine whether this situation actually led to functional specialisation for the older general hospitals. So far there are only a few clues: for example, according to the 1724 ordinance, Notre-Dame de la Charité de Marseilles admitted the poor, whether able or unable to work, as well as invalids, who had to be from Marseille or have lived there for ten years. They were expected to work according to their abilities. The target group was once again the whole of the poor. The most frequent cause of invalidity was eye problems. The differentiation of the inmates was reflected in different daily rates, which were at 5 sous for those able to work, and 7 sous for invalids.[57]

According to the Bordeaux workhouse's register of deaths for the years 1659–83, 63 per cent of the 502 deaths were women who were mainly from Bordeaux and its environments, and who thus, in contrast to the situation at the city hospital, had rarely migrated from far away. Perhaps for them the Manufacture was an attractive alternative to the city hospital.[58] Compared to the middle-age groups, children feature more prominently in the mortality numbers, as well as the over-fifties, with a peak for those aged between 60 and 69. Overall the data for Marseille and Bordeaux suggest that the workhouses served mainly for dealing with the 'old life-cycle poverty', and little scope remained for the improvement of sturdy beggars. There are no contemporary records for the patients of the Hôpital Saint-André, but in a comparison with those for the 1620s, it is noticeable that the Manufacture cares for fewer migrants from far away and fewer men. It would appear, therefore, that the Manufacture was oriented more strongly than the old hospital towards welfare for life-cycle poverty, in which old or young age, female gender and unfavourable economic situation were decisive factors. More solid information regarding medical specialisation – possibly achieved in an indirect way – in the hospital system could only be obtained via the analysis of inmate data over long time-periods and for several hospitals in one town, as well as a comparison between different towns.[59]

While the medical impulse appears to have been of little relevance, the Hôpital Général of Grenoble, founded as late as 1712, nevertheless had a special room for the chronically ill and for sick prostitutes.[60] One could interpret this as steps towards internal medical specialisation, as it is also visible in the small general hospital of Montmorillon in the eighteenth century. Contrary to the earlier usage of operating directly in the general ward, the amputations there were performed in a room especially reserved for surgical interventions.[61] Sometimes the forces of Catholic reform only developed an influence on sick care after having achieved a majority in the hospital's administrative boards. Thus the Compagnie du Saint Sacrement infiltrated the hospital administration in Grenoble during the 1640s and 1650s, until it had become the majority of members taking part in meetings of the administrative council. It is interesting to see that the active majority of those actually participating was sufficient for swaying the entire board, even without a formal majority of seats. The activating of even a small number of lay people inspired by Counter-Reformation ideas had sweeping success, because others had too little interest in poor relief. The new 'majority' introduced first (before 1662) the nursing confraternity of the Frères de la Charité, for caring for the men, later the Soeurs de Sainte-Marthe, for looking after the women at the Hôpital Général.[62]

This touches on an impulse of Catholic reform important for the hospital system, namely the innovation of nursing. As for the chronology of this development, which can be observed mainly from the second third of the seventeenth century, originating from the North of France, and spreading increasingly in the South too during the last third of the century, I refer to the research by Jones and Gutton.[63] It has become clear from the example of Bordeaux that new nursing orders were sometimes more likely to find a foothold in the newly founded institutions such as the Manufacture, than at the old city hospital, where it took until 1739. The question whether this pattern can be generalised cannot be answered at present. The renewed value of nursing within the orders, confraternities and lay associations led to new appreciation of services to the poor and the sick, on the basis of older Christian concepts of the seven corporal works of mercy. The specifically missionary intentions aiming at the moral improvement of the sick and poor, by catechisation and by guided prayer, are characteristic of the Counter-Reformation. By applying the concept of spiritual purity, stressing the connection between outward cleanliness and inward orderliness of the soul, the nursing orders succeeded in creating the necessary conditions for what, by a modern term, would be called hygiene. The evidence suggests that this can be considered an essential cause for the decline in mortality among hospital patients during the seventeenth and eighteenth centuries.

In Bordeaux, an internal regulation of 1739, highlighted the importance of the quality of food and the cleanliness of the buildings. This fact, too, suggests that the introduction of staff who were religiously motivated, and some of whom lived by the rules of an order, was causally linked to an improvement of the standards of hygiene. Regarding the influence the Counter-Reformation had on medical care, it seems plausible that, as Norberg says 'in the old regime trained nurses with some knowledge of drugs and bandages were, by definition, members of religious orders. When the directors and directresses called upon these religious, they were not trying to strengthen the role of the church in poor relief; rather they were trying to provide the poor with the best available medical care'.[64] Given that the, mainly female, nurses primarily intended to give their own life a sanctifying content, it can be assumed that the improvement of hygiene was accompanied by an accentuation of the religious character of life at the hospital.

All told, the influence of the Counter-Reformation on health care became stronger in the seventeenth century and continued to solidify until 1740; the foundation of new small, specialised hospitals addressed special needs.[65] Thus the 'exemplary character' of the Bordeaux Hôpital Saint-Charles lay in the successful harmony between the name (after Charles Borromaeus), the choice of a particularly pitiable target group and the fact that it was adminstered by a religious order. Another institution that had pioneering character in the sense of Catholic reform was the Grenoble Providence, founded in 1676 purely as a hospital for local people, because the founders active in this small institution were mainly lay women, and from the beginning the sick were cared for by a nursing order, the Soeurs de Saint-Joseph.[66] Nevertheless, the decisive path towards gaining influence presumably remained the mobilisation of lay people on the boards of trustees of the existing large institutions. Finally, the renewal of nursing can be regarded as the most effective way of imparting to the sick and poor, within the hospital routine, a concept of illness that is revalued by the Counter-Reformation and has a spiritual imprint. A spiritual understanding of purity at the same time created the prerequisites for the propagation of higher standards of hygiene.

Institutions for outdoor medical care for the poor

As early as the late Middle Ages, for example, in Flanders, community-based ooutdoor poor relief was a widespread form of assistance to the poor. In the South of France, however, it only had very shallow roots. Only for a few towns or villages of the South-East is there evidence for confraternities which, along with mutual help, are believed to have also dispensed welfare to third parties.[67]

Little is known with precision as to whether care for the poor at home was provided indirectly by the big hospitals, as the Bordeaux statutes provide.[68] The two town physicians, and later the hospital physician or the barber surgeon of the Hôpital Saint-André of Bordeaux, were commissioned to have consultation hours for the poor. However, concerning the dispensation of remedies, the statutes only contain the direction that they must not be over-priced. It remains unclear whether the hospital pharmacy offered especially favourable terms, or even free remedies, to the poor. For example, it was expressly stated as an exception that a midwife for the poor in Toulouse was paid from the public treasury, in which there was a surplus at the time.[69] The evidence suggests that initially there was no care for the house-bound poor in Bordeaux and in most other towns of Southern France during the sixteenth century.

Toulouse provides the earliest examined example of municipal home care for the poor, the municipal authorities attempting, together with representatives of the church, to close this gap in support. From 1536, the city council collected a tax from corporations and wealthy citizens, and organised church collections. At markedly fewer than 5 per cent, only a small percentage of the population was cared for, in particular women, the aged, the infirm and children. One can deduce from the only surviving parish register for the parish of St Etienne (for the years 1535/6) that almost 60 per cent of all persons and households receiving support fell under the categories 'sick' or 'disabled'.[70] In Toulouse, the tax was collected, by quarter, by the dizainiers, who were also responsible for restricting begging in their quarters. In Bordeaux, too, money was collected by the dizainiers – albeit only in times of plague.[71] What developed into municipal poor relief in Toulouse, did not lead to the same result in Bordeaux. However, the scarcity of evidence for municipal welfare even in Toulouse suggests that the institution was short-lived. It is only in 1592 that the town council of Avignon launches a similar attempt with the foundation of an *aumône générale* for the support of the housebound poor in each parish. In doing so, it continued a generous endowment by the Baronne de Lers et de Monfredin that originated from a climate of religious renewal. A Jesuit confraternity and further confraternities – for assistance to prisoners and for a Mont de Piété – that were being founded at the time played a part in this development, as well as the donor's personal acquaintance with Alexander Farnese.[72] In this case the influence of the Italian Counter-Reformation (geographically in close proximity) on poor relief is almost tangible. Nevertheless, home care for the poor in Avignon soon collapsed under the weight of the plague.

It is no coincidence, therefore, that parish relief in Bordeaux is also a result of Counter-Reformation influences. A Marian congregation of the Jesuits had existed there since 1576, the members of which visited prisons, the needy and hospitals outside their congregation. In 1604 it had eighty members.[73] Archbishop de Sourdis, already mentioned in connection with the hospital buildings, could presumably build on the preliminary work done by this pioneering Catholic order, when, beginning in 1601, he promoted the foundation of *sociétés de la miséricorde*. In 1603 they were already in existence in all parishes and were to care for the housebound poor,[74] their main supporters the wives of high judges at the parlement. Thus the focused theological and catechetical 'treatment' of this elite, pursued intensively by both the Jesuits and Surin, paid off.[75] As little as ten years earlier, the parlement judges had refused to take part in town-wide collections for the Saint-André hospital, preferring to send out their servants on a task that was considered undignified. Now, however, their wives considered the service rendered to the sick and the poor as sanctification of their lives – as defined by the revival of Christian virtues in the Counter-Reformation.

From 1611 the statutes of these associations become more strictly regulated. When drawing up wills, the clergy were to call for donations for parish relief. The town councillors were invited to be present at the opening of the collection boxes, in order to involve them in the reform work, and to confer public solemnity on it. The assembly of parish priests expected this to result in an increased readiness among the citizens to give in church collections, while the jurade feared for the returns of their own Lent collections for the Hôpital Saint-André. In 1617 a *Compagnie de la charité* was founded in the parish of Sainte-Eulalie, followed by a *Confrérie de la bonne nouvelle* in 1628. While for the charity associations the spiritual health of the sick poor was at the centre of their activities, the statutes of further *Compagnies de la charité*, founded in the 1630s in two of the parishes of Bordeaux and in four other towns in the diocese, gave equal importance to the care for physical well-being. After a medical examination, needy persons who had been resident in the parish for at least three months should be provided with remedies, linen and two daily meals. In 1635, a further *Compagnie de la charité* followed in the parish of Saint-Rémy. Around 1639 the *Soeurs grises* (of Saint Vincent de Paul) are first mentioned in the parish of Sainte-Eulalie, and in 1645 the *Confrérie Notre-Dame des agonisants*, which visits hospitals, prisons and the shamefaced poor, is formed. From 1654, the *Compagnie du très Saint Sacrement* also becomes involved in, among other things, welfare for the poor in their homes. At the same time they criticise sharply the fact that at the hospital the sick are given only food, but no moral support.[76] Because of the scarcity of evidence, it is not always possible to determine whether each of these associations was in fact newly founded or only converted. It is, however, true that in matters of parish poor relief Bordeaux is a pioneer within Southern France – even when compared to Lyons and Paris, or to the activities of Saint Vincent de Paul.[77] The spread of the Compagnies de la charité to rural areas, too, appears to have started earlier in the diocese of Bordeaux than elsewhere. A course typical for the success of the Counter-Reformation on the whole can be observed here, too: here and there individual activists, often inspired by Italian ideas, began applying exemplary measures, which were imitated in other places, often with conspicuous delay. Parish relief in the South of France, in particular, demonstrates that it often took several attempts. It is certainly worth noting that, in Bordeaux, it took a few years to re-involve Catholic lay people and the clergy as important actors in poor relief. The few active lay men and women, who before had, for example, collected goods for the town hospital, now involved themselves in the church's parish welfare, together with many newly-recruited female activists.[78]

The Counter-Reformatory impetus of the confraternities – which, given their almost exclusively female membership, could just as well be called sororities – is most clearly recognisable in the strongly spiritual form of the visit to the sick (along with its being subject to the parish clergy). Similar to the Bordeaux statutes, the 1714 regulations for Saint-Galmier (Loire) also contain detailed instructions.[79] Here, too, visiting the sick was at the centre of the activities, which were supported by a linen room.

In Bordeaux, the ladies were meant to talk about pious topics on the way to the sick (twice weekly), after joint attendance at morning mass, and confession. They were to enter with a modest, friendly and helpful countenance and, having greeted the family, serve the patient some light broth or an egg, and enquire about the illness, but also about the practice of receiving sacraments and of prayer. A questioning of the family members regarding the dogmas and commandments was planned, as well as the pious admonition of those present in the sick room to assist the patient, as God would then not let him die. At Saint-Galmier there was also the threat of sanctions; for example, if the patient refused the sacraments, no further help was to be given. The parish priest was to be informed in time about the patient's state of health when death was approaching, so that no-one would die without receiving the sacrament. The Confrérie also intended to assist the dying, in order to render possible a good death, that is an accepting, Christian death. In the case of mothers who died in childbirth, the christening of the child was provided. There is also mention of Caesarian section, which would be performed by a surgeon, in order to save at least the child when the woman was dying.

At Saint-Galmier up to two visits per day were provided. The visitors brought food and cleaned, aired and fumigated the sick room. They loaned bedlinen, and thus considered hygiene important, just as in Bordeaux. Continuous records were kept on the patient's state of health, and a weekly report was given to the Superior; in the case of acute problems this could also be done daily. The confraternity had a contracted surgeon, a *chirurgien de la compagnie*. Vigils were held for the dying, and a winding-sheet was donated for the dead, so as to allow a dignified funeral even for the poor.

At Saint-Galmier, soup was provided up to twice daily, three times in Bordeaux, together with fresh eggs and, for those able to eat it, 'some meat'. In Bordeaux, 245 grams of veal or mutton were provided, as well as the same amount of bread, one chopin (1.1 litres) of wine, or other food according to the doctor's instructions.[80] At Saint-Galmier it was all to be eaten by the patient only. This regulation was meant to avoid the handing on of patients' meals to third parties, as this could have resulted in casual family welfare. Medicinal teas are also mentioned as therapeutic means.

On the way back the wealthy ladies were to meditate on the virtues of 'poor people', and they were also to inform the Superior on any mistakes made by the doctor. At Saint-Galmier they were also meant to involve their daughters in the charitable activity from a young age, and thus recruit them for it.

What is striking on the whole is the great stress on spiritual help for the salvation of the visitor's own soul as well as for that of the sick. Moral improvement in the sense of Catholic Counter-Reformation is one of the main aims of parish poor relief, which also facilitated the formation of family traditions of involvement in it.[81] In addition, similar to indoor relief, high-quality and plentiful food played an important part. Nursing care in a stricter sense is mainly related to hygiene for the sick-bed (linen) and the sick room (airing, fumigating, cleaning). The ladies not only secured medical treatment through contracted physicians or surgeons, as well as taking part in determining the point in time (for childbirth), but they also claimed control over the doctor. The scheduled keeping of exact records on the course of the illness suggests innovations in the sphere of nursing. This mixed offer of spiritual, medical and nutritional assistance, coupled with intended catechisation and controls, certainly was the way in which the movement of the Counter-Reformation penetrated most deeply into the households and families of the sick poor, for here it not only preached, but it also offered services; it not only disciplined, but it also helped.[82]

For smaller rural communities it appears to have been common for communal welfare to be institutionally linked to the local hospital. At Saint-Galmier the latter served as a place of assembly and as linen store, and at Vic-en-Bigorre, at the foot of the Pyrenees, the Dames de la miséricorde, belonging to the local upper class, even managed to take control of the hospital. In 1729 they were present at the rendering of accounts. As usual in the taking of control over hospitals, earlier irregularities committed by the hospital administrator had given them a chance to intervene, of which they resolutely took advantage.[83]

Altogether it is very difficult to learn anything beyond the aims of parish poor relief expressed in the statutes, regarding their actual functioning. Loupès has been able to demonstrate, by using the records of visitations, that communal welfare functioned well in the mid-eighteenth century in the about ten towns of the diocese of Bordeaux that had a population of over 2,500, where one can see the beginnings of a local bourgeoisie.[84] Where the local charitable association disposed of a sick room in a house, it often created the pre-conditions for a later introduction of the *Soeurs grises*, a nursing order.[85] Otherwise the sources rarely mention more than the mere existence of an institution of the kind, which was to work locally without elaborate written records.[86] The *de facto* capacity of survival of these groups is therefore difficult to judge. However, the evidence of just 162 wills made in Bordeaux in 1675 points to the continued existence of confraternities for parish poor relief. In a dispute on parish finances the priest of Saint-Rémy made known that in his poor community of craftsmen at the end of the seventeenth century 120 families were cared for in 180 houses.[87] This suggests a certain stability of lay organisations during the entire seventeenth century, as well as considerable efficiency.

Their re-Catholicisation of poor relief and sick care was supplemented by private endowments. I have already described to what extent large individual legacies contributed to reforms in the main institutions and to the recovery of the church's initiative in poor relief in the seventeenth century. Here we are talking about minor endowments. For example, in Bordeaux they were used for providing poor, nubile young women with a trousseau. This concerns a group the potential danger to which – pregnancy and ensuing prostitution – the Counter-Reformation wanted to check by the appropriate institutions.[88] In the accounts of one such charity I have also found mentions of slaves whose freedom had been bought or (poor) Jews, who either had just converted or intended to convert to Catholicism after having received a subsidy.[89] The *Congrégation pour la propagation de la foi* (1647–85) in Grenoble, for example, overtly aimed for the reclaiming of poor 'heretics' for the Catholic faith by its combination of poor relief and catechisation.[90]

Against this background it seems appropriate to give a brief outline of Protestant communal welfare in Bordeaux. It can be used to show how the 'competition' armed itself.[91] It is particularly important, given that the even smaller Jewish community cared for its poor from the same motivations; however, there is even less information on this.[92] For the Protestants – in Bordeaux mainly merchants and their families from North-Western Europe, as well as some local nobles and migrants from the 'Protestant crescent' in Western, South-Western and Southern France – care for their sick was an even greater question of denominational survival than for the Catholics. The Protestants were well aware of this, and their community treasury was always well replenished by donations and legacies. In a social environment dominated by Catholics, and with a town hospital that had an altar for daily mass in every ward, the Calvinist minority of around 2,000, about 5 per cent of the city's population, always had reason to fear that the Catholic clergy attached to the hospital would take advantage of the emergency situation created by illness for the purpose of religious propaganda.[93]

Poor relief was one of the main topics of the Calvinist community elders during their weekly assemblies. What has survived is the second *Registre des délibérations du consistoire*, for the years 1660–70, so one can assume the existence of a similarly formalised communal poor relief beginning in 1650 at the latest. The political pressure on the Calvinists, which had been increasing since the 1620s, even suggests that the institution may have older roots, not necessarily expressed in a corresponding amount of written evidence.

Every week the elders decided on viatica for co-religionists travelling through, as well as on the payment of subsidies for housebound poor, sometimes following the report given by a member of the board, who had verified their neediness locally. These payments were often meant as help towards self-help, as one can see in the buying of tools for craftsmen, or of clothes for prospective servants. They also procured jobs for unemployed members of the community. Along with these things, assistance with living expenses for large families or orphans played a certain role; nuclear families especially often feature as receivers of alms. However, these payments were usually only supplements towards a livelihood to be sought by the person concerned.

Payments for the sick, on the other hand, could go so far as to cover the needs of the patients and their families. Since no clear pattern can be ascertained for the payments – by family size, etc. – it would appear that the Consistorium aimed for 'nourishment appropriate to the person's status', so that an impoverished merchant received more in case of illness than a harbour hand.

The great incidence of illness as the explicitly-named reason for support is illustrated by its accounting for over 37 per cent of the total payments, followed by unemployment, with just over 30 per cent, and poverty, with not quite 30 per cent. It seems that in a great number of the cases of necessity, too, illness had been the cause of impoverishment.[94] For the sick who could no longer be cared for in their household, the Consistorium first attempted to organise sick care in the home of another community member. In these cases it often fell back upon families that were under an obligation to it because of previous assistance; this stressed the mutuality of the service relationships. For those patients only who could no longer be billetted in other households, as well as for the bedridden and for those travelling through, the Consistorium kept a small ward with several beds, which was in the charge of a married couple. They would care for the linen and cook for the – usually between one and three – patients. Unfortunately the records say nothing of any further nursing care. Medical care was secured through the contracting of doctors and apothecaries. Thus the Protestants of Bordeaux combined indoor andoutdoor relief for the poor with an extensive programme of assistance towards self-help.

One can get an idea of the health problems communal poor relief had to deal with by studying another source, containing information on the 'disabilities of those persons interned under the declaration of 1724 in Aix-en-Provence'.[95] With this 'internment', problems that had previously been dealt with elsewhere – without written records – came onto the record of an institution. It is true that the beggars interned between 1725 and 1732 showed a social profile slightly diverging from the local population: they were slightly younger (up to 42 per cent were under 20), and, with 70 per cent, men were represented beyond the usual proportion. Nevertheless, the data for 167 persons demonstrate the frequency of eye problems, disabilities restricting walking and other problems of the extremities, as well as mental retardation, all of which can be considered real obstacles to the pursuit of a regular and sufficient income.

With the sphere of parish poor relief, the Catholic church of the Counter-Reformation discovered at the same time an essential gap in assistance and an effective tool for taking effect in individual households by services and catechisation. It achieved a considerable mobilisation of lay people. It was mainly women who became personally involved in the charitable associations, confraternities or charitable orders. The special significance of the Counter-Reformation's social movement lies in this reactivation of women for a public charitable task, as well as the gender-specific opportunity for sanctification of the individual's own life by an active practice of faith. As well as 'womanpower', considerable financial means were also activated for poor relief under the direction of the church, partly by withdrawing them from the official representatives.

The penetration of Catholic reform into people's minds and practices, as far as their attitudes towards the poor are concerned

This development can easily be reconstructed from wills, which are a useful indicator for the depth of penetration, social boundaries and the chronology of the success the Counter-Reformation had with the donors. They reflect not only the changing image of the poor, but also the degree of the citizens' readiness to give and their preferences.

The following is based on my own research on 508 wills made by Catholic testators in Bordeaux between 1525 and 1675, as well as on

Norberg's results, which are based on 5,012 wills made in the years 1620–1789 by Catholic and Calvinist testators.[96] Pugh's investigation of 2,218 wills from Lyons and 739, of both denominations, from Nîmes, is used to supplement the evidence.

For Bordeaux, the connection between the testator's Catholic religiosity and the aim of social welfare can be outlined broadly as follows.[97] In the sixteenth century it was common in all strata of society to bequeath something not only to the church, but also to the poor. Craftsmen as well as nobles mentioned the housebound poor or the hospital in their wills, and usually gave very small amounts. This pattern of donations can therefore be interpreted as conventional behaviour. In the course of the sixteenth century, up to the year 1600 and beyond, the readiness to donate money for the church or for the poor declined overall – albeit at first primarily to the disadvantage of the church. At the same time the pattern of donations changed: the majority of the population gave hardly anything, while a decreasing number of persons who had become wealthy gave large sums for charitable purposes. During the second half of the sixteenth century this type of legacy became more and more characteristic of the upper class. At the same time, one can at first notice, in the sixteenth century, a great enthusiasm on the part of the citizens for the centralised hospital as a new solution. However, this welfare reform appears to have lost its attraction soon after the mid-sixteenth century. The 'large institution', by now centralised, is considered less and less often, while other target groups move to the fore: personally known poor from the donor's own community or neighbourhood, from 1600 parish poor relief and private charities, as well as particularly poor prisoners (a newly-rediscovered group of recipients). At the same time domestic servants become the main recipients of bestowals from the generally well-off donors; they are directed primarily and mainly at the testator's own household.

As we can see, those citizens who were prepared to donate money had already shown preference for the poor as individuals and turned away from larger institutions during the second half of the sixteenth century, i.e. before the revalutation of charitable works by the Counter-Reformation and the widespread visual propaganda for charity towards the poor. It is possible that they took public funding of these institutions for granted, with the result that the latter had deprived themselves of financial support from the donor by their own success. However, the new pattern can also be interpreted as the desire for a more direct mutual relationship with the poor as representative of Christ and as paraclete, who could no longer be recognised behind the hospital walls. In this point it is certain that there was a readiness – well before the start of large-scale preaching by the Counter-Reformation – to give for a poor relief that was closer to the citizen; this had its effects, for example, on the development of parish poor relief and on private charities. In this respect the Counter-Reformers met already existing expectations, which could explain their, in part very quick, success.

It is interesting to follow the spread of the Counter-Reformation pattern of donations, using Grenoble as an example, against the background of the social make-up – increasingly exclusive during the course of the sixteenth century – of donators. As with parish poor relief in Bordeaux, here, too, the judges played a leading part in the acceptance of the Counter-Reformation model:[98] in 80–90 per cent of wills from 1620 onwards, they always gave for religious bequests, followed in this by the nobles, with 60 per cent, but after 1700 always over 79 per cent. In Grenoble the master craftsmen, who in sixteenth-century Bordeaux had been giving ever more rarely for the poor, were late in following this elite pattern: between 1620 and 1670 their share of wills including religious bequests rose from 26 per cent to 62 per cent, declined to only 45 per cent by 1700, only to reach 77 per cent again between 1700 and 1730. Thus the cultural pattern that had once been abandoned was only reassimilated very slowly.

In Grenoble, too, Catholic donations became part of a seigneurial ethic in the upper class (a tendency already visible in the preferential treatment of domestic servants in Bordeaux), recognisably furthered by the Counter-Reformation. By comparison, for the Protestants denominational motivation was predominant, and 59 per cent of all testators – compared to 39 per cent for Catholics – continued to leave money to the poor.[99] However, Pugh's results for Nîmes suggest that the readiness to give is highest for representatives of both denominations where the inter-denominational competition is open and therefore particularly fierce.[100]

While in sixteenth-century Bordeaux the development of bequests for the poor and those for the church ran in separate, and at times opposite, directions, Catholic religious mentality again turned towards the poor from the seventeenth century and during the first half of the eighteenth. Thus the Counter-Reformation church had successfully transformed the poor from competing recipients into partners for the church's expectations of funding. In contrast to this, the Calvinists in Grenoble as a rule decided between a bequest for the poor and one for the church: religious attitudes form the demarcation between objectives of welfare and direct support of the church.[101] It seems, however, that this was not a general pattern, since their fellow Calvinists in Bordeaux generally divided their favour equally between the treasury for the pastors and that for the poor.[102]

Neither in Bordeaux nor in Grenoble was the testator's gender a decisive variable in patterns of donation. This only changed for Grenoble in the eighteenth century, when the men showed earlier signs of 'de-Christianisation' than the women.[103] It can be stated at this point that Counter-Reformation piety was of longer duration for women, a fact that corresponded, not least, to their paramount role in communal poor relief, that is in the practice of charity.

Survey and perspectives

In the sixteenth century the church as institution had largely lost direct influence on health care and poor relief everywhere, even though individual pious donors fostered institutional change by their large donations, and representatives of the church remained involved, in a minority position, in the public administration of poor relief. Even the widespread, rather conventional, readiness to give for the poor, from religious motivations, diminished and became elite behaviour.

If one regards the Counter-Reformation as the intensification of Catholic reform towards a spiritualisation of everyday practice, and the increased, more strictly regulated participation of lay people in the life of the church, then considerable success can be noted in the sphere of welfare for the sick poor. The incentives given by the Council of Trent were accepted and developed, with greatly varying speed, by French bishops and regional synods (1585–1615). Even before 1585, and simultaneously with the reforming bishops, the Jesuits worked as 'shock troops', leaving their traces in communal poor relief in, for example, Avignon and Bordeaux in the last two decades of the sixteenth century. The realisation of the decisions of the Council of Trent consisted in the training of reformatory clergy, the targeted catechesis of the elites, and the formation of lay confraternities, which only became fully effective a generation later. It gave new impulses to poor relief (ca. 1600–30), and in Bordeaux it led to a reorganisation of communal welfare in the first decade of the new century by the imitation of Italian examples. This form of poor relief, as well as the religious nursing orders, offered an additional public role to women in particular, which at the same time conveyed spiritual meaning to their lives. Another generation later, Vincent de Paul, by his suggestions, opened up new tasks in poor relief to the Christian involvement of lay people and of the orders inspired by him (1630–65). Thus in many institutions, members of religious orders or at least staff with a strong religious motivation, took charge of nursing, improving it even in practice – in particular in matters of hygiene – by their spiritual orientation towards an ideal of purity.[104]

Through Vincent de Paul's connections at court his ideas finally found their way into the 1656 legislation on general hospitals. Its realisation – propagated not least by the Jesuits Guevarre, Chaurand and Dunod – during the following generation (1665–1700) can be considered the next phase in the development of welfare stimulated by the forces of Catholic reform. In the background, the Catholic secret societies, as well as the *Compagnies du Saint Sacrement*, often played an important part. However, in the case of the general hospitals, imperatives of public order and mercantilist hopes mingled with the religious goal of moral renewal through work and prayer. After 1700 the discussion of poor relief politics shifts more and more towards economic and fiscal aspects, with increased focus on the objective of putting the poor to some use for society,[105] but at the most this leads to an increase of methods of repression and discipline in the large institutions, spiritual aspects being simultaneously pushed back. Before independent new solutions can be developed, the institutional structure, moulded by successive impulses of Catholic reform, consolidates until the 1760s.

While in the sixteenth century the centralising tendencies of large poor-hospitals rather side-stepped the church or went against its institutional influence, both the rediscovery, or re-establishment of parish poor relief and the leading institution of the seventeenth century, the general hospital, demonstrate the church's regaining of the leadership of public opinion in poor relief. It was only in the *Dépôts de mendicité* (1764) that aspects of public order and usefulness outweighed the goal of religious improvement of the inmates.[106] It is likely that the influence of Catholic reform and of the Counter-Reformation can be seen in the self-help that is usually decisive for the sick in making use of spiritual and religious possibilities of healing, such as pilgrimages. There were often members of the clergy among the authors of the 'pharmacopoeias for the poor' and similar widely-used works. Furthermore, the Counter-Reformation developed its depth of penetration through communal poor relief, by which it was able to influence individual households by aiming simultaneously for hygiene of the body and of the soul. Finally, in the course of the seventeenth century, staff with a stronger religious motivation improved nursing in almost all hospitals, and supplemented the existing institutions by a plethora of smaller specialised ones, while some orders virtually became medical or surgical specialists. And not least, it revaluated the image of the sick and the poor among those who were prepared to give.

However, there are quite a few aspects of this topic that need further investigation. Little is known on how, with what frequency, in which media and to what effect the new, spiritual image of the sick and the poor was spread in Counter-Reformation preaching and propaganda (i.e. in the representations), in contrast to an orientation aimed primarily at their capacity to work and their usefulness. Too little is known also about the actual development and importance of, as well as the participation in, pilgrimages to saints believed to have power over illness. Could this be a further aspect of the re-Catholicisation of everyday life in opposition to the otherwise assumed secularizing tendencies? We still know too little on the medical market in France, i.e. which offerers of which services were used at what prices even by the poorer people.[107] For the South of France, the systematic analysis of lists of debtors in doctors' wills – which can be found in large numbers in notaries' registers – could bring some solutions to this question. Little is known, too, about the reception of pharmacopoeias for the poor. Finally, the difference in the importance of self-medication between town and country needs to be investigated more closely. If it is true that the Counter-Reformation exerted most of its influence via communal poor relief in towns and via the hospitals, also usually in towns, its means of influence in the sphere of sick care for the poor in rural areas would have depended almost exclusively on the local priest, whose medical function for villages also needs to be researched more extensively.[108]

Notes

1 Robert Jütte, *Poverty and Deviance in Early Modern Europe*, Cambridge, 1994, pp. 100f.

2 On the concept and its history, cf. Heinrich Richard Schmidt, *Konfessionalisierung im 16. Jahrhundert*, Munich,1992, pp. 86f., 106f.

3 See now, on a specific aspect of this topic, Daniel Hickey, *Local Hospitals in Ancien Régime France. Rationalization, Resistance*, Renewal, 1530–1789, Montreal, 1997. Françoise Hildesheimer and Christian Gut, *L'Assistance hospitalière*, Paris, 1992, pp. 51f., is less helpful.

4 Barbara Beckerman-Davis, 'Poverty and poor relief in sixteenth-century Toulouse', *Historical Reflections* 17 (1991), pp. 267–96, 296.

5 As for the regional delimitation of Southern France, I am referring to the region south of the cultural fault line (developed from quantitative social and cultural history) of the kingdom, which runs from Saint-Mâlo to Geneva. From an institutional point of view, the laws made by the monarchy in Paris were as valid there as in the North.

6 The sources for a study of poor relief and health care in Bordeaux are not exactly numerous, but a certain number of documents relating to poor relief (some registers of entry of the principal hospitals in the seventeenth century, and the account-books for several years during the same century, as well as a register of the Protestant Consistory), combined with the use of notaries' documents, allow insights, which are not forthcoming when looking only at the sources produced by the large institutions. Cf. Martin Dinges, *Stadtarmut in Bordeaux 1525–1675. Alltag, Politik, Mentalitäten*, Bonn, 1988.

7 Kathryn Norberg, *Rich and Poor in Grenoble. 1600–1814*, Berkeley/Los Angeles, 1985, p. 14: in 1591 Grenoble had 10,000 inhabitants, in 1685 22,000. Cissie C. Fairchilds, *Poverty and Charity in Aix-en-Provence 1640–1789*, Baltimore/London, 1976 (5,000 inhabitants); Jean-Pierre Gutton, *La Société et les pauvres – l'exemple de la Généralité de Lyon. 1534–1789*, Paris, 1970 (65,000 around 1550); Monique Etchepare, 'L'hôpital de la charité de Marseille et la répression de la mendicité et du vagabondage 1641–1750', law thesis, Aix-en-Provence, 1962 (45,000 inhabitants in 1610, according to Wolfgang Kaiser, *Marseille im Bürgerkrieg*, Göttingen, 1991, p. 37); Marc Venard, 'Les oeuvres de charité en Avignon à l'aube du XVIIe siècle', in: *Dix-septième siècle* 90/91 (1971), 127–46 (26,000 inhabitants in 1616, according to Kaiser, *Marseille*); Colin Jones, *The Charitable Imperative. Hospitals and Nursing in Ancien Régime and Revolutionary France*, London/New York, 1989 (mainly on Montpellier and Nîmes); Beckerman-Davies, 'Poverty and poor relief', Toulouse: 40,000 inhabitants around 1550, pp. 267–96; Joseph Verlay, *Mendiants et Bourgeois à l'hôpital de Vic-en-Bigorre. 1568–1861*, Tarbes, 1987; Pascal Herault, 'Les pauvres et l'amputation à la Maison-Dieu de Montmorillon (en Poitou) aux XVIIe et XVIIIe siècles', in: *Bulletin de la Société française d'histoire des hôpitaux* 69 (1993), 23–33. I did not have access to: Patricia Delubac-Khelifaoui, 'Les chirurgiens barbiers à Marseille', medical thesis, Université Aix-Marseille II 1987; Arielle Delachapelle, 'Histoire de l'hôpital de Sète', Thèse de médecine, Université Montpellier I 1985.

8 See Klaus Hurrelmann, *Sozialisation und Gesundheit. Somatische, psychische und soziale Risikofaktoren im Lebenslauf*, Weinheim/Munich, 1988, pp. 112ff., and Heiner Keupp and Bernd Röhrle (eds), *Soziale Netzwerke*, Frankfurt, 1987, on the importance of social networks for coping with illness nowadays.

9 For more detailed information, cf. Martin Dinges, 'Frühneuzeitliche Armenfürsorge als Sozialdisziplinierung? Probleme mit einem Konzept', in: *Geschichte und Gesellschaft* 17 (1991), 5–29.

10 Robert Jütte has calculated that the consultation of barber-surgeons in Early Modern Cologne was more or less representative for the entire

population; cf. *Ärzte, Heiler und Patienten*, Munich, 1991, p. 105; cf. Robert Jütte, 'A seventeenth-century barber-surgeon and his patients', *Medical History* 33 (1989), 184–98. Comparable research for Southern France has yet to be done.

11 Martin Dinges, 'Self-help and reciprocity in the parish relief system', in: Peregrine Horden and Richard Smith (eds), *The Locus of Care: Communities, Caring and Institutions in History* (forthcoming).

12 *Les Anciens Statuts de la ville et cité de Bourdeaus*, Bordeaux, 1593, 77 (This printed version is identical with the 1542 statutes): '. . . malades & impotens à gagner leur vie; dés [sic] qu'ils seront gueriz, seront desrollez . . .'

13 Mireille Laget and Claudine Luu, *Médecine et la chirurgie des pauvres au XVIII siècle*, Toulouse, 1984.

14 For a good outline, on the basis of material from Northern France, see: François Lebrun, *Se soigner autrefois: Médecins, saints et sorciers aux 17ème et 18ème siècles*, Paris, 1983, pp. 113ff, cf. note 19. See Marie Hélène Froeschle-Chopard, *La Religion populaire en Provence Orientale au XVIIIe siècle*, Paris, 1980, on the change in the iconographic programme in the churches of Provence; on the Italian Counter-Reformation saint, cf. Peter Burke, 'Wie wird man ein Heiliger der Gegenreformation?', in: his *Städtische Kultur in Italien*, Berlin, 1986, pp. 54f., 62. (English translation: *The Historical Anthropology of Early Modern Italy*, Cambridge, 1987). For seven of the fifty-three persons canonised during the seventeenth and eighteenth centuries, mercy and charity were the most outstanding features. With four of those being men, they are not as strongly over-represented as usual in comparison to the women.

15 Dinges, *Stadtarmut*, p. 307; Martin Dinges, 'La culture matérielle des classes inférieures à Bordeaux aux XVIe et XVIIe siècles', *Bulletin de la Société Archéologique de Bordeaux* 77 (1986), 85–94.

16 Lebrun, *Soigner*, pp. 22f; cf. Françoise Loux and Philippe Richard, *Sagesses du corps*, Paris, 1978, pp. 172f., who are less optimistic about people's prayer practices.

17 Dinges, *Stadtarmut*, pp. 221f.; Annick Pardailhé-Galabrun, *La Naissance de l'intime. 3000 foyers parisiens XVIIe–XVIIIe siècles*, Paris, 1988, pp. 355–65, confirms that impression. The inventories show the sparing use made of water in personal hygiene before 1750, but not much about medical practices.

18 Unfortunately, for Southern France during the Counter-Reformation, there is no systematic analysis of autobiographies such as Jens Lachmund and Michael Stollberg, *Patientenwelten. Krankheit und Medizin im Spiegel von Autobiographien*, Opladen, 1995.

19 There is, however, no systematic quantitative study about the changing role of saints related to health and healing, nor about the participation in pilgrimages. Froeschlé-Chopard, *Religion*, 52, 58, 60 seq. finds in her statistics about the dioceses of Vance and Grasse, healing saints as regularly as saints in the chapels. Only very little parishes did not have at least one 'specialist' saint for this purpose, some had three chapels with healing saints. St Roch, like other plague saints, became more important during the seventeenth century because of the recurrent epidemics. For eastern France, Louis Châtellier, *Tradition chrétienne et renouveau catholique*

dans l'ancien diocèse de Strasbourg (1650–1770), Paris 1981 indicates the imprtance of pilgrimages to healing saints. In Marienthal, one of the largest local pilgrimages, healing miracles represented 85 per cent of the 118 cases registered from 1651 to 1681. But it is impossible to situate more exactly the 'renouveau' of this practice in comparison to earlier centuries because of the local concentration of pilgrimages during the Counter-Reformation and a lack of quantitive information. Odile Maisse, 'Le temoigne des fidèles: Les récits de miracle de Saint-Nicolas-de-Port au début du XVIIe siècle', *Revue d'histoire de l'Église de France*, 75 (1989), 117–88, notes 173 miracles during the century with a peak between 1605–26; 17.3 per cent concern healing. Beyond these first indications, measuring the changing importance of healing saints in Counter-Reformation France is an open question. (Thanks for bibliographical information to L. Châtellier, P. Veit, G. Chaix.)

20 I calculated comparative figures for Venice basing myself on: Brian Pullan, *Rich and Poor in Renaissance Venice*, Oxford, 1971, p. 375 (1552: 0.46 per cent; 1593: 0.93 per cent; 1640: 1.62 per cent). On the problems in the second half of the eighteenth century, cf. Philippe Loupès, 'L'hôpital Saint-André de Bordeaux au dix-huitième siècle', *Revue historique de Bordeaux et du Département de la Gironde* 21 (1972), 79–111, 98f.

21 Concerning lepers in South-Western France, cf. Françoise Bériac, *Histoire des lépreux au moyen âge: une société d'exclus*, Paris, 1988.

22 On the issue of plague hospitals and the role of these temporary constructions in European plague confinement, see Martin Dinges, 'Süd-Nord-Gefälle in der Pestbekämpfung. Italien, Deutschland und England im Vergleich', in Wolfgang U. Eckart and Robert Jütte (eds), *Das europäische Gesundheitssystem. Gemeinsamkeiten und Unterschiede in historischer Perspektive*, Stuttgart, 1994, pp. 19–51, especially pp. 28f.

23 Beckerman-Davis, 'Poverty and poor relief'.

24 As there is only a single register of entry and little evidence about the exact periods of construction of the hospital, it is difficult to know the number of inmates at any given point of time; cf. Dinges, *Stadtarmut*, pp. 406f.

25 Dinges, *Stadtarmut*, pp. 373f.

26 Statuts, 70, 77.

27 Cf. Fairchilds, *Poverty and Charity*, p. 81; also Statuts, 77.

28 There is only one register of entries for the year 1620. The composition of inmates was very similar in the eighteenth century; cf. Loupès, L'hopital Saint-André de Bordeaux', p. 87.

29 Dinges, *Stadtarmut*, pp. 91f.

30 Statuts, 74, 77. Regarding the occupation of the physicians at the hospital, there is only mention of 'chargé auprès de l'hôpital', and not of 'dans l'hôpital'. Concerning city physicians, Léon Lallemand, *Histoire de la charité*, vol. 4, 2, Paris 1912, pp. 364ff., gives examples only for Northern France, which distorts the general picture. Cf. Toby Gelfand, 'Public medicine and medical carriers in France during the reign of Louis XV', in Andrew W. Russell (ed.), *The Town and State Physician in Europe from the Middle Ages to the Enlightenment*,

Wolfenbüttel, 1981, pp. 99–122, especially pp. 99f. and 108f.
31 Thus Fairchilds, *Poverty and Charity*, p. 49.
32 Comparable to the situation in Aix, ibid., pp. 52f.
33 Dinges, *Stadtarmut*, p. 407; cf. Loupès, L'hopital Saint-André de Bordeaux', pp. 101f.: in the 1760s there were, for 330 patients, 56 staff, including four barber-surgeons (*chirurgiens*), 24 *soeurs grises* and 16 *serviciaux*.
34 Fairchilds, *Poverty and Charity*, p. 81.
35 Dinges, *Stadtarmut*, p. 395. The names for the wards (also for 1739) are less informative: St Louis (the holy French king, who cured the scrofulous), St Paul, St Guillaume, St Joseph, Sts Cosmas and Damian, new ward, large ward for women, and ward for the scrofulous.
36 Fairchilds, *Poverty and Charity*, p. 81. For the location of the Saint-André Hospital in a swampy area, with humid wards, partly below ground-water level, cf. Dinges, *Stadtarmut*, pp. 394f.
37 Fairchilds, *Poverty and Charity*, p. 82; for the following see p. 85.
38 Dinges, *Stadtarmut*, p. 395.
39 Colin Jones, 'The Daughters of Charity in the Hôtel-Dieu Saint-Eloi in Montpellier before the French Revolution', in: Jones, *The Charitable Imperative*, pp. 122–61, especially 126f.; see below for other examples.
40 Loupès, L'hopital Saint-André de Bordeaux', p. 96.
41 Cf. Jones, Chapter 10, in this volume, and Colin Jones, Charity and Bienfaisance. The Treatment of the Poor in the Montpellier Region 1740–1815, Cambridge, 1982, p. 102. Fairchilds, *Poverty and Charity*, p. 82: in Aix 10–17 per cent of all patients who were admitted, died in the hospital (1780–83). Loupès' calculation, L'hopital Saint-André de Bordeaux', p. 97, for the Hôpital Saint-André is a mortality rate of 10–13 per cent during the better conditions in the 1760s, and 14–18 per cent in the overcrowded hospital at the end of the century.
42 Herault, 'Les pauvres et l'amputation', pp. 23–33.
43 These are interesting facts related to the medical ethics of the seventeenth century.
44 This is not meant to deny that they followed medieval precursors, but the specialisation of this order in this task, which is performed in a general hospital for the poor, is a newer phenomenon.
45 The percentage is difficult to calculate with exactitude, because the many payments in kind from the hospital's possessions would need to be converted into money and added to the total budget. On the problems with hospital budgets, cf. Dinges, *Stadtarmut*, pp. 423f., and Alain Croix, *La Bretagne aux XVIe et XVIIe siècles. La vie – la mort – la foi*, vol. 1, Paris, 1981, pp. 685f.
46 Cf. 'Régime des malades de l'Hôtel-Dieu de Lyon', *Bulletin de la Société française d'histoire des hôpitaux* 56 (1988), 35–7.
47 Still fundamental: J. Imbert, 'Les prescriptions hospitaliéres du Concile de Trente et leur diffusion en France', *Revue d'histoire de l'eglise de France* 62 (1956), 5–28, especially p. 27.
48 Bishops' visitations of hospitals and inquiries about charities spread from the South-East to other parts of France; see Marie-Hélène and Micahel Froeschlé-Chopard, *Atlas de la Réforme pastorale en France de 1550–1790*, Paris, 1986, pp. 81 seq., 206 seq.

49 Charles Higounet (ed.), *Histoire de Bordeaux*, vol. 4, *Bordeaux de 1453 à 1715*, Bordeaux, 1966, pp. 369f.

50 Concerning the debate about social disciplining through institutions, cf. Martin Dinges, 'The reception of Michel Foucault's ideas on social discipline, mental asylums, hospitals and the medical profession in German historiography', in Colin Jones and Roy Porter (eds), *Reassessing Foucault. Power, Medicine and the Body*, London, 1994, pp. 181–212, especially 195f.

51 Raymond Darricau, 'L'action charitable d'une Reine de France. Anne d'Autriche', in: *Dix-septième siècle* 90/91 (1971), 111–25.

52 On this point, see Jones in Chapter 10, this volume.

53 Etchepare, 'L'hôpital de la charité de Marseille', p. 26.

54 Jean-Pierre Gutton, *La Société et les pauvres en Europe (XVIe–XVIIIe siècles)*, Paris, 1974, p. 130; Fairchilds, *Poverty and Charity*, p. 36; Charles Joret, 'Le Père Guevarre et les bureaux de charité', *Annales du Midi* 1 (1889), 340–93.

55 Norberg, *Rich and Poor*, p. 88.

56 Gutton, *La Societé et les pauvres*, p. 301.

57 Later the estimates are lower for both. Etchepare, 'L'hôpital de la charité de Marseille', pp. 27, 76, 127; there is no information about medical care in the budget, for example on p. 134.

58 Colin Jones suggests this for the case of Nîmes, in 'The social functions of the hospital in eighteenth-century France: the case of the Hôtel-Dieu of Nîmes', in: Jones, *The Charitable Imperative*, pp. 48–86, especially p. 55.

59 The first elements of an analysis of inmates (albeit for the North of France) suggest that the concentration of general hospitals on new target groups was only partly successful, with the result that they often developed as duplicates of the old general hospitals, with a high percentage of infants, elderly and bedridden patients, but without acute cases. Cf. Marie-Claude Dinet-Lecomte, 'Recherche sur la clientèle hospitalière aux XVIIe et XVIIIe siècles: l'exemple de Blois', *Revue d'histoire moderne et contemporaine* 33 (1986), 345–73; Etchepare, 'L'hôpital de la charité de Marseille', pp. 127f., lists the rations and length of stay for the inmates of the Marseille general hospital for the years 1724 to 1734. They demonstrate that from the start the '*pauvres invalides*', i.e. the incapacitated, were the majority, and that their percentage grew progressively over the years, so that in 1734 the incapacitated poor residing in the institution were four or six times as many as those able to work. Cf. Robert M. Schwartz, *Policing the Poor in Eighteenth-Century France*, Chapel Hill, 1988, pp. 44f.

60 Norberg, *Rich and Poor*, pp. 83f.

61 Herault, 'Les pauvres et l'amputation', p. 28.

62 Norberg, *Rich and Poor*, pp. 32, 85.

63 Cf. Colin Jones, 'Vincent de Paul, Louise de Marillac, and the revival of nursing in the seventeenth century', in Jones, *The Charitable Imperative*, pp. 89–121. With the exception of special cases, the propagation of the Soeurs de la charité only began to increase in Southern France from the 1690s; see the map in Jones, 'The Daughters of Charity', p. 128. Cf. Gutton, *La Societé et les pauvres*, pp. 412–17.

64 Norberg, *Rich and Poor*, p. 86. I would, however, hesitate to speak of 'professionalisation' in relation to this early period and to these tasks. Fairchilds writes, concerning Aix, that it was not clear whether the personnel belonged to a religious order; this may be a further indication of the actual confusion between religious sisters and nurses.

65 Cf. Fairchilds, *Poverty and Charity*, p. 82.

66 Cf. Norberg, *Rich and Poor*, p. 83.

67 Jütte, *Poverty and Deviance*, pp. 129f. This evidence is confirmed by recent research on confraternities in the South-East, where parish relief associations seem to be very unequally distributed. See Roger Devos, 'Chapelles, autels et confréries du diocèse de Genève à la fin du XVIIIe siècle', in Marie-Hélène Froschlé-Chopard (ed.), *Les Confréries, l'Eglise et la cité, cartographie des confréries du Sud-Est*, Grenoble 1988, pp. 83–96, 84 with only one parish charity in 782 parishes at the end of the eighteenth century. Bernard Montagnes, 'Les confréries du diocèse d'Aix au début du XVIIIe siècle', in Froeschlé-Choppard, *Les Confréries*, pp. 167–79, 175, on the other hand finds nineteen rural and two urban *Misericorde* associations for poor relief in ninety-six parishes during the seventeenth century. There are no mentions of such confraternities in the other dioceses under research in this book. Louis Pérouas, 'Les confréries dans le pays creusois à la veille de la Révolution', in: Froeschlé-Chopard, *Les Confréries*, pp. 233–8, 235 finds only some confraternities dedicated to healing Saints in this region.

68 According to *Statuts*, 77, the hospital administrators were to provide the shamefaced poor with alms in their homes; this may have included medical care.

69 Beckerman-Davis, 'Poverty and poor relief', p. 291.

70 My own calculations, following Beckerman-Davis, 'Poverty and poor relief', p. 289.

71 Dinges, *Stadtarmut*, pp. 352f.; cf. *Statuts*, p. 75.

72 Venard, 'Les oeuvres de charité, pp. 140f.

73 Dinges, *Stadtarmut*, p. 443. For the Jesuit sodalities, cf. Louis Châtellier, *The Europe of the Devout. The Catholic Reformation and the Formation of a New Society*, Cambridge, 1987.

74 Dinges, *Stadtarmut*, pp. 437–41, for the following.

75 On Surin's correspondence with the Bordeaux elite, see Michel de Certeau (ed.), *Jean-Joseph Surin. Correspondance*, Bruges, 1966.

76 Dinges, *Stadtarmut*, p. 442, note 25.

77 Cf. the account in Gutton, *La Societé et les pauvres*, pp. 371f.

78 See Dinges, *Stadtarmut*, p. 440, note 16, on the disputes about collections.

79 Dinges, *Stadtarmut*, p. 440; for a further example of statutes (of 1714), see 'La confrérie de la charité à l'hôpital de Saint-Galmier (Loire)', *Revue de la société française d'histoire des hôpitaux* 74 (1994), pp. 43–5.

80 In considering these quantities of wine, one has to keep in mind that at the time it did not even have half of the alcoholic content of today's wine, and that it was considered an important source of calories, and thought to have a therapeutic effect. On the portion of wine within the calories provided by hospital food, see Dinges, *Stadtarmut*, p. 417.

81 In the sense of the concept of lay involvement as propagated by

Châtellier, *Europe*, as an important element in the creation of Catholic Europe.

82 It is only under this condition that disciplining can have a chance of success. Cf. Martin Dinges, 'L'Hôpital Saint-André de Bordeaux au XVIIe siècle: objectifs et réalisations de l' assistance municipale', *Annales du Midi* 99 (1987), pp. 303–30, especially 317, 324, and Dinges 'Self-help and reciprocity', Part 5.

83 Verlay, *Vic-en-Bigorre*, p. 74.

84 Philippe Loupès, 'L'assistance paroissiale aux pauvres malades dans le diocèse de Bordeaux au XVIIIe siècle', *Annales du Midi* 84 (1972), 37–61, especially 51.

85 Loupès, 'L'assistance paroissiale', p. 55.

86 The documents on which the accounts were based, which would make it possible to reconstruct the day-to-day activities, are hardly ever preserved; cf. Fairchilds, *Poverty and Charity*, p. 94.

87 For the evidence see Dinges, *Stadtarmut*, p. 442.

88 On this topic see further evidence in Gisela Bock, 'Frauenräume und Frauenehre. Frühneuzeitliche Armenfürsorge in Italien', in: Karin Hausen and Heide Wunder (eds), *Frauengeschichte, Geschlechtergeschichte*, Frankfurt/M., 1992, pp. 25–49.

89 See Dinges, *Stadtarmut*, pp. 463f. The Italian influence is directly visible in the endowment by the clergyman von Campo-Knieffel.

90 Norberg, *Rich and Poor*, pp. 65f.

91 For more detail see Martin Dinges, 'L'assistance paroissiale à Bordeaux à la fin du XVIIe siècle – L'exemple du consistoire protestant', *Histoire, économie et société* 5 (1986), pp. 475–507, and Dinges, 'Self-help and reciprocity'.

92 See Jean Cavignac, 'L'assistance chez les juifs portugais de Bordeaux au XVIIIe siècle', in: *Actes du 108e Congrès national des sociétés savantes, Colloque sur l'histoire de la sécurité sociale* (Grenoble, 1983), Paris, 1983, pp. 27–35, for the late eighteenth century.

93 Data for the last third of the seventeenth century. On the development of the Protestant population, cf., most recently, Philippe Benedict, *The Hugenot Population of France, 1600–1685*, Philadelphia, 1991.

94 Dinges, *Stadtarmut*, p. 147.

95 Fairchilds, *Poverty and Charity*, p. 114.

96 For the examples, cf. Dinges, *Stadtarmut*, pp. 481f., Norberg, *Rich and Poor*, p. 116; cf. Wilma Pugh, 'Catholics, Protestants and testamentary charity in seventeenth-century Lyons and Nîmes', *French Historical Studies* 11 (1980), 479–504, especially 480f.

97 Cf., in more detail, Martin Dinges, 'Attitudes à l'égard de la pauvreté aux XVIe et XVIIe siècles à Bordeaux', *Histoire, économie, société* 10 (1991), pp. 359–74.

98 Norberg, *Rich and Poor*, pp. 126f. Given that Norberg's analysis only begins with the year 1620, the period of origin of the pattern remains open. The data for Bordeaux suggest a date around or before 1600.

99 Norberg, *Rich and Poor*, pp. 142, 155; this also corresponds to the results found by Pugh, *Charity and Bienfaisance*, p. 499; cf. Raymond Mentzner, 'Organizational endeavour and charitable impulse in six-

teenth-century France: the case of Protestant Nîmes', *French History* 5 (1991), 1–29.

100 Pugh, *Charity and Bienfaisance*, pp. 480, 483f., 499, 503. She finds altogether higher readiness to give donations than in Bordeaux, where there was a clear Catholic predominance. The amounts rose most sharply after a change-over in denominational power in Nîmes.

101 Norberg, *Rich and Poor*, p. 145.

102 Dinges, *Stadtarmut*, p. 446.

103 Norberg, *Rich and Poor*, p. 252. Table 6.1, in Fairchilds, *Poverty and Charity*, p. 134, shows the same overall tendency, although it is of a slightly earlier period, less exclusive from the point of view of social stratification (given that it is based on a general collection), and not differentiable by gender. The same tendency can be seen in Bordeaux and its environments: Loupès, 'L'assistance paraoissiale, p. 42; cf. Jones, *Charity and Bienfaisance*, pp. 87f.

104 Gutton, *Europe*, p. 174.

105 Gutton, *Europe*, pp. 160f. There is an example for Southern France in Christine Menges, 'Répression et prévention en matière d'assistance au XVIIe siècle: le "Mémoire pour le soulagement des peuples" du premier président de Buisson d'Aussone (1687)', *Annales du Midi* 105 (1993), pp. 349–63.

106 On the long preparatory phase see Thomas McStay Adams, *Bureaucrats and Beggars. French Social Policy in the Age of Enlightenment*, Oxford, 1990, pp. 49f.

107 There is no study comparable to Lucinda McCray Beier, *Sufferers and Healers. The Experience of Illness in Seventeenth-Century England*, London/New York, 1987.

108 Some information is given in Lebrun, *Se soigner*; an interpretation of the Counter-Reformation as an urban phenomenon is given by José Antonio Maravall, *La Cultura del Barroco*, Barcelona, 1981; but see, more recently, Louis Châtellier, *La Religion des pauvres. Les sources du christianisme moderne. XVIe–XIXe siècles*, Paris, 1993.

13

HEALTH CARE AND POVERTY RELIEF IN COUNTER-REFORMATION CATHOLIC GERMANY

Bernd Roeck

Translated by Carey McIntosh

The attempt to summarise the history of health care and poverty relief in Counter-Reformation Catholic Germany is complicated by an array of evident difficulties. The first factor to name would be the current state of research on the subject, which lacks both comparative summaries[1] and newer studies of certain regions or cities. Although some cases have been especially well investigated, of which the primary example is certainly Cologne, the only large Catholic city in Germany,[2] conditions in Protestant regions have been on the whole much better researched.

The emphasis of most studies has been on the late Middle Ages, while a long-term perspective has barely been considered in most works. In addition, the 'municipal perspective', the examination of state institutions, has tended to dominate the discussion. The disciplining effects of public relief and an analysis of official strategies have been emphasised, whereas little – too little[3] – attention has been paid to the less obviously visible, the 'silent' mechanisms that became important for coping with poverty and disease. These subtle structures, networks such as family, household and neighbourhood, provided psychological support that at least partially immunised against the consequences of hunger and disease. As such they should be interpreted as important factors contributing to social stability, which were sometimes but not always specific to one confession. For the concentration on the 'state', which can lead to a supposition of exclusively functionally orientated behaviour patterns, must not be allowed to obscure the deeply religious character of the period under investigation. Although true not only for the Holy Roman Empire, this observation has special relevance there: the analysis of municipal poverty relief in confessional-era Germany must bear in mind the fundamental religious and moral competition between territories or cities that often took place in compact geographical areas, even within individual cities[4] or in regions such as the especially fragmented states of the South-West.[5] This competition led to a greater variety in proffered salvation, to the adoption of increasingly publicly-controlled systems of ritual and accordingly the suppression of traditional, private practices for coping with one's environment. Confessionalisation was, in other words, simultaneously Christianisation: the suppression of forms of magic not officially sanctioned by the state. In its capacity as a public institution, the Church aspired along with the state to achieve a monopoly of competence in magic. This fundamental tendency, which can be especially well observed in Germany, of course did not begin only with the Reformation. It was, however, certainly encouraged by the Reformation and the reactions against it. The Church's outward claim to exclusivity, a precondition for the wars of religion, corresponds to its inward claim, over its own subjects. This is what has been imprecisely called 'suppression of folk culture',[6] an aspect of the confessionalisation process.

To date the consequences of this process for the psychological mechanisms mentioned above have been only sporadically researched. It is known that the conflicts centred around systems for understanding the world, which clearly also had a role in stabilising and legimitising authority, occasionally had destabilising effects. On the other hand, it is not enough to consider that the riots and revolts characteristic of this period were rooted in the mentalities of the time; one must also look for causes of the revolts that *failed* to break out. This question leads us back not only to the increasingly internalised norms found in the great confessions, but also to the stabilising functions of public and Church institutions of which those for poverty relief were a part.

In the twofold crisis of systems for interpreting the world – the struggle between the confessions and the struggle for a religious conditioning of 'subjects' – welfare institutions of both the secular and spiritual powers fulfilled an increasingly important function. The achievement of a monopoly in magic by Church and state corresponded to growing expectations from the conquerors: their responsibility for seeing to earthly salvation, rather than solely that in the world beyond, grew.

This was expressed in an increasing array of laws and regulations pertaining to caritative matters. Public institutions increasingly demanded this competence for themselves, and they wanted credit for their charity; they desired political profit from the socially stabilising effects of their *caritas* – and at the same time (one would have to prove the opposite) they wanted to do justice to their responsibility as a Christian, moral authority before God. This was another aspect that produced a competitive relationship between Church and state. The transfer of poverty relief to institutions meant competition between the secular and spiritual spheres, with the addition in the sixteenth century of the confessional competition that was especially important in Germany. It should be observed, however, that this competition did not necessarily result in specifically confessional forms of relief. It is probable that it contributed to a greater intensity of relief measures, though this ought to be more closely researched.

This question is difficult to answer because the developments sketched here – in Germany as well as in other European countries – coincided with or were affected by economic and social processes that can also be observed before the Reformation and that can only be cursorily referred to here. It is impossible to definitively describe what connection there might have been between these long-term trends and the history of relief institutions; only the analysis of individual cases ought to be of help. For what we are really seeing is the relationship between theory and practice, specifically, what possibilities exist for maintaining ideological ambitions in times of scarce resources. There is a theory that care for the poor was intensified in the sixteenth century, and that this was one of the consequences of an increasing religiousness evoked by the religious controversy of the time and the growing desire for discipline in a rapidly changing society.[7] This theory must, however, take the fact into account that according to all we know, poverty also increased during this time. The factors contributing to this general worsening of economic and social conditions are known: population growth and the consequential reduction of available resources, a miniature ice age, and a decline in real wages.[8] Except for the climatic changes with their inestimable consequences, these trends were already in effect before the instability caused by the religious tremors became relevant. Certain characteristics of structured relief mechanisms, which begin to appear especially in the regulations concerning begging and the poor in the Early Modern period, should therefore be interpreted not necessarily as the result of a transformed spiritual orientation but primarily as a necessary response to prevailing socio-economic problems. The oldest extant legal ordinance for the poor, for instance, the begging ordinance in Nuremberg from circa 1370, shows the trend toward a rationalisation of poverty, the exclusion of the 'false' poor, and the inclusion of pedagogy and discipline.[9] A council decision in Cologne in 1435 indicates developments in the same direction.[10] Even before the Reformation, all poverty was not created equal. On the other hand, it is certainly true that the confessional rift in the sixteenth century accentuated the differences regarding the way relief was handled and attitutes toward poverty and begging.[11] Especially in the cities, the trend toward a rational organisation of welfare was unmistakable even in the fifteenth century. The primary concepts were centralisation and control, which at the same time meant intrusion into what had been competencies of the church. Finally, caritative institutions acted as a magnet for the poor streaming from the country into expanding cities, which in turn encouraged the general trend toward indigence. In Germany, the police ordinance from 1530 and its successors legally secured preferential treatment for the native poor at the cost of newcomers.[12]

Whether for Protestant or for Catholic Germany, it is impossible to accurately judge the quantitative relevance of groups receiving welfare. Estimates diverge widely.[13] Not even tax rolls enable a definitive identification of the poor, not to mention the fact that, by including only taxpayers, they naturally omitted the 'stray riff-raff', 'foreign beggars' and vagrants so notoriously mentioned in our sources. In the sixteenth century, however, precisely these people are most likely to have been the majority of the poor. And no matter how interested we might be in determining what specifically confessional aspects might have been relevant to the distribution of poverty, this question is impossible to answer. Reasonably reliable figures are only available for the publically assisted, 'authentic', notorious poor, and even then only in urban settings. In 'normal' times, the proportion of people receiving regular or occasional assistance from municipal or Church institutions seems to have fluctuated between 6 and 10 per cent,[14] but the urban lower class was generally a much more significant group than these figures might suggest. Fischer considers 60–64 per cent of all households in late-medieval Freiburg as having belonged to the category of primary poverty, and another 10 per cent to secondary poverty.[15] Similar figures can be named for a city with, however, an extremely unfavourable economic monostructure, namely Augsburg in the early seventeenth century – a much later point in time.[16] Augsburg was confessionally mixed, if quite predominantly Protestant.

Global estimates are not so dramatic. Maschke estimates the proportion of indigents in the entire population at the close of the Middle Ages to be 10–20 per cent,[17] a figure that one may or may not choose to believe. Of great importance for any quantitative estimate is, of course, how one wishes to define poverty.[18] It is well known that such definitions, both by people of the times and by modern historians, diverge widely.

The influence of the Reformation on the history of poverty relief and health care is qualified, for one, by the material forces that arose from negative economic and social developments. But it should not be forgotten that Bog and Fischer have brought weighty arguments against a monocausal interpretation. Bog explains the changed structures in urban poverty relief *politically*, as an aspect of the city magistrates' increased competencies in the process of becoming an 'authority', meaning, among other things, in connection with the increasing presence of the state at all levels of society.[19] Whether this was a development 'relatively independent of economics', however, is certainly a question worthy of debate, and this is exactly the point where Fischer's treatment of Bog's theories begins.[20] Supported by his findings in the cases of Basel and Freiburg im Breisgau, he points to social shifts within urban societies. According to Fischer, a lack of economic growth substantially contributed to increasingly rigid social structures, the aggravation of social tensions, and thus to the formation of anti-begging policies. As important criteria for these urban social 'shifts', Fischer names the flight of wealthy citizens and the influx of groups from surrounding rural areas. He accurately describes the sum of the measures concerning welfare as *social policy*, ('planned measures . . . that were aimed at certain people in, absolutely and relatively, particularly difficult situations').[21] The trend toward objectivising the concept of 'neediness' continued throughout the sixteenth century. It was expressed in the often extremely detailed criteria catalogues of alms ordinances, a development that at least in principle took place similarly in cities and territories of different confessions.

Behind all these measures toward the organisation of welfare, the again tendentially supra-confessional ideal of a Christian, well-ordered community is palpable. In its service were increasingly differentiated police ordinances and measures to ensure proper moral conduct, which admittedly developed much more clearly or at least earlier in Protestant than in Catholic Germany. The moral competition between authorities, also acting according to their own Christian conscience, had significant drawbacks for some social groups. The question was one of justification before God: 'right living' protected from God's punishments, which posed a threat to the entire community, even when provoked by the mistakes of individuals. The city (or state) as 'salvation community'[22] considered itself to be in a position of collective responsibility before God, and one of the authorities' most important duties was to do everything in their power in order to ensure that their subjects led a Christian life. Wars, epidemics, famines, even deflation, a phenomenon not rationally explicable to the inhabitants of the sixteenth century, were primarily to be explained by people's sinful, 'bad' lives. In order to extirpate all evil, this was the place to begin, which meant intervention against all things depraved, irregular or evil. The crusade against 'witches' is only the especially dramatic articulation of such thinking. In the 'guilty' poor, one found morally responsible outsiders who literally had no business being in a well-ordered city, in a Christian land. They were, when at all possible, expelled from the city and at times even branded to ensure that they did not return.

The poor stood in the way of an ethical state ideal, which, by the way, found an analogous aesthetic expression in geometrically ordered ideal cities. These also tolerated no crooked lines or deviation. In the ideal cities of the times, above all in Thomas More's Utopia, there is no laziness; it follows that there can be no poor responsible for their own fate. The problem of indigence, the proliferation of beggars, and especially the mass poverty of the non-sedentary so typical of the 'long sixteenth century' formed the backdrop of pleas in utopists' and countless other works damning idleness and laziness and preaching the duty of labour. The argument ran that since God Himself had been the one to impose the duty of labour and who expected its fulfilment, it must be God's adversary, the Devil, who tried to keep people from serving God through their work. As far as such convictions were concerned, the confessions stood in general agreement with each other.[23] God was the founder of labour, thus the Devil the lord of laziness and idleness. Johannes Muthesius, a preacher from Joachimsthal, propagated this opinion, which also spread through Catholic areas, apparently especially after the Council of Trent. The Bavarian court secretary Ägidius Albertinus incorporated popular Protestant imagery for demonising idleness into his teachings on the Devil. He devised a differentiated, hierarchical phenomenology 'which' – as Paul Münch emphasised – 'in the intensity with which it attacks idleness was hardly to be dinstinguished from the pathos of Protestant literature'.[24] Nevertheless, literature by Protestant authors clearly predominated in what Münch concisely calls the 'campain for industriousness'.[25] And Catholic preachers during the Counter-Reformation such as Abraham a Sancta Clara tended to fall back on late-medieval topoi when attacking laziness. Not the Devil but the fool (such as in Sebastian Brandt's 'Ship of Fools') became the pejorative metaphor. Such differences were, however, slight. In condemning laziness there was only agreement, and the stereotype of the 'lazy beggar' provided a category whose fate was conveniently neither the responsibility of the state nor of the Church, and that the authorities therefore did not have to accept as their concern. In this sense their admonishment to industry and hard work automatically freed them of responsibility; it made living with mass poverty before one's eyes easier to endure. It also gives us an idea of what kind of causal relationship might be seen behind a phenomenon that its contemporaries could not otherwise explain to themselves. This line of reasoning also provided arguments for justifying why some needy went uncared for despite the commandment of *caritas*, Christian brotherly love; why the use of scarce resources was restricted, e.g. according to the principle of indigence.

The idea that poverty has its ultimate source in human immorality, in the hidden will of God exacting the consequences of this state, can also be found in the writings of Vives, the most important Catholic theorist on poverty relief.[26] It came to have a measure of influence in Germany. The main principles of Early-Modern welfare were taken from the spirit of Christian humanism, a spirit that was Catholic at least in its theoretical core, and it is here that we may begin to grasp the differences from the Protestant conception. Vives believes in the reformability of society, that it can be improved, even in the possibility of a return to the happy natural state of the lost Golden Age. And although the structure of society is the result of original sin and thus a corrupted version of what was initially a good state, the Church nevertheless exists therein as carrier and dispenser of mercy.[27] It will help mankind reform this earthly society into an ideal one using Christian virtues – especially through love. This spontaneous, directly practised Christian brotherly love is 'the driving motivation of, and its intensification the goal of, all care for the poor':[28]

> *Verum omnia superat incrementum amoris, quod fiet communicandis ultro et citro beneficiis, candide ac simpliciter, sine suspicione indignatis, et nunc praemium illud coeleste, quod paratum esse ostendimus eleemosynis, quae ex Charitate profiscuntur.*[29]

This is the concept of the righteousness of works classically formulated. Morally, good behaviour towards the needy has three functions: it sanctifies the individual and brings him heavenly rewards, it contributes to the sanctification of the society in which the individual acts are performed, and it brings that society a bit closer to earthly perfection. But Vives' work does not remain confined to these ideas. The goal is not individual assistance for the individual in order to obtain some diffuse reward from God, but the eradication of poverty altogether. In this respect his text is utopic; on the other hand he has fairly clear and at least partially realistic ideas about how to master the problem of poverty as a question of social policy. He wants welfare to assist the poor in helping themselves, to make them capable of work. His admiration, based on scholastic traditions, for the duty of labour is the rationale behind his call to strictly separate the employable poor from those who are not capable of labour and to define categories of poverty according to which assistance should be administered. Begging should be replaced entirely by publicly organised relief; the medieval distinction between permitted and non-permitted begging disappears; his text does not refer to mendicant orders. Conversely, work must be found for the willing and those convinced to be willing. This is a core element of his argumentation. For example, masters in the trades should be required to employ a certain number of the poor in their works. These passages of Vives' fundamental tractate will be relevant again at a later point.

Those unwilling to work, meaning those whose situation is considered to be their own fault, should be reformed through forceful measures. This implies not only the encouragement of forced labour but simultaneously the prevention of waste. Such opinions, whether or not inspired by Vives' text, found practical application in various ways, not least of which were the laws against luxury[30] that saw their great rise in popularity in the sixteenth century, or the simultaneous arrival of prisons and workhouses.[31] The individualisation of poverty relief, the strict distinction between alms for the 'worthy' and the 'unworthy', for locals and 'foreigners', also defines the structure of welfare during the entire period. One could inscribe Vives' words '*Adhibeantur congrua singulis remedia*' as a kind of motto over the times, equally valid for Catholic and Protestant spheres. Vives nevertheless warned against distributing alms with overly fearful care, which love would not allow for. He and other Catholic theorists of the sixteenth century[32] considered *caritas*, as the basis of almsgiving and the motivation for good works, to be of decisive importance. Good will counted, even when the occasional wrong person should enjoy its fruits.

This attitude is significantly unlike the Protestant approach. No less revealingly, opinions diverged at least in theory about the question of state participation in care for the poor, although Catholic opinion on this point was not entirely unified. Vives considered welfare to be one of the authorities' basic responsibilities, while most other Catholic theologians rejected public participation entirely or wanted to allow it only in very reduced measure.[33] Thus there were certain, if not fundamental, differences from Protestant attitudes. No one could fail to see the reality that had been developing before and during the sixteenth century, and this everyday reality demonstrated that Church and secular institutions strongly overlapped in the area of welfare.

In practice, new laws were declared – beginning in the 1630s in Protestant cities and from the middle of the century increasingly in Catholic cities and territories as well – in response to the general worsening of the situation and obviously influenced by guidelines the theorists had been formulating.

A well-researched example of a Catholic poor ordinance is from 1587 in Fulda.[34] Its preparation probably more or less goes back to the governor Eustachius I von Schlitz gen. von Görtz, who had been steward of the prince-bishop Julius Echter, a zealous counter-reformer. It reflects a situation that is in many respects typical. Catholic institutions – a seminary, provostaries, a Jesuit college – were faced with a citizenry that was already predominantly Protestant. The Catholic authorities' goal was to force the Protestants back into the Roman Church, and the caritative system was seen as a means toward this end. This admittedly required restrained, differentiated policy-making, which was expressed in various regulations of the ordinance such as the process for selecting beggars worthy of receiving alms. Representatives of the (predominantly Protestant) town council and the clergy were expected to participate. The purpose of this inqisition was to separate the 'worthy' from the 'unworthy' poor and to eliminate the fraudulent. Excluded from receiving alms were those capable of work and foreigners, who were supposed to make way for the local needy. Their moral history was also investigated, and – a decisive and touchy point – their Christian attitudes: the beggars should go to church in order to confess and receive the sacraments, so that others would sense 'that they are true Christians and have the spirit of Christ in them'.[35] Although this said nothing about the *confession* of those entitled to assistance, these 'rubber-band clauses' were in practice used to favour Catholics. That the 'poor people belonging to the Augsburg confession should be excluded from alms' was the council's complaint in a petition to the governor two weeks after the regulation was made public.[36] Conflicts also arose concerning control of the Common Chest. There were complaints that the parish's God's Chest, donated long ago by the citizens, had been united with the Jesuits' chest, and that the Jesuits used the contents to support their students instead of the truly needy. The council called for a renewed separation of the chests so that poor citizens could also be helped. The Common Chest should also be used to support Protestants.

This point apparently continued to be a source of conflict, which was resolved only in 1603 with the city's re-Catholicisation. Control over the Common Chest remained with the Jesuits, who became a fixed institution of Fulda's social policy.

The Fulda beggars' ordinance otherwise included many elements that can also be found in Protestant ordinances of the time: aside from the tendency toward categorising the poor, the attempt to centralise their care as well, which was most clearly demonstrated in the establishment of a body for determining the 'respectable poor'. Increasing bureaucratisation was expressed in the abolition of beggars' markings, which had to be worn much longer in other places, and in the registration of beggars. Positions of scholastic poverty theory, especially Thomas of Aquinus' idea that begging is a means of practising Christian humility, can be found in a passage of this ordinance. It should be clear from the above that this ordinance, while infused with a Catholic spirit, includes traces of a modern work ethic. On the whole, it describes a perception of social order that postulates poverty as an integrative element, even as one necessary for the non-poor's achievement of spiritual salvation.

It should admittedly be observed that the Fulda ordinance analysed here was written in the late 1680s and thus represents a relatively late stage in post-Reformation begging policy. Modernising tendencies prevail, despite the continuing existence of obviously traditional elements. For instance, individual begging and thus the individual distribution of alms was not absolutely forbidden, which should not imply that such bans were standard practice in Protestant ordinances, at least not when the continued existence of Catholic institutions in those territories had to be taken into account.[37] Examples to the contrary were Strasbourg, where begging was forbidden in 1523, Basel, where this was the case in 1530, or (Catholic) Freiburg, where begging was banned, if only in 1582.[38] Not begging *per se* but most likely the lack of order, excesses and the unmanageable proportions associated with the influx of outsiders were the target of a beggars' ordinance in an important South German residential city, Catholic Munich.[39] The most important relevant ordinances were declared in 1562 and 1572, and a third in 1599 after laborious consultation and only after it had been approved by the princely central office. These regulations were prompted by an increasingly difficult social situation; the ordinance from 1572 was directly influenced by the terrible hunger crisis of 1571/72. In Munich as well, the trend toward centralising welfare can be observed. Alms should be brought to collections organised by the city in favour of the 'respectable poor' distinguished by their alms sign, and donations should be distributed to the hungry. One can also find the idea of supplying the needy but healthy with useful activities. The ordinance from 1562 provided that poor children be sent to spin wool and thread; similar suggestions were made in other places, such as Münster.[40] The ordinance from 1572 even threatened those who resisted its measures with forced labour or prison.

Many beggars' ordinances, some of Catholic origin, aim to prohibit at least outsiders from begging, sometimes under the threat of eviction from the city or branding. The territorial states, although such solutions were more difficult to impose there than in the cities, also developed similar provisions. The copious mandates of this sort that Duke/Elector Maximilian I the Bavarian showered over his subjects during his long reign are documents of an early-absolutistic desire for control and order, and should be seen in the context of extensive police laws that encompassed all spheres of life. He declared about fifteen such mandates and land decrees between 1597 and 1642;[41] one can only speculate about the actual degree of influence they might have had on daily reality.[42] In a large Early-Modern city such as Augsburg, beggars were thrown out at one gate only to come in by another.[43] And although free begging had been made illegal there in 1541, i.e. while Protestants still controlled city government, compliance with this rule was negligible.

Ordinances thus often expressed expectations that were then ignored in practice. Cologne would seem to offer a good example of this. Here as well, countless regulations were decreed against begging but were resisted by the traditional attitudes of the citizens.[44] Certainly it was not only here that the language of the ordinances – in many ways similar to corresponding regulations in other cities – contrasted with everyday practice. Illegal begging was threatened with draconian punishments, and as in other places, alms signs were only awarded to certain categories of the indigent, after a detailed examination of each individual case. The citizens of Cologne, however, considered begging to be an obviously legitimate means of acquiring property and giving to be an opportunity to do a good deed.

Let us now consider the special case of a mixed Catholic and Protestant city.[45] Augsburg provides the example of a predominantly Protestant community dominated by a Catholic elite and home to several Catholic welfare institutions. Care for the poor, regulated by ordinances in 1522 and 1541, none the less was and remained fundamentally under Protestant influence. The responsible almsmen, accompanied by servants, were supposed to personally collect donations; appeals for donations to the church were also made. In 1541 free begging in the city was drastically restricted, although these regulations were again practically ignored. The council had at most very concealed counter-reformatory ambitions; anything other than a 'lukewarm' attitude would have been practically unthinkable in light of the city's confessional structure. It is telling for the council's precarious situation that as late as 1625 collectors suggested that while appeals for alms donations should be made publicly from church pulpits, they should not include any mention of the authorities.

Toward the end of the sixteenth century, the unusual situation arose in Augsburg that care for the poor in a Catholic-dominated city was to a great extent financed by Protestant almsgivers. Figure 12.1[46] shows to just what extent this was true: the 'towers' indicate alms collected from Catholics and Protestants in church collections in the various city thirds between 1583 and 1596. Unambivalent is the dramatic decline between 1586 and 1591, which was due to a Protestant sermon boycott: the council had forced politically loyal preachers onto the citizens after unrest in the city prompted by the introduction of the Gregorian calendar in 1548. Figure 12.2[47] offers a no less impressive example for the effects of political measures on the Augsburg Protestants' caritative activity. It shows the decline in donations to the Church after the imposition of the Restitution Edict of 1629, the renewed increase after the Swedish invasion and, of particular interest, the disproportional increase around the turn of the year 1634/35. Afterwards the city experienced an extremely difficult siege. Hunger and disease costed thousands of lives: of Augsburg's pre-war population of around 45,000, only 16,422 inhabitants remained to witness the city's passage into Catholic hands. This situation made the increase in almsgiving around Christmas time in 1634 all the more remarkable. The people offered sacrifice to

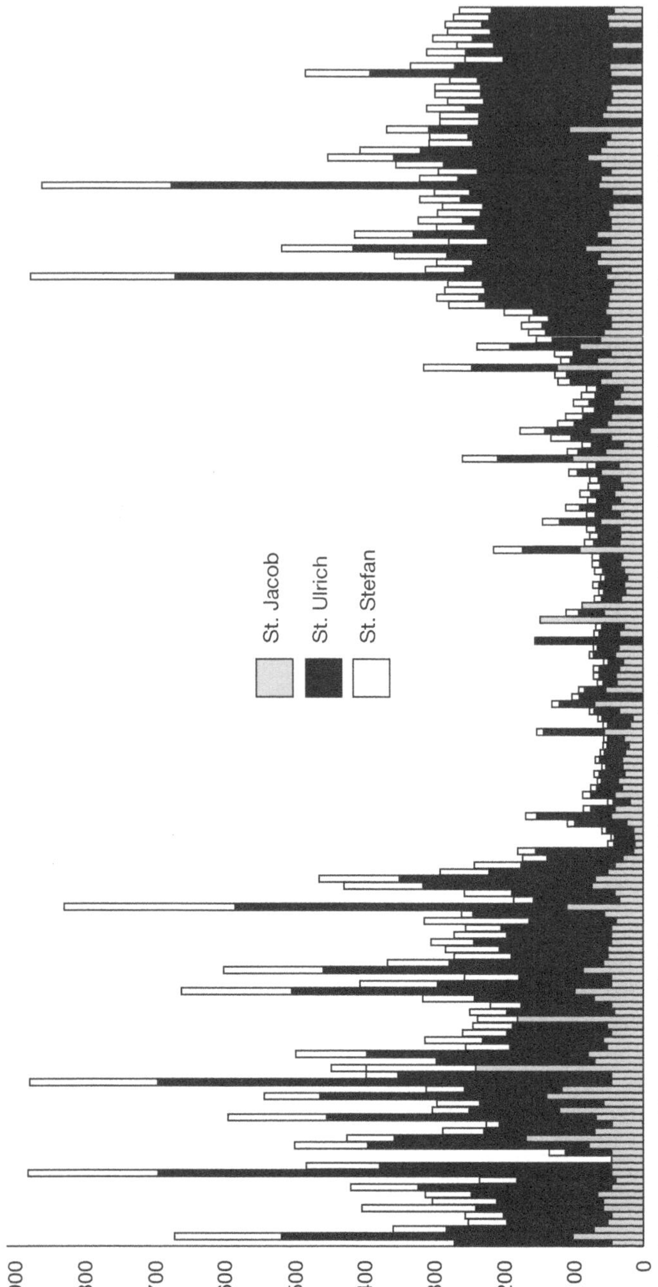

Figure 13.1 Church spending in Augsburg 1583–1596
Source: After Roeck 1989

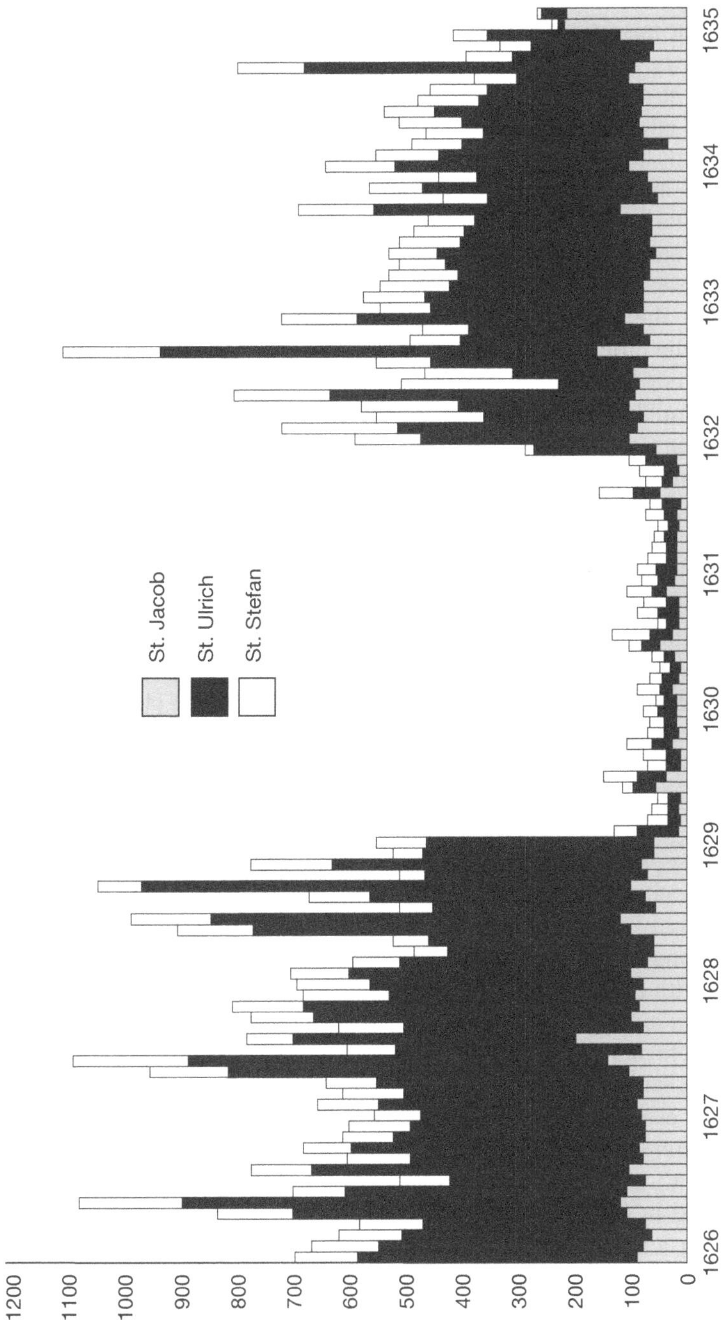

Figure 13.2 Church spending in Augsburg 1626–1635
Source: After Roeck 1989

a vengeful God; it would seem that when confronted with such extreme misery even the Protestant citizens had returned to old ideas about the righteousness of work.

We have established that theological theory, city and territorial-state laws and finally everyday practice rarely coincided. Centralisation, the consideration of individual cases and the principle of indigence became no less important for Catholic than for Protestant welfare. Conditions in Bavaria as well as in Catholic cities at the end of the sixteenth century demonstrated strong similarities to those in Protestant Germany. A certain hesitation to blindly accept the neat idea that begging had been generally allowed in Catholic cities but forbidden in Protestant ones[48] is appropriate. Beggars were unwelcome everywhere and the authorities tried what they could to be rid of them. The central difference that did exist between Catholic and Protestant cities and states was the existence of beggars' orders.

In general it is probably accurate that the centralisation of welfare, not to mention its development into a codified system, was not seen in Catholic areas as being any less desirable, but was more difficult to carry out there than in Protestant areas. A greater variety of welfare institutions and their benefactors is thus perhaps the most important characteristic distinguishing Catholic areas from Protestant ones. This resulted if nothing else from the unwillingness of clergical institutions – for example, in Freiburg, Cologne or Munich – to relinquish their control over the resources intended for welfare, and above all their desire to use these resources for purposes specific to their confession. Fulda was only one of many cities where this was the case. This was expressed, for example, by the welfare institutions run by city monasteries, and by charitable foundations (which also appeared frequently in Protestant areas and often remained under independent administration).[49] The tendency in the latter half of the sixteenth century to combine foundations with confessional,[50] 'missionary' aims or to redefine originally confession-neutral or even pre-Reformation foundations according to confessional politics is occasionally all too clear.

An especially well-known example of the latter case is the Fuggerei sponsored by Jakob Fugger the Rich, which was the only foundation of its kind in Germany.[51] This miniature ideal city erected in one of the city's poor quarters, in its way an ordered utopia amidst the surrounding chaos characterised by increasing poverty and social tension, carried on the tradition of late-medieval benefactor piousness. The first signs of this great undertaking date from 1514. Poor 'craftsmen, daily-wage workers and others' could stay there, 'so that they would not publicly seek alms'. For modest (if not merely symbolic) rent, the poor could lead a 'private' life with their families and even take advantage of health-care institutions (e.g. for syphilitics). The most important thing that every one of this settlement's residents – in the early seventeenth century around 300 people – had to do in return was to pray 'one pater noster, Ave Maria and one credo' daily for the founders' salvation.[52] Although we know of no written decree to this effect, over time a strict practice developed that only Catholics were to be taken in. The Fuggerei quickly became a Catholic enclave in an otherwise predominantly Protestant under-class quarter; it became a counter-reformatory institution.

The Fuggerei was paralleled in many other, less important foundations in Augsburg. Warmbrunn has documented 91 such bequests between 1548 and 1649. This private activity boomed with 22 bequests (6 Catholic and 16 Protestant) during the aforementioned decrease in donations to the Church prompted by the calendar controversy,[53] thus achieving a certain compensation for the general decline in church donations during this time. In this way, the confessional controversy brought about a return to traditional, decentralised forms of charity. Such a confessionally mixed city demonstrated other significant differentiations. Only institutions for Protestant citizens received public alms, where most of the financial resources for caritative purposes were concentrated, while the orphanage was remembered primarily by Catholics.[54]

One should also keep welfare institutions in mind, which in the Counter-Reformation age were established in ways clearly dictated by confessional politics. The Julius Hospital in Würzburg, established between 1576 and 1580, is a prominent example of this. It was a 'bastion of the Counter-Reformation' and apparently a Catholic response to the establishment of 'High Hessian State Hospitals', which had begun receiving both the poor and the mentally and physically ill in 1535.[55] The Julius hospital was intended by its founder, Julius Echter von Mespelbrunn, to take in pilgrims, orphans, the sick, cripples and also pregnant women from the entire area under his reign. Hospitals had always been the centre of the church's care for the poor and the ill.[56] In its seventh and twenty-second sessions, the Council of Trent had passed regulations for the hospitals foreseeing that they – except for hospitals belonging to the Knights' Orders or those otherwise exempt – would fall under the bishop's jurisdiction. These resolutions were consistent with the Provincial Synodes and the laws of the Empire.[57] Bishop Julius

Echter emphasised this special, episcopal competence with a relief mounted on the hospital's gate tower in 1578 showing him in an attitude of prayer.[58] Here he has lain away the insignia of wordly power and clergical rank – his bishop's staff, sword and gloves – and is now merely and individual carrying out a deed of compassion. The subjects of his *caritas* are portrayed in the background: the poor, the sick, orphans and pilgrims. The accompanying inscription:

TIBI . DERELICTVS . EST . PAVPER

defines the hospital's purpose and simultaneously an expectation. The text continues:

IN . PRAECE . PAVPERVM . SPEM . HABVI

the bishop hopes for heavenly rewards from the prayers of those receiving the benefit of his good works.

It is certainly probable that this motto is an expression of the bishop's conscience; however it clearly also portrays the image he desired for this fairly pompous establishment. The architecture alludes on the one hand to the tradition of the medieval 'spital', while expressions of rank – especially two powerful towers – amplify the triumphal gesture. That its propagandistic effects were directed not only against the neighbouring Hessian Protestants is indicated, for one, by the fact that the establishment was erected on the site of a former Jewish bath. Baptisms of Jews were arranged; the hospital benefited from the publicity surrounding these conversions.

The erection of hospitals in Catholic Germany was otherwise not necessarily a direct consequence of the resolutions in Trent (the next best example would be the expansion of the Citizens' Hospital in Salzburg). Often enough, such activity was simply prompted by the need to renovate dilapidated establishments.[59] Care for the poor was gradually reorganised in early absolutistic Bavaria, and it is in this context – as well as that of the lord's personal piousness – that the construction of hospitals in Munich in the first quarter of the seventeenth century should be seen.

Relief for the poor and the ill in Counter-Reformation Catholic Germany had many facets and could be felt at diverse levels of society. Although its most pronounced manifestations were hospitals, poor houses and orphanages,[60] the significant role of brotherhoods, private foundations and monks' and nuns' orders should not be underestimated. These were complemented by simple citizens' 'good works', the feudal lords' assistance, the guilds and the many-faceted, often subtly effective mechanisms of local care for the poor and ill. It is in this context that the urban policy of care for the needy should be mentioned, which was intended to provide especially the poor with the most necessary basic foodstuffs.[61] Dating back to the Middle Ages, this policy was now carried on in a perhaps more highly developed but fundamentally unchanged fashion. This should not, however, obscure such details as the subsidising of rye achieved by keeping the price of 'luxurious' wheat artificially high.

It should also be remembered that poverty relief and a 'social policy' focusing on prevention often existed side by side. This included the creation of opportunities for employment, a topic that has received little attention in the discussion about poverty relief in Germany. Not to be confused with the topic of 'forced labour', which we do find in alms ordinances from Cologne to Munich,[62] this was rather the chance for daily-wage workers and craftsmen of all kinds to find work at public construction sites. An Augsburg city-council resolution emblematically described the motivation for constructing an enormous town hall – the largest of its kind in Central Europe – as creating work for the local poor. The corner-stone carried the inscription that the building had been erected:

URBIS VINDEL. PARTIAE ORNAMENTO ATQ.
SUBLEVANDAE OPIFICUM PENURIAE.[63]

Similar motives can be demonstrated for numerous other construction projects of the time; suggestions can be found as early as in the writings of Vives.[64] Thousands of people must have found work in *Germania sacra* at Counter-Reformation construction sites. Admittedly, the one or the other magnificent Baroque building bursting with gold and colour was certainly primarily intended as a tribute to its benefactor's fame, and one may with good reason attribute the abbots' and other patrons' claims that their projects should provide for 'people without work or bread' to a guilty conscience.[65] An eighteenth-century abbot classically expressed this reasoning when he noted that many of his monastery's subjects would suffer need and deprivation were it not for the work created by the House of God's construction projects. The large population of the times, he continued, had to be fed somehow, and one '*ratio motiva*' behind such projects was a wish to employ the people.[66] Churches, monasteries, hospitals and hospices in Counter-Reformation Germany thus not only formed parts of an affirmative culture by paying tribute to their patrons' religiousness and brotherly love, but their construction was also a perfectly concrete measure against poverty and need. Although exact figures are not available, it can be said that a 'construction boom' probably took hold at the end of the sixteenth century, only to be disrupted by the Thirty Years War. This was followed by a second boom of unparalleled dimensions, especially in the German South and the Habsburg crown lands. Strangely enough, the disciplines of economic and social history have yet to treat these developments and their consequences. There can be no question that the flattening out of this boom in the middle of the eighteenth century had drastic consequences, especially for the rural population. Neither rural trade nor the manufactures just appearing at the time were in a position to take in the newly jobless. The slowdown of this construction frenzy, which was at its roots still genuinely counter-reformatory, thus encouraged the formation of a rural pauper underclass and with it the 'industrial reserve army'.

Notes

1 See Wolfgang von Hippel, *Armut, Unterschichten, Randgruppen in der Frühen Neuzeit*, Munich 1995, with many references; Wolfgang Fischer, *Armut in der Geschichte. Erscheinungsformen und Lösungsversuche der 'sozialen Frage' seit dem Mittelalter*, Göttingen, 1982; Franz Ehrle, *Geschichte und Reform der Armenpflege*, Freiburg im Breisgau, 1891; Georg Ratzinger, *Geschichte der kirchlichen Armenpflege*, 2nd edn, Freiburg im Breisgau, 1884; Gerhard Uhlhorn, *Die christliche Liebestätigkeit*, vol 3, 2nd edn, Stuttgart 1895; Christoph Sachße and Florian Tennstedt, *Geschichte der Armenfürsorge in Deutschland. Vom Spätmittelalter bis zum 1. Weltkrieg*, Stuttgart, 1980; Brian Pullan, 'Catholics and the poor in Early Modern Europe', *Transactions of the Royal Historical Society*, 5th series 26 (1976), pp. 15–34; Ingomar Bog, Über Arme und Armenversorgung in Oberdeutschland und in der Eidgenossenschaft im 15. und 16. Jahrhundert, in: his *Oberdeutschland. Das Heilige Römische Reich des 16. bis 18. Jahrhunderts in Funktion*, Idstein, 1985, pp. 56–72; C. Schott, *Armenfürsorge, Bettelwesen und Vagantenbekämpfung in der Reichsabtei Salem*, Bühl, 1978; Adalbert Nagel, *Armut im Barock. Die Bettler und Vaganten Oberschwabens*, Weingarten 1986, pp. 11–19; Maria Ackels, 'Das Trierer städtische Almosenamt im 16. und 17. Jahrhundert: Ein Beitrag zur Analyse städtischer Unterschichten', *Kurtrierisches Jahrbuch* 24 (1984), pp. 75–103.

2 Robert Jütte, *Obrigkeitliche Armenfürsorge in deutschen Reichsstädten der frühen Neuzeit. Städtisches Armenwesen in Frankfurt am Main und Köln*, Cologne/Vienna, 1984; Franz Irsigler and Arnold Lassotta, *Bettler und Gaukler, Dirnen und Henker. Außenseiter in einer mittelalterlichen Stadt*, 2nd edn, Munich, 1989.

3 Martin Dinges, 'Frühneuzeitliche Armenfürsorge als Sozialdisziplinierung? Probleme mit einem Konzept, in: *Geschichte und Gesellschaft* 17 (1991), pp. 5–29.

4 See Paul Warmbrunn, *Zwei Konfessionen in einer Stadt. Das Zusammenleben von Katholiken und Protestanten in den paritätischen Reichsstädten Augsburg, Biberach, Ravensburg und Dinkelsbühl von 1548 bis 1648*, Wiesbaden, 1983; Etienne François, *Die unsichtbare Grenze. Protestanten und Katholiken in Augsburg 1648–1806,* Sigmaringen, 1991.

5 See Jürgen Sydow, *Städte im deutschen Südwesten. Ihre Geschichte von der Römerzeit bis zur Gegenwart*, Stuttgart, 1987; H.C. Erik Midelfort, *Witch Hunting in South Western Germany 1582–1684*, Stanford, CA, 1972.

6 Robert Muchembled, *Culture populaire et culture des élites dans la France moderne. XVe-XVIIe siècles,* Paris, 1978.

7 Winfried Schulze, *Deutsche Geschichte im 16. Jahrhundert*, Frankfurt a. M. 1987, p. 13.

8 Dieter Saalfeld, 'Die Wandlungen der Preis- und Lohnstruktur während des 16. Jahrhunderts in Deutschland', in: *Beiträge zu Wirtschaftswachstum und Wirtschaftsstruktur im 16. und 19. Jahrhundert*, Berlin, 1971, pp. 9–28; Ingomar Bog, 'Wachstumsprobleme der oberdeutschen Wirtschaft 1540–1618', in: F. Lütge, ed., *Wirtschaftliche und soziale Probleme der gewerblichen Entwicklung im 15.–16. und 19. Jahrhundert*, Stuttgart, 1968, pp. 44–89; Peter Clark, ed., *The European Crisis of the 1590s,* London, 1985; Hartmut Lehmann, 'Frömmigkeitsgeschichtliche Auswirkungen der "kleinen Eiszeit",' in: W. Schieder, ed., *Volksreligiosität in der modernen Sozialgeschichte*, Göttingen, 1986, pp. 31–50; Georg Schmidt, 'Die frühneuzeitlichen Hungerrevolten. Soziale Konflikte und Wirtschaftspolitik im Alten Reich', *Zeitschrift für Historische Forschung* 18 (1991), pp. 257–80, especially pp. 263ff.

9 Willi Rüger, *Mittelalterliches Almosenwesen. Die Almosenordnungen der Reichsstadt Nürnberg,* Nuremberg, 1932, pp. 68ff. On the generally common 16th-century practice of differentiating between 'real' and 'false' poor, see Robert Jütte, 'Poor relief and social discipline in 16th-century europe', *European Studies Review* 11 (1981), pp. 31ff.; Pullan, pp. 15ff. and Hans Scherpner, *Theorie der Fürsorge*, Göttingen, 1962, pp. 66ff.

10 Irsigler/Lassotta, 'Poor relief and social discipline', p. 18.

11 For summary see von Hippel, pp. 48, 105ff. (with the most important literature); aside from the summaries (note 1) also see Otto Winckelmann, 'Über die ältesten Armenordnungen der Reformationszeit (1522–1525)', *Historische Vierteljahresschrift* XVII (1914/15), pp. 187–228, 361–400.

12 See I. Friedrich Battenberg, 'Obrigkeitliche Sozialpolitik und Gesetzgebung. Einige Gedanken zu mittelrheinischen Bettel- und Almosenordnungen des 16. Jahrhunderts', *Zeitschrift für historische Forschung* 18 (1991), pp. 33–70, here pp. 46ff.

13 For figures see Bernd Roeck, *Eine Stadt in Krieg und Frieden. Studien zur Geschichte der Reichsstadt Augsburg zwischen Kalenderstreit und Parität*, Göttingen, 1989, pp. 481ff., footnote 637.

14 See von Hippel, *Armut, Unterschichten, Randgruppen*, p. 87; Jütte, pp. 15–17. In Munster at the end of the 16th century, between a fifth and a

third of its 10,000 inhabitants were poor; see Alwin Hanschmidt, 'Zur Armenpolizei der Stadt Münster im ausgehenden 16. Jahrhundert', in: *Civitatum communitas. Studien zum europäischen Städtewesen, Festschrift Heinz Stoob zum 65. Geburtstag,* vol. 2, Cologne/Vienna 1984, pp. 655–82, here p. 659.

15 Fischer, p. 55.

16 Roeck, pp. 481ff., 948ff.

17 Erich Maschke, 'Die Unterschichten der mittelalterlichen Städte Deutschlands', in: E. Maschke and J. Sydow, *Gesellschaftliche Unterschichten in den südwestdeutschen Städten,* Stuttgart, 1974, pp. 1–74, especially p. 58; also see Volker Hunecke, 'Überlegungen zur Geschichte der Armut im vorindustriellen Europa', *Geschichte und Gesellschaft* 9 (1983), pp. 480–512, p. 489; Ackels figures 27.5% of Trier's population to have been poor (at the begin of the 17th century; see p. 101).

18 Roeck, *Zur Armenpolizei der Stadt Münster*, pp. 384ff., 480, 619; von Hippel, *Armut, Unterschichten, Randgruppen*, pp. 3–7.

19 Ingomar Bog, 'Über Arme und Armenfürsorge in Oberdeutschland und in der Eidgenossenschaft im 15. und 16. Jahrhundert', in: *Jahrbuch für fränkische Landesforschung* 34 (1975), pp. 983–1001, especially pp. 983, 994.

20 Fischer, *Armut in der Geschichte*, pp. 165ff.

21 Ibid., p. 161.

22 See Karl Frölich, 'Kirche und städtisches Verfassungsleben im Mittelalter', *Zeitshrift der Savigny-Stiftung für Rechtsgeschichte, Kanonistische Abteilung* 22 (1933), pp. 188–287, especially p. 286; Heinz Schilling, 'Die Konfessionalisierung im Reich. Religiöser und gesellschaftlicher Wandel in Deutschland zwischen 1555 und 1620', in: *Historische Zeitschrift* 246 (1988), pp. 1–45, here p. 34.

23 See Paul Münch, *Lebensformen in der frühen Neuzeit. 1500–1800*, Frankfurt a. M./Berlin, 1991, pp. 358–66.

24 Ibid., p. 366; also see I. M. Battafarano, 'Armenfürsorge bei Albertinus und Drexel. Ein sozial-politisches Thema im erbaulichen Traktat zweier Schriftsteller des Münchner Hofes', *Zeitschrift für Bayerische Landesgeschichte* 47 (1984), pp. 141–80.

25 Similar views were expressed even before the Reformation, e.g. by Geiler von Kayersberg; see Scherpner, *Theorie der Fürsorge*, p. 62.

26 For summary see Scherpner, *Theorie der Fürsorge*, pp. 80–88; Roland Stupperich, 'Das Problem der Armenfürsorge bei Juan Luis Vives', *A. Buck*, ed., Juan Luis Vives, Hamburg, 1989, pp. 49–62; see Armando Saitta, ed., Ludovico Vives, *De subventione pauperum*, Firenze 1973. For other Catholic writers see C. Göttler, *Die Kunst des Fegefeuers nach der Reformation. Kirchliche Schenkungen, Ablaß und Almosen in Antwerpen und Bologna um 1600*, Mainz, 1996, pp. 31–45.

27 Scherpner, *Theorie der Fürsorge,* p. 80.

28 Ibid., p. 81.

29 Vives, II, p. 84.

30 See Liselotte Constanze Eisenbart, *Kleiderordnungen der deutschen Städte zwischen 1350 und 1700. Ein Beitrag zur Kulturgeschichte des deutschen Bürgertums*, Göttingen, 1962; Veronika Baur, *Kleiderordnungen*

in Bayern vom 14. bis zum 19. Jahrhundert, Munich, 1975.

31 See H. Stekl, '"Labore et fame". Sozialdisziplinierung in Zucht- und Arbeitshäusern des 17. und 18. Jahrhunderts', in C. Sachße and F. Tennstedt, (eds) *Soziale Sicherheit und soziale Disziplinierung. Beiträge zu einer historischen Theorie der Sozialpolitik*, Frankfurt a. M., 1986, pp. 119–47; Bernhard Stier, *Fürsorge und Disziplinierung im Zeitalter des Absolutismus. Das Pforzheimer Zucht- und Waisenhaus und die badische Sozialpolitik im 18. Jahrhundert*, Sigmaringen 1988 (with a discussion of the 'concept of discipline'); D. Weber, 'Zucht- und Arbeitshäuser am Niederrhein', in: *Düsseldorfer Jahrbuch* 60 (1986), pp. 78–96; H. Eicheler, 'Zucht- und Arbeitshäuser in den mittleren und östlichen Provinzen Brandenburg-Preußens. Ihr Anteil an der Vorbereitung des Kapitalismus', *Jahrbuch für Wirtschaftsgeschichte 1970/1*, pp. 127–47; Rudolf Endres, 'Das "Straf-Arbeitshaus" St. Georgen bei Bayreuth', in: *Jahrbuch der Sozialarbeit* 4 (1981), pp. 89–105; G. Fumasoli, *Ursprünge und Anfänge der Schellenwerke. Ein Beitrag zur Frühgeschichte des Zuchthauswesens*, Zurich 1981; D. Marzahn, 'Das Zucht- und Arbeitshaus. Die Kerninstitution frühbürgerlicher Sozialpolitik', D. Marzahn and H.-G. Ritz, (eds), *Zähmen und Bewahren. Die Anfänge bürgerlicher Sozialpolitik*, Bielefeld, 1984, pp. 7–68; H. Schlue, '*Die* Geschichte des Bonner Zuchthauses und des Bonner Arbeitshauses', dissertation Bonn 1957; M. Sothmann, *Das Armen-, Zucht- und Werkhaus in Nürnberg bis 1806*, Nuremberg, 1970; W. Traphagen, *Die ersten Arbeitshäuser und ihre sozialpädagogische Funktion*, Berlin, 1935; H. von Weber, 'Die Entwicklung des Zuchthauswesens in Deutschland im 17. und 18. Jahrhundert', in *Abhandlungen zur Rechts- und Wirtschaftsgeschichte. Festschrift Adolf Zycha zum 70. Geburtstag,* Weimar, 1941, pp. 427–68; Günther Rhiemeier, *700 Jahre Armenfürsorge in Lemgo*, Lemgo, 1991, pp. 174, 191–6.

32 For summary see Jütte, p. 34.

33 Ibid., p. 38.

34 See Battenberg, 'Obrigkeitliche Sozialpolitik und Gesetzgebung'.

35 Ibid., p. 61.

36 Ibid., p. 63.

37 Examples (Butzbach, Jülich-Kleve) are mentioned in Battenberg, 'Obrigkeitliche Sozialpolitik und Gesetzgebung', p. 68.

38 Fischer, *Armut in der Geschichte*, pp. 270, 274, 316.

39 See Ingo Schwab, 'Zeiten der Teurung. Versorgungsprobleme in der zweiten Hälfte des 16. Jahrhunderts', in: Richard Bauer, (ed.), *Geschichte der Stadt München*, Munich, 1992, pp. 166–88, here p. 187; and generally Christine Rädlinger, 'Armenwesen und Armenanstalten in München vom 14. bis zum 18. Jahrhundert', in: *Oberbayerisches Archiv* 116 (1992), pp. 15–106.

40 Hanschmidt, *Zur Armenpolizei der Stadt Münster*, p. 678.

41 For complete list see Hubert Glaser, *Um Glauben und Reich. Katalog der Ausstellung in der Münchner Residenz,* Munich, 1980, Vol. II, p. 296.

42 Also see Martin Dinges, *Stadtarmut in Bordeaux, 1525–1675. Alltag, Politik, Mentalitäten,* Münster 1988, p. 264.

43 Roeck, *Eine Stadt in Krieg und Frieden*, pp. 156, 805ff.

44 Irsigler/Lassotta, 'Poor relief and social discipline', pp. 20ff.

45 See Roeck, *Eine Stadt in Krieg und Frieden*, passim.
46 Ibid., p. 172.
47 Ibid., p. 724.
48 Hanschmidt, *Zur Armenpolizei der Stadt Münster*, pp. 657ff.
49 See Otto Winckelmann, *Das Fürsorgewesen der Stadt Strassburg vor und nach der Reformation bis zum Ausgang des sechzehnten Jahrhunderts. Ein Beitrag zur deutschen Kultur- und Wirtschaftsgeschichte,* Leipzig, 1922, p. 196; Marlene Besold-Backmund, Stiftungen *und Stiftungswirklichkeit. Studien zur Sozialgeschichte der beiden oberfränkischen Kleinstädte Forchheim und Weismain*, Neustadt a. d. Aisch, 1986; Ronnie Po-chia Hsia, 'Civic wills as sources for the study of piety in Muenster, 1530–1618', *Sixteenth Century Journal* 14 (1983), pp. 321–48; Ackels, p. 82.
50 See Jütte, p. 317; Besold-Backmund, *Stiftung und Stiftungswirklichkeit*, pp. 98ff. Interesting is her observation that starting at the turn of the 17th century in the small Frankish city of Weismain, anniversary foundations – which aimed 'directly' at their benefactors' salvation – were increasingly replaced by foundations for the poor (p. 359); in 16th-century Forchheim a large number of 'Seelgeräte' were founded, whose effectiveness for salvation, according to the benefactors, depended primarily on charity for the poor (ibid.).
51 See Marion Tietz-Strödel, Die *Fuggerei in Augsburg. Studien zur Entwicklung des sozialen Stiftungsbaus im 15. und 16. Jahrhundert*, Tübingen 1982; Hermann Kellenbenz, 'Fuggersche Sozialpolitik', in H. Pohl, (ed.), *Staatliche, städtische, betriebliche und kirchliche Sozialpolitik vom Mittelalter bis zur Gegenwart*, Stuttgart, 1991, pp. 66–88, here pp. 66ff.
52 Pohl, *Staatliche*, p. 66.
53 Warmbrunn, *Zwei Konfessionen in einer Stadt*, pp. 314–316.
54 Ibid., p. 315.
55 See Dieter Jetter, *Das europäische Hospital. Von der Spätantike bis 1800*, Köln 1986, p. 118; *Das Juliusspital in Würzburg*, vol 1 (Alfred Wendehorst), *Kulturgeschichte*, Würzburg, 1976 (here p. 14ff.), vol 2 (Friedrich Merzbacher), *Rechts- und Vermögensgeschichte*, Würzburg 1979; Walter Heinemeyer and Timan Pünder, *450 Jahre Psychatrie in Hessen*, Marburg 1983.
56 Many references in Jetter and von Hippel. See especially Ulrich Knefelkamp, *Das Heilig-Geist-Spital in Nürnberg vom 14.–17. Jahrhundert. Geschichte, Struktur, Alltag*, Nuremburg, 1989; B. Kurg-Richter, *Zwischen Fasten und Festmahl. Hospitalverpflegung in Münster 1540–1650*, Münster 1994; A. Mischlewski, 'Alltag im Spital zu Beginn des 16. Jahrhunderts', in A. Kohler and H. Lutz, (eds), *Alltag im 16. Jahrhundert. Studien zu Lebensformen in mitteleuropäischen Städten*, Vienna, 1987, pp. 152–73; W. Kögel, 'Das Heiliggeistspital als zentrale Institution des Wohlfahrtswesens im mittelalterlichen München', dissertation, Munich, 1952; W. Moritz, *Die bürgerlichen Fürsorgeanstalten der Reichsstadt Frankfurt am Main im späten Mittelalter*, Frankfurt a. M., 1981; S. Reicke, *Das deutsche Spital und sein Recht im Mittelalter*, 2 Vols., Stuttgart 1932; Marie-Luise Windemuth, *Das Hospital als Träger der Armenfürsorge im Mittelalter*, Stuttgart 1995.

57 Ratzinger, *Geschichte der Kirchlichen Armenpflege*, pp. 463–5, 469–72.
58 Jetter, *Das europäische Hospital*, pp. 121ff. (with illustration).
59 This was for example, the case with the Heilig-Geist-Spital in Augsburg, see Bernd Roeck, *Elias Holl. Architekt einer europäischen Stadt*, Regensburg, 1984, pp. 232, 249.
60 See finally Rhiemeier, pp. 174–80 and Markus Meumann, *Findelhäuser, Waisenhäuser, Kindsmord. Unversorgte Kinder in der frühneuzeitlichen Gesellschaft*, Munich, 1995.
61 See Dietrich Ebeling, 'Versorgungskrisen und Versorgungspolitik während der zweiten Hälfte des 16. Jahrhunderts in Köln', in: *Zeitschrift für Agrargeschichte und Agrarsoziologie* 27 (1979), pp. 32–59; Franz Irsigler, 'Getreidepreise, Getreidehandel und städtische Versorgungspolitik in Köln vornehmlich im 15. und 16. Jahrhundert', W. Besch, K. Fehn and D. Höroldt (eds), *Die Stadt in der europäischen Geschichte, Festschrift Edith Ennen*, Bonn, 1972, pp. 571–610; Bernd Roeck, *Bäcker, Brot und Getreide in Augsburg. Zur Geschichte des Bäckerhandwerks und zur Versorgungspolitik der Reichsstadt im Zeitalter des Dreißigjährigen Krieges*, Sigmaringen, 1987 (with further references).
62 See Jütte, p. 322; Rädlinger, 'Armenwesen und Armenstalten' pp. 58–60.
63 See Bernd Roeck, 'Wirtschaftliche und soziale Voraussetzungen der Augsburger Baukunst zur Zeit des Elias Holl', in: *Architektura* 14 (1984), pp. 119–38; Bernd Roeck, 'Konjunktur und Ende des süddeutschen "Klosterbarock". Umrisse eines wirtschafts- und geistesgeschichtlichen Forschungsproblems', in Dieter Albrecht Karl Otmar, Freiherr von A and Winfried Schulze *et al.*, *Europa im Umbruch, 1750–1850*, Munich, 1995, pp. 213–27.
64 Vives/Saitta, *De subventio pauperum*, pp. 60ff.
65 Roeck, *Eine Stadt in Krieg und Frieden*, pp. 221ff.
66 Ibid., p. 221, footnote 40.

INDEX

For Product Safety Concerns and Information please contact our EU representative GPSR@taylorandfrancis.com Taylor & Francis Verlag GmbH, Kaufingerstraße 24, 80331 München, Germany